To Anne

SOUNDING THE SOUND BODY

May you Sound
from the Depths of your
Heart!

Rinchenma
August 2000

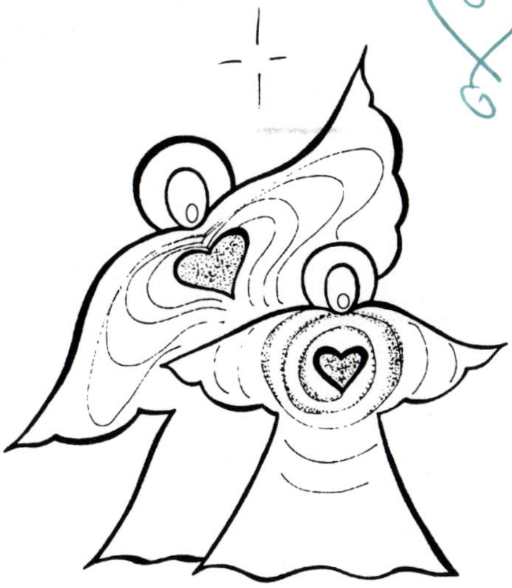

*"Lift up your hearts and sing.
The magic lies within."*

On Wings of Angels
Eugene, Oregon

SOUNDING THE SOUND BODY

Transformation through the power of Inner Sound

Vocal Power. Understanding Your Name. Healing with Voiced Sound.

RINCHENNA K'HARDO (Voice Shaman)

Illustrated by Nancy Jo Graham

Library of Congress Catalog Card Number: 98-91611

ISBN 0-9664881-0-5

Forthcoming books by Rinchenna K'hardo:

Sounding the Bones
Seeing with the Inner Eye

Also, a demonstration cassette on the various voice exercises in this book is planned. Those interested in such a tape and others inquiring about sound workshops, seminars, private name-consultations and special event "Soundings" can write to Rinchenna at:

Rinchenna K'hardo
#235-1400 Candlelight Dr
Eugene, OR. 97402
e-mail rkhardo@aol.com

ACKNOWLEDGMENTS

To the intuitive genius of Shirlee Kiley and Rochelle Gordon, whose articles on names (appearing in several early 80's Dell Magazines) fired my zeal to do further research and make subsequent discoveries of my own. To David Wallechinsky and Irving Wallace for compiling "The People's Almanac" (volumes One throughThree), which gave me the tools to launch my early research into names. To Musicologist Don Campbell (whose brilliant idea of releasing the voice through sounding the vowels I combined with my understanding of the *meaning* of the vowels). To my dear friend and tireless editor Marge Stoddard..for doing double-duty. To artist/illustrator Nancy Joe Graham for our collaboration on this project (her exquisite "singing angels" set the tone for this work). To the many friends and clients who gave me feedback when I analyzed their names. To the endless patience of my late husband Roger Sweum who encouraged my investigations. To the spiritual, mental support and challenging suggestions of my Jazz musician son, Ricky Sweum - and to my eldest son, Damon Permezel who, supplied me with a much needed, decent computer so I could write efficiently (plus frequent "How's the book coming along?" progress-proddings!). To my long-suffering, ever-patient, friend and neighbor Pat Giles, who unstintingly gave (and gives) me expert technical support (through all my quavering computer escapades) and who tirelessly "scanned" many of the images for this book and scurried on request through the Internet, looking up biographies for my research and finally editing them. To my Mother, my sister Margot and daughter Lynden in Australia and to Dixie (my other daughter in Canada) who keep me in their hearts. Also, my deepest thanks extends to long time associates and friends Cathy Brenner and Christine Courchaine for unflagging moral support, general encouragement and seminal suggestions. To Douglas Bloch in Portland for nagging me to record what I know for the benefit of posterity. To Jessica Morrell for generously teaching me basic writing skills. To Gunter Benz for his friendship and future vision of my work; to Jan Burch for her singular 'processing;' and to the insistent urgings, inspiration, healing touch and compassion of Joene Bone and Bobbie Sinclair. To Nancy O'Fraley with Virginia and Steve Scoggins, who set the countryside on fire with healing sound and Crosses of Light; to all my very patient students and others I may have touched and hopefully inspired through sound workshops and seminars in Australia, Canada and the USA, to you all, I am forever grateful.

Also, words can't express my gratitude to Mary at Western Printers for her expert and patient advice in the final production stages of this book - plus, I owe an additional debt to Catherine Harris of Eugene's Perelandra Books, whose timely talk on the "hard facts" of the publishing business faced me in the right direction.

Rinchenna K'hardo.

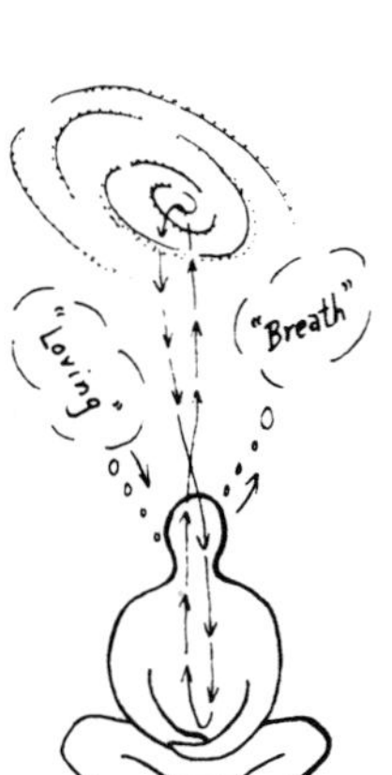

CONTENTS

CONTENTS

HOW TO USE THIS BOOK

Please don't think of this as a "read-through" book, but a "how-to" reference about taking charge of and empowering your voice. It explains how to sing and speak your own releasing sounds, including the intonation of the name given you at birth (or the new one you've changed it to) and how it relates to the amazing alphabet of sound-symbols from which your name was formed.

You'll also find tools for you to basically know who you are--on both an intimate and a vast scale; tools that will free your speaking and singing voice and if you so desire, help develop a personal healing method for yourself and others. If you want, you'll be able to set up sound-healing groups and to use specially voiced sounds to make a difference in communities, nature, governments and difficult situations.

The book caters to many different tastes and levels of awareness, encompassing all of human nature from the mundane and material to the mystical and spiritual. Be selective. You may not want to heal with sound, open your Throat Chakra or train your singing voice, but who *wouldn't* want to know the secret meaning hiding in the letters of their name[1] and the names of those they know (or even don't know)?? If so--choose those Chapters. Also, you should be interested in opening to the power of your speaking voice by practicing the Releasing Exercises. Perhaps the meditations and the esoteric practices may not be your "cup-of-tea"....but you'll still find other things to catch your interest and pique your curiosity. Hopefully, the more mystically inclined may just intrigue and challenge themselves, as well as learn how things fit together within the human and universal sound panorama. *In addition, you can tailor the various energy exercises, meditations and mantras into a personalized Spiritual Practice for your own expansion and transformation.*

For those wanting to try this new kind of Spiritual Practice begin with Chapter 11, "Sounding and Charting Your Name" and continue with Chapters 16, "Special Meditations," 17, "Energy Exercises," 20, "Advanced Vowel Sounding," and 21, "The Sacred Symbols" (with the meditations appropriate for the letters in your name).

As to the chapters dealing with the alphabet meanings themselves, they are far from complete; it has been incredibly difficult to condense 18 years of research into a mere one and a half pages for each letter (in Chapters 6 and 8). There's so much more I could have included and I make no apology for the crammed information in "More Letter Meanings A to Z." Almost daily I discover new letter nuances with no room left in this book to include them....so please use this as a good beginning-guide - and by no means the "last word."

The Bibliography at the end of the book, though not as large as I might have made it, none-the-less contains a spectrum of subjects (beginning with sound) that relate to the understanding and enrichment of consciousness (including our interdimensional heritage) necessary at this crucial time in history when what we do with the power of our mind and voice could make the difference between the restoration and transformation of life on this planet--or its inevitable ending.

The "soundings" I perform with my own voice (described in the book) are not fixed like precise frequency patterns from electronic sound-machines, or pre-arranged music aimed at specific energy-centers, physical conditions or body organs (though these methods have their own value). My voice is spontaneous and in direct response (through entrainment), to the total organism of the person I happen to be sounding for *at that moment in time* and what I subsequently sing for them (on any other occasion) always changes in response to the further needs of that person.

You also have the intuitive and latent power to sound in this fashion and the choices as to how you develop and use this material will be up to you. My fundamental responsibility is over--I am now satisfied that the basic tools are in your hands. DO IT!

Rinchenna K'hardo,
Spring of 1998.

---

[1] expanded from an original concept by Shirlee Kiley and Rochelle Gordon, who wrote "Personal Power is in Your Name." A Dell Book.

1.....THE WAY OF A VOICE SHAMAN

People frequently ask me to explain what I am, what I do and when it all began. These are not easy questions to answer, except possibly the last. Shamans come in several varieties, and the phenomenon is ubiquitous throughout all native peoples, in every country on the globe and with traditions that go back thousands of years. Essentially they were (and still are), the psychic, mystical healers for the tribe and used specific and personal gifts and sometimes crystals, herbs and other sacred objects that had been imbued with power by frequent use and intention. One shamanic ability is that of 'journeying' - the power to alter consciousness and enter other dimensions with the purpose of rescuing, releasing or healing.

I class myself as a Western urban shaman and in addition to using sound, I am an empath; that is: when working, I often feel and directly experience in my own body, the sensations, emotions and mental states of others. This guides me to ask certain questions and to put my attention on particular areas of their body and Life Field. After aligning with someone else's Field (or the group energy of a roomful of people), I receive information that then translates through me as sounds, tones, speech and song (often in languages unfamiliar to me and in both male and female voices). Although in an altered state, I am fully aware at all times allowing the process to unfold. Yet this is only part of what happens. As to how and when it all began? - I will explain with a story from my youth:

"We have a Singer unto the Lord here.....stand up and sing!!"

All ears attended to the Preacher's extraordinary words. The meeting hall was packed yet hushed, while the song of cicadas drifted through the wide open windows. Although evening, the heat of the Australian summer day lingered. I sat fanning myself with a hymnal in the midst of some out-of-town visitors. The silence in the room deepened, but no one stood. After a few moments the statement was repeated, this time louder.

"There's a Singer unto the Lord <u>here</u> .....***stand up and SING!!***"

Heads began to turn and ripples of whispering broke out. "What does he mean?" "Who is it, do you think?" "What's happening?" The room buzzed with questions as the Preacher stood quietly in front of us - waiting. For no apparent reason my heart started pounding and my breathing became alarmingly erratic, a strong throbbing pulsed through my chest - and then I heard it - a single clear note rang out and sustained itself.

"Where did *that* come from?" I wondered through my discomfort; then it rang clear again, high and sweet. "Oh my God !" I realized in disbelief, "It's in my head, it must be **me**!" Gripping the back of the chair in front for support, I pulled myself up unsteadily - I could hardly stand, yet was totally unable to remain seated! Meanwhile, unchecked by the hymnal, the perspiration gathered on my face and scalp. I began to drip. The now silent roomful of people regarded me expectantly and the Preacher looked triumphant. A smile widened his face, but I felt acutely embarrassed. The energy from my chest now rose into my throat and the one pure note still sang in my head.

"Don't be afraid," his voice spoke kindly. "Let it come out, *trust* - just open your mouth and sing!"

The power filling me became overwhelming; I stopped resisting and surrendered to it. Sound came soaring out of my throat like a bird freed from its cage! Other notes followed, cascading in unbelievable tones. All pressure gone, I sang like one transported, oblivious to everything but the joy of hearing - of *being* the sound. From those opening notes a beautiful song followed in a language unfamiliar to my outer mind, yet strangely known to my heart. When the song finally died away, I sat down, astounded! From that moment, my life changed forever. Unwittingly, I had been initiated into the realm of a Voice Shaman, although in that belief-system it was not recognized or developed as such. It took many years in the future to find out what really had happened--my Throat Chakra had been opened!

More than forty years have now passed since that amazing night. To say the least, life has been eventful! I married twice, produced four wonderful children, studied and taught music, art, Yogas and mystical disciplines, entered widowhood, embraced croneship, changed names and citizenship's but throughout everything the Sound prevailed, demanding I use it and penetrate its mysteries. As these enigmas unfolded I discovered the secret potential of the human voice--that when the outer voice releases the inner sounds, it functions like a frequency tool bringing healing and integration. The final revelation came when I found out the "sound code" for personal names: that letters within a name are actually symbols - symbols for the sound patterns revealing who we are and what we have come to accomplish.[1]

Sound is also another frequency of light, an audible frequency. With our limited sensory perception, sight and sound are separated, but on refined levels of awareness they merge. I once observed (with great wonder), the marvel of sound translated into moving patterns of light and color as I lay listening to music in the early morning sunshine--relaxed and alone for the first time after a night of non-stop activity (during which I had counseled a house full of people). In me, the temporary power to "see" sound was partly due to sleep deprivation and partly due to the extended time of being intensely focused in Spirit.

There are of course, certain people naturally gifted with extrasensory seeing who perceive the form of sound as a matter of course! To them, sound is always both audible and 'visible.' I love having these Light See-ers present in my workshops; they bring wonderful input to group sound work and on occasion, some have even created on-the-spot color sketches of what they observe while everyone else is singing.

My purpose in writing this book is much more than giving you information about your names; I want to fill you with desire, the desire to sing and sound--to activate your Sound Body and reclaim your secret vocal powers. Then, we can begin re-tuning the earth and the people of the earth to their ancient resonance and balance......and eventually restore our Light Being bodies through the power of higher Spirit.

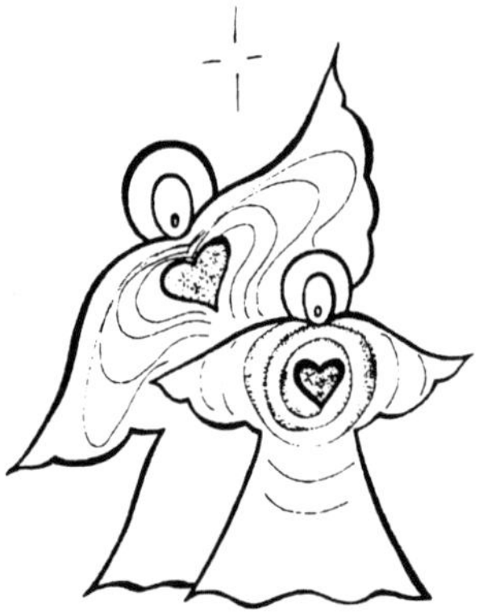

1 Thanks to Shirlee Kiley and Rochelle Gordon - see Acknowledgments.

2..... THE SOUND BODY

Sound Body? - what do I mean by a Sound Body? YOU are a sound-body--that comprises all of your emanations beginning at the microscopic cellular level to the vast, invisible, life Field surrounding your solid physique; it includes the ordinary speaking-singing voice and the dormant sounds and songs of the inner voices, which added together form the marvel of your entire sound spectrum. Our Western culture does not prepare us to accept a fully actualized vocal palette, so we go through life oblivious to our true potential as Sounder-healers, power speakers and life-changing singers. These remain the most hidden and neglected parts of vocal expression. Not withstanding, its partial use has been retained by a few shamanic and group ecstatic traditions in which healings and interventions intuitively "sing themselves" from these superconscious channels. The transcendent level of inner sound allows us to reunite with our Spirit (the life-force energy), and reconnect to the ground of being--our Source.

Lacking a direct interaction with Spirit, we can no longer 'sound' our inner voices. But in spite of our cultural bias, this could now be changing. TV media productions in recent years ran shows about several End of Age prophecies and presented a wide scope from the Bible, the writings of Nostradamus, the oral traditions of the Hopi Indians and other indigenous peoples, up to the more modern prognosticators of doom (including a large body of environmental scientists and astrophysicists), who all insist the "last days" are upon us unless we become an earth-responsible Global Community. Millennium Fever perhaps? Perhaps not! Although many of their predictions seem dire and terrifying, an underlying positive theme exists amongst a few spiritual dreamers and workers, who see this as a challenge and an opportunity for transformation with the emergence of a strain of superconscious, super physical beings, who will help during these chaotic times and even deflect or change some of the present destructive patterns. Signs of their emergence: the restoration of spiritual awareness along with the power of sound and the human voice. In the different traditions these super beings hold many names...Sons of God, Rainbow Beings and Children of Light are some. A modern visionary, Barbara Marx Hubbard calls them "Universal Humans" and postulates the creation of a new society from a "whole centered, Spirit centered" consciousness. I definitely see a 'singing branch' developing and my favorite term for them is **Sounders**, or **Light Singers**.

Already many Sounders (to-be) are having first encounters with interdimensional sound as their Throat Chakras begin to open spontaneously. Sometimes it takes a strong group energy to trigger the inner voices (as in my own case), or working closely with another person (like giving or receiving a massage) has been known to do it. Recently a new electronic activator emerged in the form of a "Sound Table," namely, a professional massage table fitted with several implanted speakers, each set to resonate various key points on the body. A certain lady had been using such a table while listening to a tape of her own personalized tone frequency (called Bio-Tuning).[1] One day, she became confused to hear an unknown language being spoken and sung along with her personal "tone." At first she thought her expensive Bio-Tuning tape had become damaged; *finally, she realized the voices were coming from her own head and not due to some anomaly on the tape!* The combined technology of the sound table together with the electronic "tone" enabled her inner voices to be heard for the first time and undoubtedly, she was also spiritually and emotionally ready for the experience! Later that week, through the prompting of a mutual friend, she asked me what I thought had happened to her. I explained about the inner sounds and offered to facilitate her process; I also remarked that her unusual encounter showed she was ready to consciously open her Throat Chakra--it was time to use her power voices. She was more than willing! I stood in front of her as a catalyst and while my own inner voices swelled into sound I encouraged her to do the same. She did--and immediately received a forceful release, singing-speaking her inner sounds with freedom, joy, and (I might add), some suprise! Such personal break-throughs occur frequently when I conduct Sound Seminars, the strength of the group

---

[1]Sound tables and Bio-Tuning can be obtained from Dr. Jeffrey D. Thompson, D.C., B.F.A. 1(800) 349-7358.

energy then provides the catalyst; I have also watched a collective sound-release elevate an entire group into higher dimensions of sound and expanded awareness.

What precisely *are* these "other" voices? To comprehend their place in our lives, you need to realize we live in more than one dimension. The non-physical power centers (Chakras) with their energy meridians, cannot be examined with X-rays or scalpels. Unseen by eyes (yet responsive to touch), their precise locations in the body have none-the-less been known for centuries in the East and form the basis for the practice of acupuncture and other related healing systems now accepted and somewhat respected in the West. The same general invisibility applies to our Life Field (aura), although this **can** be seen by those with extrasensory perception and has been partly recorded on film by Kirlian photography. *Attached to this veiled and extended body are sub-selves from our* ***other*** *physical lifetimes who choose to be reborn along with us.* They appear to reincarnate **not** as the primary consciousness (that's us!), but as memory frequencies in the Life Field or attached to certain key points in and on the body. Specific traumas, can cause confusion as to which soul has the primary consciousness (i.e., the one that *should* be in charge of the physical body); when this occurs, you have the phenomenon known in clinical terms as "multiple personalities.[2]"

During individual sound-balancings, I encounter these past-life entities in a person's Field; each has a 'voice' capable of singing or speaking through me--and not necessarily in English! These usually *unknown* languages (although there have been some dramatic exceptions!) can assert a marked beneficial effect on the mind, emotions and occasionally the physical body of the person receiving the Sounding. *And yes, "multiple personalities" have been successfully integrated through 'sound balancing."*

Though largely unrecognized, this multilevel co-habitation appears to be the normal state of the human organism, which (unwittingly) strives each lifetime, to unite all these 'selves' into a hidden, transcendent Self through higher Spirit, thus beginning a greater evolutionary design. I like to call it, the ultimate game-plan! *Having for the most part lost the ultimate game-plan, multiple sub-selves attach to a single body for several reasons:* to re-tackle unresolved past problems (get in another shot, so to speak!); to learn vicariously through the present life experiences of the host personality (you!); to access previously gained knowledge (past-life skills and abilities) and use them afresh in the present life. Some of them seem determined to catch up on eating--having lived a 'hungry' past-life or died of hunger--and so the host (you again!) may develop an uncontrollable eating pattern. Then others return *precisely* to find the lost game-plan and alert the outer self to its transcendent possibilities. It's common to be aware of the polarized sub-selves, the ones you have to wrestle with (and re-educate), who seem in conflict with the others that aid and support you. We generally know these more hidden and secret parts of our personality as persistent inner tendencies, 'intuitions' and inexplicable urgings.

When you first open the Throat Chakra and begin to talk in "tongues," the phenomena known as glossalalia, it is usually your past-life sub-selves (these inner 'others' who share your total being), who are speaking and singing! At first, you may find yourself voicing only one or two languages, more tongues will emerge as you access the rest of your inner selves.

Another group of voices come from a different level in the Life Field (sub-selves usually cling closer to the body). This other group only periodically sing and speak; they claim to accompany us through many lifetimes and present themselves as guides, guardians (Angels?), and even teachers to facilitate our latent creative abilities and healing talents. Their underlying concern **is** the lost game-plan--to restore the human race to its highest physical and spiritual evolution. From them we receive the occasional intuitive push in the right direction, if not a shout in the ear when we refuse to notice their promptings! And when *they* sound through us, their voices always seem to lecture and advise or give special encouragement and instruction.

The last inner voice level (at least from my present experience), links you directly to your highest Spirit, the life-force energy itself. There are techniques for *consciously* doing this as part of opening the Throat Chakra in Chapter 14; but often when I'm alone, the connection happens quite spontaneously. An unmistakable sensation will call me to drop whatever I'm doing and enter fully into

---

2 This term has recently come into disrepute due to the activities of various spurious practitioners. A true multiple personality is when the host soul regularly exits the body and another personality takes control and lives an entirely different lifestyle with even different illnesses--which disappear when the host soul re-enters the body!

what I can only call "The Inner Presence." The ensuing sounds always transport me into blissful expansion and later, when the last ecstatic note has sung itself to silence, I always know one thing for certain....."This is who I really am, a Sound Being, empowered to sound my own completeness!"

As if this wasn't enough! - we are however, not alone on this planet, we share it with Devic beings from a dimension that interpenetrates our own and who connect (through some mysterious stewardship), to the natural realms of earth forms, animals and the higher pursuits of humans. These enigmatic intelligences also express in sound frequencies. On rare occasions, Devas of healing, art, music and even the nature Devas from the surrounding countryside will communicate with us - or through us to others (during personal Soundings and earth celebrations and rituals). Their songs have a unique, ethereal beauty, often with several overtones sounding simultaneously. At first (when you begin sounding in the Spirit), it's hard to accept (or even believe) that so much sound could be pouring from one throat--and that the throat in question could be your own! This Devic experience takes place so seldom, you don't really have much of an opportunity to get used to it, but when it happens.....it's something you'll not easily forget.

To do a Sounding for someone else, you begin by aligning with that person's Life Field (described fully in Chapter 15); then instantly your sounds become dual in nature. Not only do your inner voices sing and speak (whenever inclined), but the sub-selves of the person you're sounding for will also speak and sing through **your** throat.[3] In effect, you have assumed the role of a sound-surrogate and in the shamanic tradition, you "journey" empathetically into the other person's present and past, directly experiencing their emotional, mental and physical states (as well as their voice frequencies). Part of this process involves actually *seeing* events and *feeling* emotions from past-life traumas that relate to their present-life problems. Another aspect of this work involves releasing entities and other interdimensional life forms that may have become attached or trapped in the other person's Life Field. During all of this, you are speaking and chanting (or singing) with a multitude of inner voices, some of which you have never heard before--and will probably never hear again! Each person you do a Sounding for may feel a different effect and receive a different benefit depending on their needs, but the ideal culmination results in a re-balancing of their total system--their Life Field, mind, emotions and physical body. For more practical information read Chapter 15 entitled "Healing with Sound and Sound Power Groups."

In the next Chapter we'll consider how the physical body is actually a musical instrument, a sounding board upon which we 'sound out' out lives and if we choose, a way of returning to our Spiritual Essence through the voice.

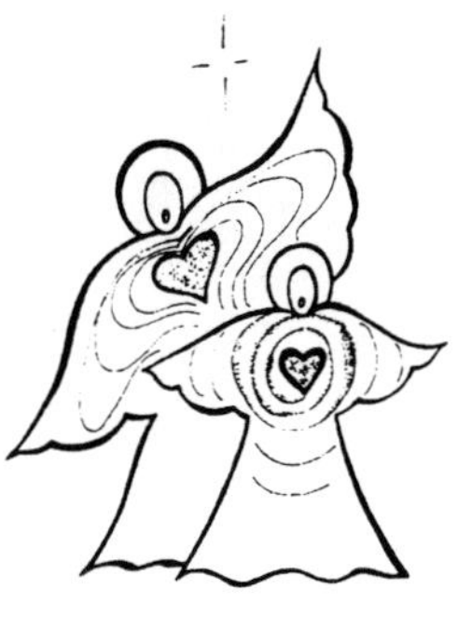

3 See "Case in Point" plus a second example from page 119-122.

3.....THE BODY - A MUSICAL INSTRUMENT

Did you know the physical body is actually a musical Instrument? Most instruments need careful tuning before playing their best and that includes us - the human instrument. We tend to think of the vocal cords in the throat as the only part that could do with a 'tuning.' *Not true at all!* Your entire body forms a complex, sensitive device capable of compelling speech and exquisite song; every part of you (not just the throat) adds up to how well or how badly you speak or sing.

The voice you have or don't have results from childhood conditioning. When you were very small were all of your sounds acceptable? Could you (without attracting disapproval or shaming) scream and holler and even bang your fists on the table when you were angry - in other words, were your emotions understood, respected and put in perspective for you by your parents (or parent figures)? Further more, as you grew older, could you express your needs and feelings with all their consequent noises - not just the joyful and happy ones, but all the sounds of sadness, calamity and fury that from time to time seized your young heart? Some of us grew up in environs of systematic sound suppression and endured shriveling reprimands, far worse than the mere: "Shut up you brat!" - "Stop all that crying and carrying-on, **at once**!"

When children, many of us never had permission to be *heard*, we were always being shamed and our feelings discounted. Also today, there's a whole breed of non-singers, convinced they must be tone-deaf and tuneless, because early in life, their enthusiastic and innocent attempts at singing caused pained and startled looks to appear on the faces of family members, peers and mentors; in school choir their teachers usually said: "To spare us all--could you *please* just 'mouth' the words?" These and other examples of negative conditioning make it difficult and well-near impossible for some people to vocalize with confidence and power.

Discouragement (or outright repression) isn't the only thing that throws a spanner in your vocal cords: your country of birth, the milieus of your childhood and youth, the time in history you were born into--all of these shape and 'tune' the type of sound instrument you become and form a background control through which you struggle to express yourself.

In spite of all this past conditioning you **can** *re-tune your body to sound freely!* **The exercises in this book will help you re-discover, explore and express all of your lost 'voices.'**

Now for a detailed look at the body instrument itself: yes, you **do** possess those crucial vocal cords in the throat, but even if they're perfectly healthy, they can't guarantee a superlative speaking or singing voice, unless you know how to breathe correctly and control the flow of tone. Your lung power begins with the intercostal muscles between the ribs, these let your chest expand sideways as well as upward creating a strong elastic cage. Then separating the lungs from your digestive tract is a large muscle membrane called the diaphragm; when depressed/relaxed, it allows for full lung expansion and when contracted/tensed, it helps expel the air and control the voice. (What voice student has not heard the constant exhortation of some teacher - "*Remember to use your diaphragm!*"?) The final breath support, believe it or not, is the belly, or more specifically, the girdle of layered muscles keeping the gut from falling out. Besides your lungs, the basic foundation for breathing and vocal strength comes from these three forces: an expandable rib cage, a flexible diaphragm[1] and powerful belly muscles. Furthermore, don't expect to sound your best if you sag your shoulders and depress your chest. Lungs need room to breathe; the underlying foundation for breath and voice rests on how we stand or sit--our good or poor posture!

Further components that create and modulate tone in our complex physical instrument include the (obvious) lips, tongue and teeth, then the (less obvious) soft and hard palate, followed by the sternum (the flat bone between the ribs), the various sinus resonators in the cheek bones, nasal septum and forehead, the resonating spaces in the mouth, windpipe and pharynx (the space connecting mouth, throat and nose, where you begin to swallow). The dome of the skull acts as the upper resonator,

---

[1] Refer to page 103 "The Diaphragm" also, The Diaphragm "Bellows-Breath" Release.

conducting the sound around and **out** of the head....depending on where you direct it. And finally, the feet--your posture begins there in your shoes. Try and think of how you place each foot with its feeling of solidness, then extend that feeling up through the legs to your spine, giving you a culminating sense of being grounded and poised in space. The chest, arms and head can now relax and 'float' allowing your songs to soar.

You might professionally train this body-instrument in a variety of ways to create an expert speaker (or actor) through the study of elocution, or a singer in one of the many vocal styles ranging from Jazz to opera. **However, none of these training methods releases the inner sounds.** You need no previous study to magnificently sing or speak with these 'other' voices. When the special energy center (Chakra) in the throat opens, the inner voices sing **you**! They arise of themselves requiring only that you listen and monitor; your role is to trust the energy and permitt it to sound.

First of all, you need to release the conditioned fears that prevent you from becoming a free and effortless sound instrument. Here I would like to quote from Kristin Linklater's book, "Freeing the Natural Voice."

"Blocked emotions are the fundamental obstacle to a free voice."

The following chapter gives you tools to release blocked emotions, enabling you to retune yourself and begin using your Sound Body.

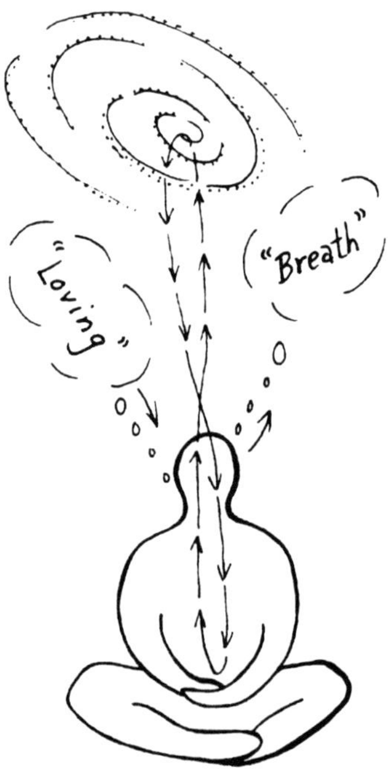

And I mean REALLY releasing the voice!

This work is important, but it's going to take some courage on your part, so give yourself permission to do it!

The first essential:

Find a secluded, preferably sound-proof place to work in. Your moving car is not always a good location because of the overwhelming emotions that sometimes come up. My best sound release work happened in the seclusion of the bathroom while sitting on the toilet! Some other ideas: a large walk-in closet that will hold you and a chair, a small back room (close the doors, windows and drapes), a secluded cabin in the woods, or bribe a night janitor for the use of an empty classroom or office suite!

Should you decide to try this when the house is empty or even if you conveniently live alone, first warn the neighbors that you will be doing some 'sound therapy' sessions and **not** to call the police if they hear blood curdling sounds issuing from your direction!

YOU ARE READY!

You've found the perfect spot to make all the noise you want, but it's not just a throat block you're unblocking, it's your **whole body!** Think of it as a rusty, unpracticed instrument and you need to unlock it all, not just your throat!

First give yourself a good stretch, then stand and shake everything that can possibly be shaken, followed by two or three very deep breaths. Let the breath out with a forced noisy sigh or even a groan or two. See what feelings come up after the sighings and the groanings. Whatever else happens, the sounds must connect to your feelings! Settle yourself in a comfortable position. You may want to sit or lie on the floor, seat yourself on a chair or even remain standing. To get yourself in the habit of breathing deep into the belly, rather than the upper chest, try sounding while lying flat on your back. I still like to do my basic releasing exercises in that way. But first, release the upper body.

Releasing the upper body.

Begin with the shoulders: - move, rotate and shrug; thump them with your fists and feel how tight they are - loosen all those responsibilities sitting on them!

Extend the movement up into the neck and throat: - move the head from side to side and any which way you want, feel the gratings and grindings of how you've calcified your self expression. Several times tuck your chin in and strongly stretch the back of your neck.

Now take the movement into the face (the Mask of Identity). Increase the blood supply by moving and contorting the cheek, brow, eye and forehead muscles.

Next, stretch the mouth in all kinds of shapes: open it very wide, purse the lips, stretch them wide again, purse your lips once more and then make an enormous grin with the lips parted; 'play' with your lip muscles. Move everything and feel your face come alive.

Place your attention on your jaw: With the back of your hand, repeatedly pat the area directly below the chin. Now slightly press the same area and tense-relax this muscle several times against your fingers. Next try moving your jaw from side to side - little movements, then **big** ones. Finally, stretch your chin out belligerently and allow any feelings of anger come into the area. Relax and repeat till you've connected with the emotions in your jaw and throat. (If you don't feel any do it anyway, it's an excellent tension releasing exercise.)

Finish with the following movements: scowl fiercely and *feel* the scowl. Relax and 'soften' your eyes, smile tenderly and gently. Discover a still, peaceful place deep inside you. Stay there for a moment and take a few quiet breaths, before calling up joy and beaming it across your face in your biggest and most wonderful smile! (Notice how your feelings change as you deliberately change your muscle tension?)

Note: A large number of different voice exercises are given in this Chapter; don't think you have to do them all each day--do only what you can comfortably manage or feel particularly attracted to.

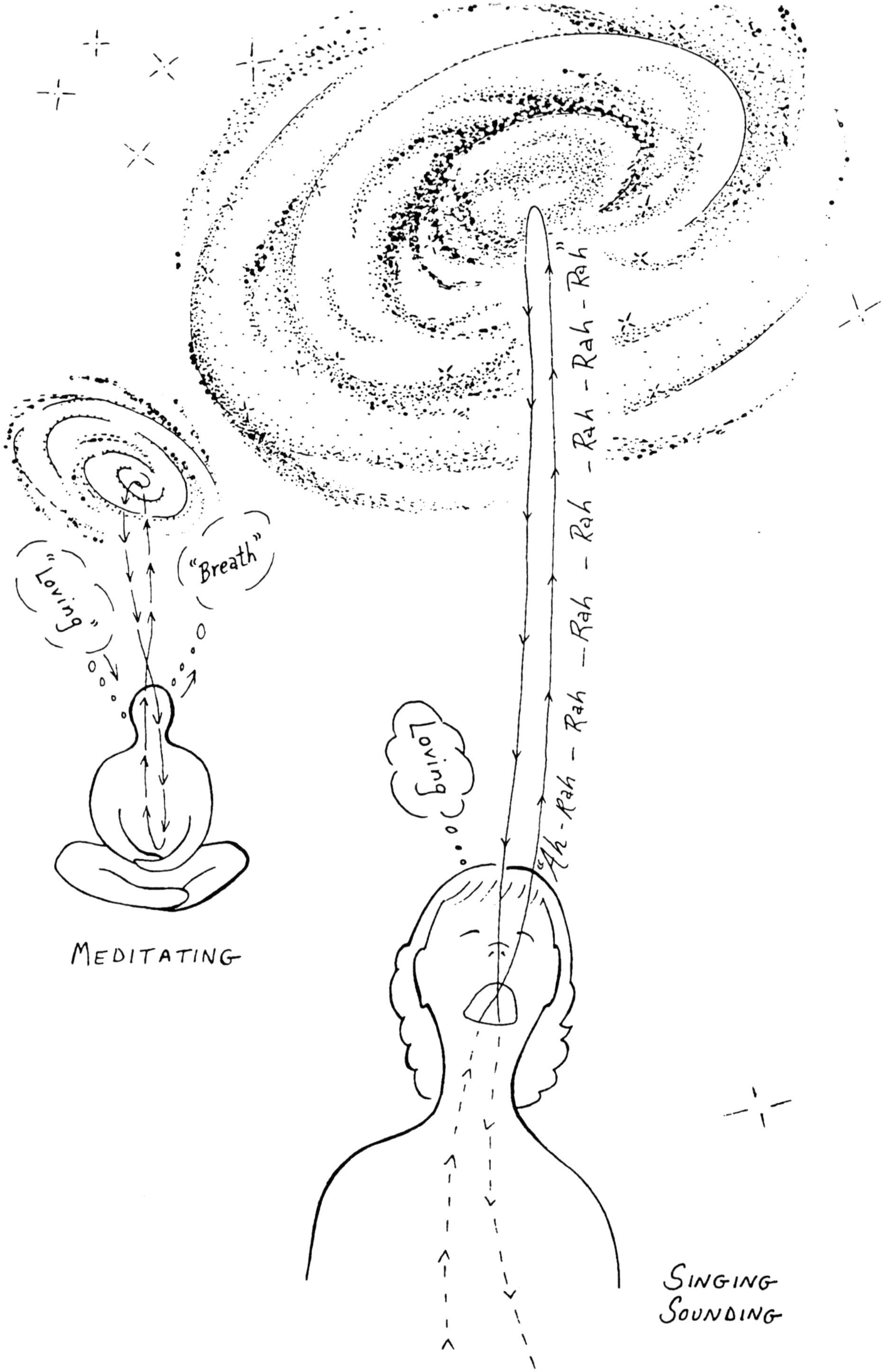

MEDITATING

SINGING
SOUNDING

But Before the Voice comes the Breath!

You may soon notice after a vigorous session with sustained notes, that you become a bit light-headed. The deeper breathing increases the amount of oxygen normally available to the brain. Most of us breathe so improperly we suffer from oxygen starvation. You'll eventually accustom yourself to the improved oxygen supply and the symptoms will disappear.

To further strengthen the lungs try blowing across the tops of glass bottles. There's a special knack to it which I'll leave you to discover for yourself, unless you did it for fun as a child, then you'll know the trick! I suggest the narrow necked, wine, pop and liquor-store bottles. Experiment with different heights; the taller the bottle, the deeper the tone. Larger bottles present a greater challenge; they take more huff and puff to make a really good sound and of course your lungs, intercostals and torso muscles receive a better workout. Eventually, you might think of looking for some Pan pipes (many music stores now sell exotic instruments). Most people find Pan pipes difficult to blow (if they haven't first conditioned themselves on bottles)! It takes the same precise breath angle along with enormous force and volume to produce a note on the pipes and your first attempts could make you *extremely* light-headed and dizzy. It has a similar effect to singing a long **"Aaaaaaaaaaeeeeeeeeeeee"** but much stronger. The sudden increase in air volume immediately floods the blood (and your brain) with massive amounts of extra oxygen. Regular practice on Pan pipes gradually diminishes the light-headed reaction; you'll also acquire more lung capacity and a stronger mid-section. In others words, you'll improve the muscle support for speaking and singing. You'll find Pan pipes worth the effort to practice, they produce wonderful reedy tones in a haunting pentatonic scale. I also suggest you "play" them with your diaphragm (the same goes for the bottles) - strongly contract your mid-section as you blow each note (or series of notes) into the pipes or bottles; in that way, you'll begin to build and condition those key support muscles. However, don't overdo the 'contractions' or you'll have a sore middle the next day! **While on the subject of increasing your lung capacity (and consequently your health), please realize if you happen to smoke cigarettes, that in the long run, it becomes counterproductive to all you are trying to achieve with your voice.**

THE GALACTIC BREATH

Eventually, you may want to try a more advanced way of breathing: let's presuppose the essential nature of the Life Force is Love - and that you can draw that Love into you with the breath. When most people breathe in it's with an upward movement filling only the chest cavity; the subsequent out-breath usually has a 'downward' motion, as though the breath discharges into the ground. This same breathing pattern patterns the *chemical* process of respiration, which is: when you breathe IN, gasses exchange in the lungs and when you breathe OUT, toxins expel from the body.

In galactic breathing, this outer physical/chemical process continues, but with a big difference: you now additionally activate the non-physical meridians of the Energy Body (familiar to practitioners of the centuries-old Martial Arts and Eastern medicine) and enable an energetic interaction between the two systems. Now, not only do you engage your lungs and circulatory system, but you begin to receive the subtle Life-force (Ki, Prana, Chi), as well. The physical sign of receiving the Ki is the presence of the bliss-current. But first you have to reverse the usual directional pattern of the breath. **Now** *when you breathe in, the breath is figuratively taken down through the top of your head, drawn deeply into the lower lungs and* ***belly*** *and then expelled up and out the top of the head again - an entirely different way of directing the breath!*

Stop reading for a moment and try several of these breaths to see how different they feel.

It requires some getting used to--but there's more to come. Having accustomed yourself to this new breathing, get ready to take it one step further:

1) Next, I want you to visualize the glowing center of the Milky Way Galaxy, resplendent in the blaze of its countless billion suns. Our own miniature solar system spins in one of its outermost spiral arms (incomprehensible light-years away from the brilliant galactic core)....yet we were originally spawned by (and are part of) its majestic energy.

2) When you exhale and direct the breath through the top of your head, take it *way* out, into interstellar space. Then direct it to the ultimate omega-point in the center of our spiral galaxy.

3) Finally, breathe in and draw down the golden light from that central radiance into your belly. *Try several of these breaths and compare the difference again.*

The Galactic (Love) Breath.

1) This time when you breathe IN and fill your belly with golden light, repeat mentally:

"Loving....."

2) This time when you breathe OUT and send the breath back up to the galactic core, say mentally:

"Breath."

"Breath" is a traditional word for higher Spirit and when you think "breath" while directing the *physical* breath (out the top of your head to the cosmic center), you're actually invoking and activating your own higher Spirit to reconnect to **its** original source. This reconnection immediately opens inner pathways via the Energy Body meridians to receiving the galactic Love energy (particularly in response to the powerful word "loving"). You'll soon find yourself experiencing gentle waves of bliss with tinglings and discharge from the soles of the feet--especially, when (with the IN breath), you also sweep the energy through your belly and down into the magnetic core of the planet. You then become the re-connecting rod between the earth and its distant genesis in the hub of the galaxy!

After mastering the Galactic Breath technique, you'll need to sustain it with a formal time set aside to practice this new way of breathing. Then you'll catch yourself during the day "remembering to breathe." Soon you'll be doing both - a few moments of daily formal breath meditation (with the golden light visualization, plus the "Loving breath" mantra)....**and** finding it easier to reverse the breath-direction during your normal day. When you remember to breathe galacticaly, you'll notice how the "loving" breath instantly brings bliss and joy into an otherwise hectic schedule! Do the Galactic Breath in any position, sitting, standing, walking, lying down.

Applying Galactic Breathing to the Voice.

The galactic breath not only enhances us physically (with health, strength, energy), it immediately empowers the voice--and I cannot stress strongly enough the benefits of applying this new way of breathing to singing; **a dramatic voice improvement can come from this breath practice alone!**

Incorporate it into all of your voice exercises and songs. The silent inspiration (of the breath) marks the pause in your vocalizing where you mentally interpolate the word "loving." Then allowing your voice to soar, you mentally direct the words/sounds to the galactic Center through the top of your head. Or if that's too distracting from your usual singing style, commence your song (or vocal workout) with two or three silent galactic breaths to establish a mode of connectedness. **A very strange way of singing, yes?!!** Yet in this singing/speaking manner, you constantly enliven yourself with Ki from the Life Force while your thoughts and mood become suffused with bliss and love. In the nature of 'cosmic-energy,' you might call it the "Descent of Love".....or the descent of Spirit into matter.

Meditate on photos and drawings of spiral galaxies especially ones that astronomers regard as parallels to our own Milky Way. Several beautiful ones are illustrated in Carl Sagan's book "Cosmos."

Now, with breath primed and ready - it's time to release your voice.

THE FIVE MAJOR RELEASING LETTER-SYMBOLS.

These letters happen to be the vowels in our language: A,E,I,O,U (more about them in Chapter 6 and 21). Symbols usually represent other more hidden meanings and <u>some</u> of these meanings are given here in the form of affirmations; keep these in mind while you're speaking or singing the letters. *Sound the symbols, and feel the feelings, the sounds will integrate the feelings.*

The First Releasing Letter -- identity-affirming "A," with the same sound as "play." **Now *you* say it -- "A" -- "Aaaaaaaaaaaeeeee."**

Letter **"A"** *affirms identity.* "I am ME - I'm perfect just the way I am!"

1) Begin by speaking the "A" several times in a variety of ways, as a question - **"Aaae??"**- a reprimand - **"Aaee!!"**....an approval, a defiance. Try different pitches, even alter the shape *inside* your mouth as you're sounding it. Connect **how** you say "A" with feelings and memories. Widen and stretch your mouth and sound it exaggeratedly, gutturally, harshly, loudly. Now relax your face and say **"Aee"** softly, sweetly and lovingly.....try reversing or mixing-up the order. These are suggestions only, let your intuition lead and your feelings 'feel.' Screech and holler the **"A"** if that's the way the energy goes.

Do the above again, <u>**while adding**</u> a "Y" to the "A" -- **"Aeeeyay,yay,yay,yay,yay,yay, yaaaaeee..."**

Letter **"Y"** *possesses assertive force.* "I am free to do it MY WAY!"

2) Now move the voice out of speech and into song. Sing the **"Aee...yay, yay,yay,yay"** and after a while, sound a *very* extended and powerful **"Aaaaaaaaaeeeeee"** -- a single glorious note with an **"eee"** at the end.

Finally, pause, close your eyes and feel the new energy coursing through you as a result of sounding this letter.

The sound of **"A"** brings up identity issues as well as *strengthens* identity. Practicing daily will not only increase your breath capacity and quality of tone, but you could even begin to feel quite marvelous! Remember to include screams and yells if a sudden need to scream and yell comes up. Don't limit yourself to only 'pretty' sounds. Open and let the tone go exactly where **it** wants--high, low, harsh, sweet, masculine, feminine--*forget your gender!* Express those squashed feelings and your voice will unfold and reclaim its power. By 'voice' I mean speaking as well as singing.

<u>*With* **each** *of the subsequent vowels, observe the* **same** *instructions given in the above paragraphs numbered 1) through 2). Remember to begin each new vowel by first speaking and then singing it and finish by pausing and feeling its effect in the body.*</u>

"A" also has another way of being spoken, **"AH"** (as in 'car'). **Now you try it -- "Aaah."** It has an aspirant, **"H,"** at the end of the sound.

The letter **"H"** *potentiates ambition and vision.*
"My life has a purpose, I have come to do something."

<u>**After a while add**</u> an **"R"** to the **"AH," -- "Aaah...rah,rah,rah,rah,raaaaaah."**

The letter **"R"** *brings identity and ideas together.*
"I think, therefore I am."

The combination of letters **"R"** ***and*** **"AH"** *represent mental, physical and visionary power.*
"I am the Master of my life, what I decide, I do."

If, up until now, your life has been *less* than the **"RAH"** potential, you may stir up old anger and disappointments when making these particular sounds. Feel free then, to literally **roar** with rage! You'll find **"Ah...rar,rar,rar, RAAAARRR"** releases anger! The flood-gates could open and all kinds of tormenting memories might gush out. Let them wash over you and "sound" them away. Most of us were raised to 'stuff' our frustrations or be punished, and if we dared voice *our own* hopes and dreams, we were often ridiculed. Now call up any offending faces and defiantly **"Rar,rar,rarrr"** at them! Connect your rage to the source memories and they will soften and release through the sound.

The Second Releasing Letter -- verbally-affirming "E" with the same sound as in "see." **Sound it yourself -- "Eeeee."**

Letter **"E"** *releases limitless communication.*
"I speak and express whenever, however I want to!"

Now add a "Y" to the **"E"** -- **"Eeee,yee,yee,yee,yee,yeeeeee."**

The letter **"Y"** *combined with* **"E"** *powerfully embodies individual self-determination.*
"I speak and express myself -- MY WAY!"

The Third Releasing Letter -- creatively-affirming **"I"** with the same sound as in "high." **Say it now -- "Iiiiiiiiiieeeeee."**

Letter **"I"** *inspires ecstatic, creative expression.*
"I am the tool of inspiration, I draw attention where it's needed."

Now add the sound **"Y"** to the **"I,"** --**"Iii...yie,yie,yie,yie,yie,yiiiiiieeeee."**

Letters **"Y"** ***and*** **"I"** *together produce unique creativity.*
"I create and perform IN MY OWN SPECIAL WAY!"

The Fourth Releasing Letter -- emotionally-affirming **"O"** with the same sound as in 'flow.' (It also assumes two possible endings, an **"O"** with **"h"** at the end, or an **"O"** with a **"w."**)

Letter **"O"** *embodies emotional nurturing.*
"All of my feelings are O.K, I don't have to hide them (or from them) anymore."

Letters **"O"** *and* **"H"** *together create emotional strength and vision.*
"Self-contained, I nurture myself, I create my own remarkable future."

After *speaking* the **"O"** in a variety of ways, now *sing* a series of long, drawn-out **"Oh's."**
Now add the **"w"** to the **"O,"** as in **"O....wow,wow,wow,wow."**

Letter **"W"** *relishes life with enthusiasm!* "What a fabulous challenge life is!"

Letters **"O"** ***and*** **"W"** *combined say:* "I delight in the magic and wonder of life."

Your work with **"O"** may foster painful memories. When I first sounded this letter, I was shocked by its strong emotional charge--I almost fell apart, *"painful memories" was putting it mildly!!* Fortunately, I remembered to let the sounding of the **"O"** release my feelings AND I certainly shed some tears! (Keep a good supply of Kleenex handy.) For some of us, let's face it, life has NOT been magical and wonderful and a tremendous amount of pain and grief might surface, along with lamenting and deep sobbing. Try not to hold back tears, they will wash away the sorrow, especially if you feel the emotions fully. Sing the **"O"** with a long, wailing, keening sound. When you've let go some of your pain turn it into a glorious wolf-call (howling to the moon and telling the world, "Beware! - I howl my power!"). If fear comes up in any part of the process, you might want to enlist a trusted friend (or two) as backup support. (My most consistent and comforting backup support was a large cuddly stuffed bear!) In the end, I promise, you *will* sing the **"O"** with new found joy and wonder!

The Fifth Releasing Letter -- expansion-affirming "U" (the same sound as in "through"), you make it with the lips pursed together in a closed **"Oooooo."**
Letter "U" means expansion and manifestation, giving and receiving.
"I create total abundance, I see my life as limitless."

Now add **"W"** to the **"U"** -- **"ooowoo,woo,woo,woow,woooooooo."**

Letters **"U"** ***and*** **"W"** *together mean expansion and enthusiasm.*
"I live each moment to the fullest - I encourage you to do the same!"

Now add the autonomous and singular **"Y"** to the **"U,"** -- **"Yoo,yoo,yoo,yoo,yoo, yooooooooo."**

Letters **"Y" "U"** ***and*** **"W"** *together have the energy of sovereignty, generosity and enthusiasm.*
"I see the adventure and challenge of life, and we're here to enable each other to fly!!"

THE RESONATORS

In addition to the five vowels (your primary releasing sounds), there are two additionally important letters, "M," "N" as well as the combination of "NG." These create humming frequencies that vibrate the throat, nasal passages, jaws, septum (nose bones), hard and soft palate (inside the mouth behind the upper teeth), and the sinuses in the face and the skull itself. *You'll learn several ways to send humming waves of vibration through these areas, for shaking lose old blocks and releasing the voice.*

Hearing the Inner Resonance.

It's very important--and encouraging, to also practice the resonators (and even the other open tones) with your hands held over your ears. Not only will you thrill to the richness of tone, but hearing it will connect you more deeply to your inner-voice...and the free and glorious sounds you will soon be making as a matter of course.

The "M" Resonator.

Letter "M" is one of the Goddess or Mother sounds; whether you're male or female, the energy reflects the desire to create a perfect home or 'nest' for yourself. **"MA"** *means being united with your own self-nurturing feminine power (regardless of gender). Its sound resonates this power in the body. If your relationship with your own mother was unsatisfactory, it then becomes the cry for the mother you never really had and releases the pain of that inner ache--leading to your own 'self-mothering.'*

1) Lightly close your lips (but **not** your teeth), flatten your tongue into the lower jaw and hum **"M"**. Try different tones with your tongue in this position, you'll feel a strong vibration at the back of your throat and up to the top of the skull. The higher notes will tickle your soft palate and nose - even to the corners of your eyes.

2) Next press your tongue against the back of your front teeth and hum (but still **don't** put your teeth together). This brings the vibration forward. Now alternate the two tongue positions given in **1)** and **2)** *and with your hands over your ears, listen to the differences in resonance.*

3) At last you can *forget* your tongue and put **your teeth together**. Behind closed lips hum into the teeth, feeling them vibrate. Now make minute movements with your teeth, tapping them lightly together or alternately biting down firmly and then releasing as you hum. (Experiment with the above suggestions; hum little melodies and try other mouth positions with letter **"M."**)

4) Finally add the open **"Maaaaah,"** and then rapidly, **"Ma,ma,ma,ma,ma, maaaaaah"** -- with as many **"Ma's"** as you feel like doing, this can be spoken or toned.

The "N" Resonator.

Letter **"N"** *contains the energy of discernment, balance and responsibility, but in this exercise you'll use the frequency to balance yourself with a self-affirming, self-empowering* ***denial*** *- a "Nah,nah, nah, ney,ney,ney,* ***NO!*** *" -- to all the times you have been thwarted in your life-- when your essential self and its needs were denied, either by yourself or by others. With these sounds you reclaim the power to give yourself what you need (and want), and you'll say* **"No"** *to self denigration and* **"No"** *to all those responsibilities that are really not yours. So begin. Curl your upper lip into a defiant snarl and first speak - then sound* **"Nah, nah,"** **"Ney, ney"** and **"No, NO!"** *Claim your ability to discern and satisfy your needs in a balanced way.*

Variations:

1) Part the lips, remember to snarl if you feel like it and place the tongue firmly on the hard palate directly behind the top teeth. Then clamp your molars (back teeth) together and sound "N" (remember to keep your lips open). It will project through the nose with a strong nasal resonance. **"Nnnnnnnnnnnnnnnnn."** Do it several times on different pitches. The snarl really helps!!

2) Repeat variation one, but cover your ears to more fully feel and hear the resonance.

3) Again, hold your teeth together and this time sound **"Nnnaah-nnnaah-nnnaah,"** several times. Then do it faster, **"Nah,nah,nah,nah,nah,"** for as long as you want culminating (still *with your teeth clenched together and lips open),* in an extended **"Naaaaaaaaaaaaaaah."**

4) Then, open your mouth and sing **"Nah,nah,nah,nah,nah"** any way you wish, making a final long **"Naaaaaaaaaaaaaaaaaaaah."** (Also do variations **3)** and **4)** but substitute **"Ney"** instead of **"Nah."**)

Finally, letter **"N"** *has the amazing facility of bringing us bit-by-bit into balance on all levels of our being. For this more healing quality of* **"N"** *sound the letter in a steady, resonating tone with the mouth relaxed, teeth together and the tongue resting behind the front teeth.* **"Nnnnnnnnnnnnnnnnnnnnnn."** *Vary the pitch as you desire.*

The "NG" Resonator.

1) You can regard this one as a 'drone' frequency. It resonates like the steady hum of a beehive **and occurs at the endings of many words as 'ong' 'ung' and 'ing.'** When sustained in a vocal exercise, you'll experience an almost tickling feeling in your nose and soft palate; also the very back of your tongue will vibrate (extending up into the nasal passages and sinuses) creating a strong 'opening' sensation in the area. You'll notice a lingering feeling there long after the sound has ended. Resonating higher notes on **"NG"** vibrates the top of the skull. While sounding it, try pressing and releasing the *back* of the tongue intermittently on the roof of the mouth (next to your back molars), this alters the drone resonance and releases tension from the root of the tongue. You need to keep making the 'closed' **"NG"** sound and not the more 'open' **"UNG"**......that's the *next* exercise!

2) Establish the **"Ng"** drone at the back of your throat, then vary it by sounding **"ung,ung,-ung,ung"** repeatedly. First, do it rapidly and then slowly with a long drone at the beginning and the end of the shorter **"ung, ung, ung's."** Vary the exercise by using **"ing"** instead of **"ung."** With **"ing,"** you'll feel a completely different 'stretch' on the back of the palate and into the nasal sinuses.

The letter **"G"** *represents another element of balance, the balance between work and play, and between physical and spiritual beauty. Also, the* **"NG"** *drone relates directly to a Hatha Yoga voice technique called "Brahmarie" (The Bee) used traditionally in India for "sweetening, beautifying and strengthening the voice."*

BRAHMARIE (The Bee)

The exercise is in two parts.

Part One. (The hardest part.)
Try and constrict the back of your throat and breathe in at the same time! It's a similar feeling to when your air passages are partially blocked, as though suffering from bronchitis or asthma - or you've nearly choked after something went down the wrong way!! It sounds like a high, gasping, wheezing whine, as though barely enough air is getting through to sustain you; however, *this* time you have to do it on purpose! The way we were taught to perform it at the Yoga Ashram in Val Moren (Canada) was to open our mouths and 'suck' in the air for as long as we could - while trying to make the required gasping, whining sound. It was *supposed* to sound terrible but if you hurt your throat (which I often did), then that meant you were **not** doing it correctly!

Part Two. (The easiest part.)
Having just finished your labored **in**-breath, **close your mouth and clench your back teeth together** while you release the breath in a high pitched, sustained **"humming"** sound against the teeth--like the hum of a bee. Repeat **Part One** and **Two**, once or twice a day.

The Modified Brahmarie.

I now find it vastly easier to begin the exercise at part one with my mouth shut and my teeth already clamped together. You then make the same ghastly, rasping noises in the back of your throat while drawing the air in through your nose instead of your mouth - flowing effortlessly into the second part of the high pitched "bee" drone. If you begin by practicing my modified method first, you'll find it simpler when you come to try the traditional Brahmarie - yes, you should try them both (with mouth shut or open), to see which is best for you. Each method has its merits.

You have now completed the basic releasing exercises for the three resonators and the five vowels. If you can manage one practice session a day, you'll begin to notice a considerable difference in how you feel and how you speak and sing. When you have released most of the painful emotional energies, your voicings will become more re-charging than dis-charging--and you won't sound quite so blood curdling to the neighbors!

Practice Sheets follow for the vowels .

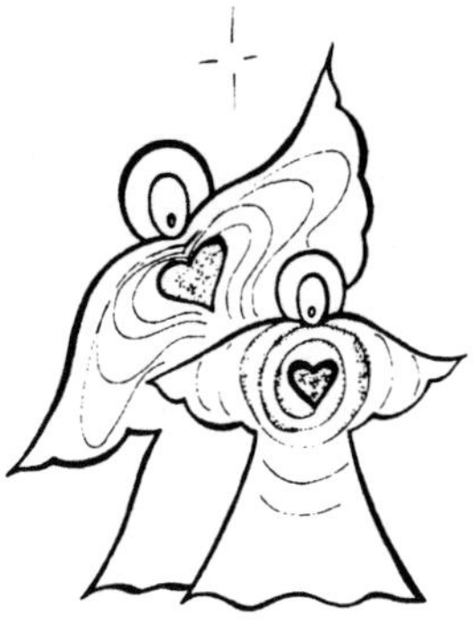

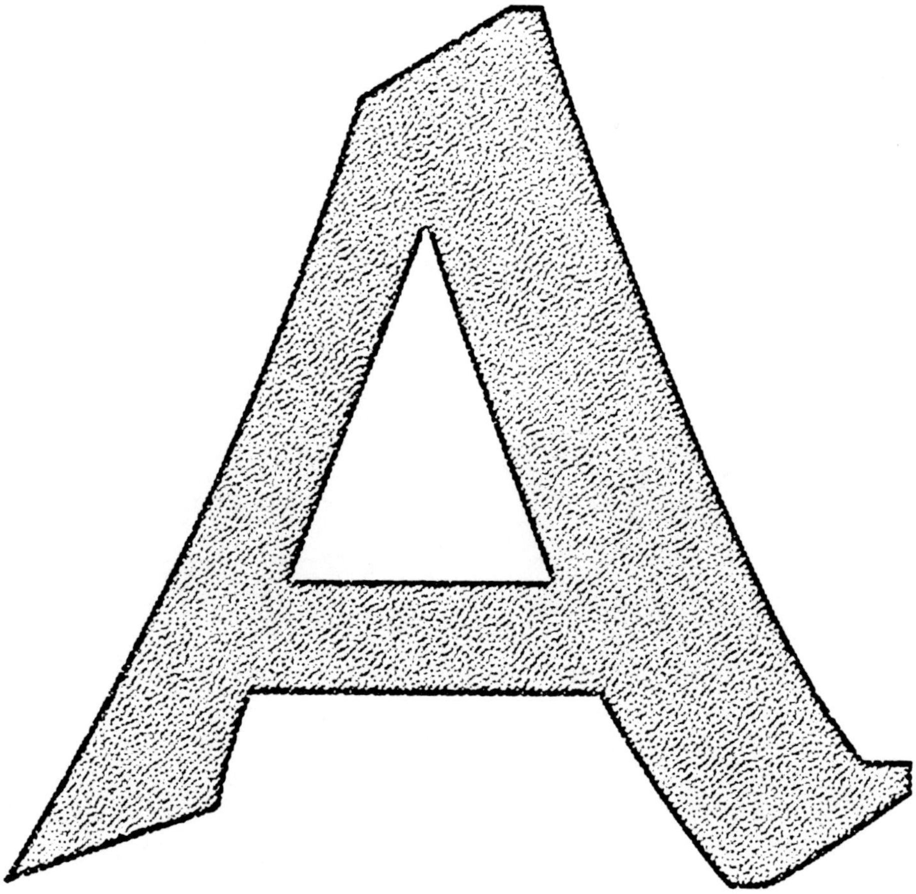

"A" -- "Aaaaaaaaaaaeeeee."

"A" *affirms identity:*
"I am ME -- I'm perfect just the way I am!"

Now add "Y" to "A" -- "Aeeeyay,yay,yay,yay,yay, yay,yaaaaeee..."

Letter **"Y"** *possesses assertive force:*
"I am free to do it MY WAY!"

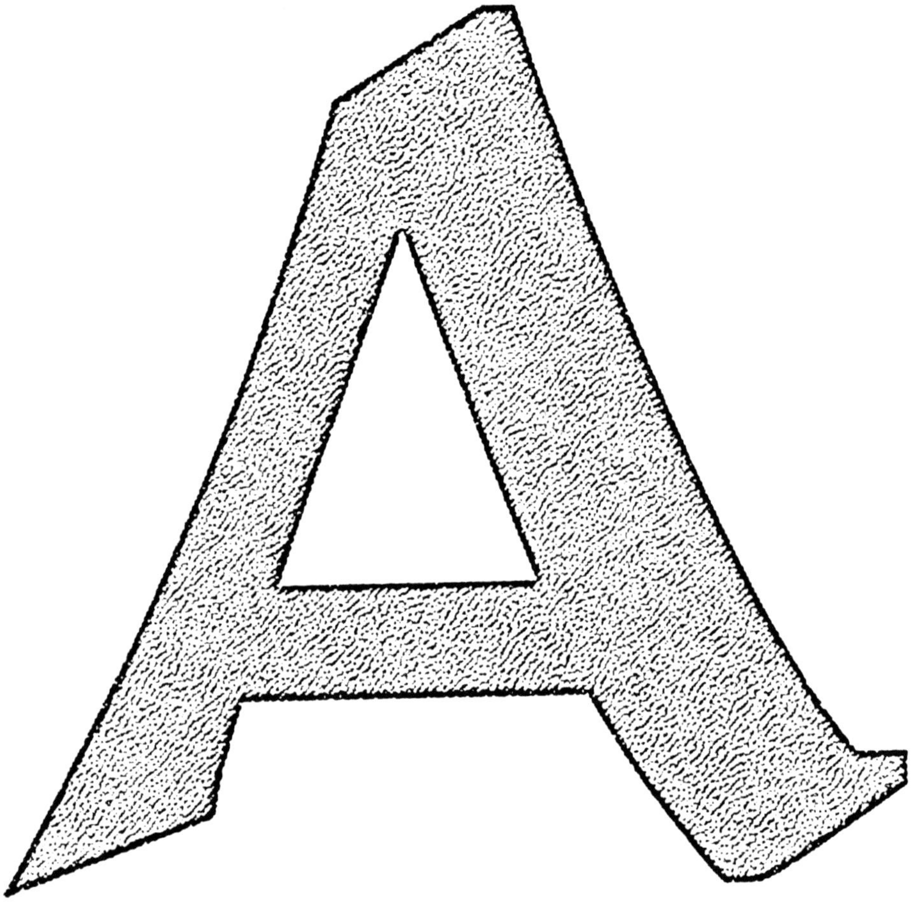

"AH" (as in 'car') -- "Aaaaaaaaaaaaaaaaaaaaaaah."

The letter **"H"** *potentiates ambition and vision:*
"My life has a purpose, I have come to do something."

Now add "R" to "AH" -- "Aaah...rah,rah,rah,rah,raaaaaaaaaaaaah."

"R" *and* **"AH"** *combined--mental, physical and visionary power:*
"I am the Master of my life, what I decide, I do,"
"I have the power and the strength, to always follow through."

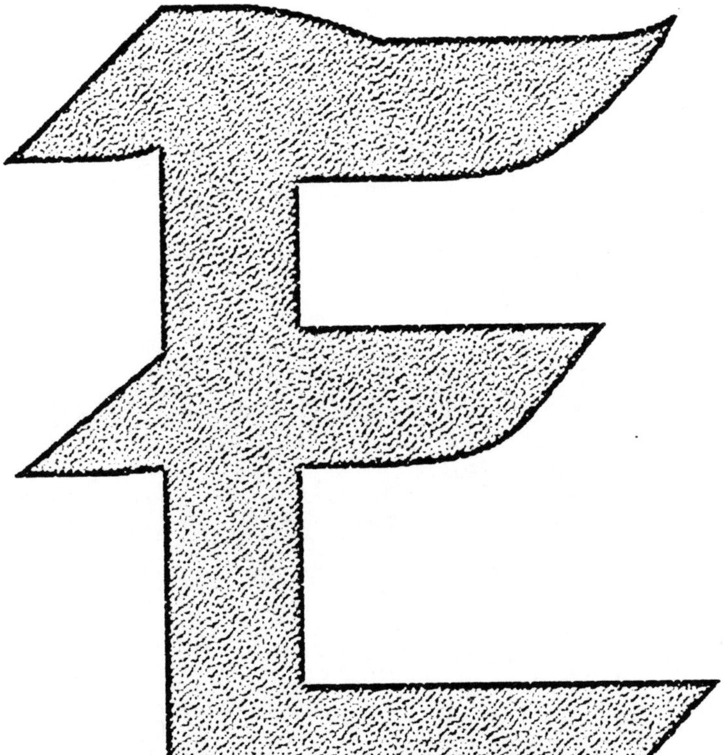

"E" -- "Eeeeeeeeeeeeeeeeeeeeee."

"E" *releases limitless communication:*
"I speak and express however--whenever, I want to!"

Now add "Y" to "E" -- "Eeee,yee,yee,yee,yee,yeeeeeeeeee."

"Y" *combined with* **"E,"** *embodies individual self-determination:*
"I speak and express myself -- MY WAY!"

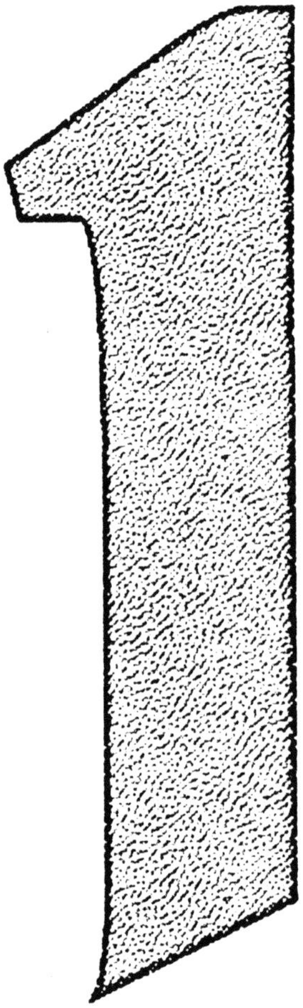

"I" -- "Iiiiiiiiiiiiiiiiiiiieeeeee."

"I" *inspires ecstatic, creative expression:*
"I am the tool of inspiration - I draw attention where it's needed."

Now add "Y" to "I" --"Iii...yie,yie,yie,yie,yie,yiiiiiiiiiiieeeee."

"Y" *and* **"I"** *together produce unique creativity:*
"I create and perform -- IN MY OWN SPECIAL WAY!"

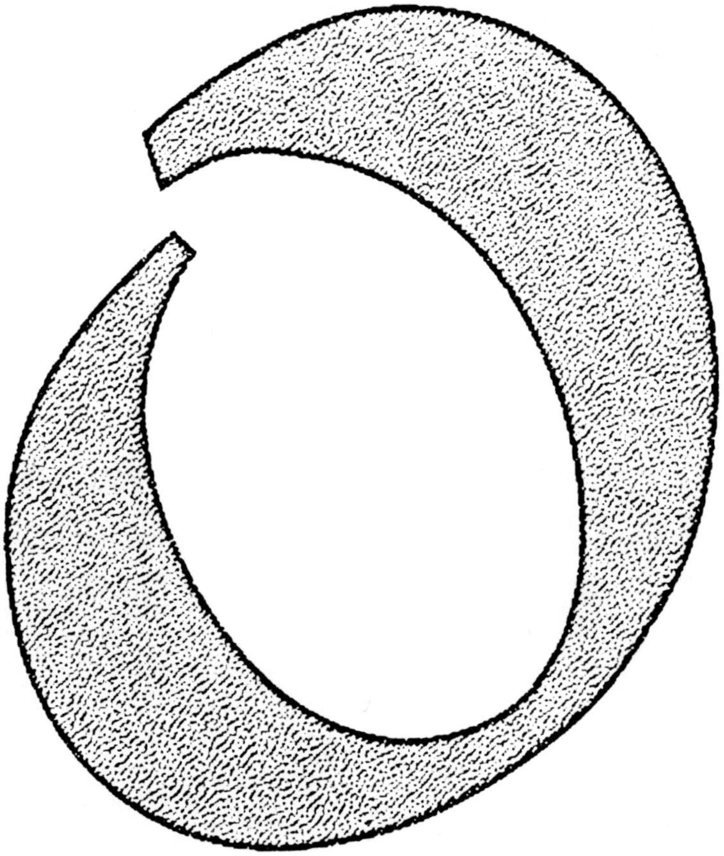

"O" has two possible endings, an "O" with "h" at the end, or an "O" with a "w."
Make some long, drawn-out "Oh's" -- then "O...wow,wow,wow,wow,wow."

"O" *embodies emotional nurturing:* "All of my feelings are O.K.,
I don't have to hide them (or from them) anymore."

"O" *and* **"H"** *create emotional strength and vision:*
"Self- contained, I nurture myself -- I create my own remarkable future."

"W" *relishes life with enthusiasm!* "What an fabulous challenge life is!"
"O" *and* **"W"** *combined say:* "I delight in the magic and wonder of life."

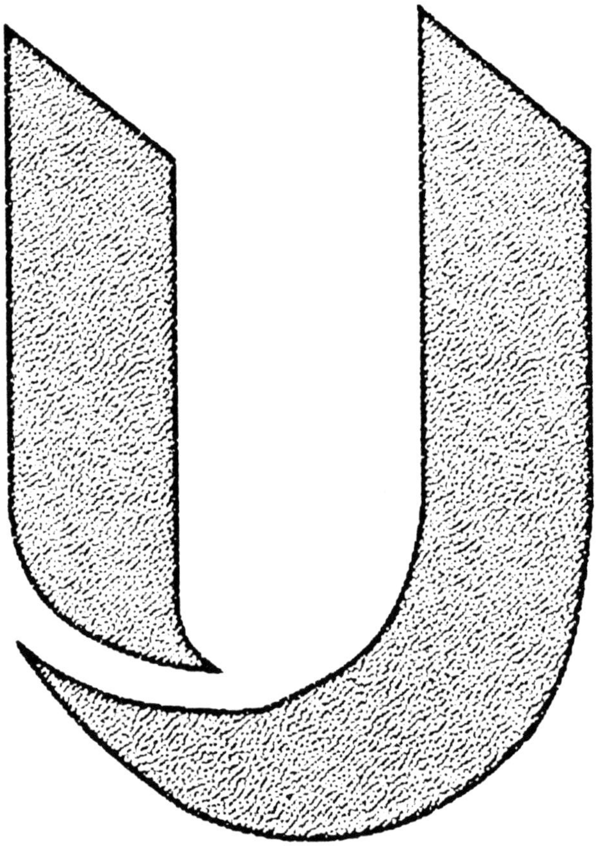

"U"-- make with the lips pursed together in a closed "Oooooo."

"U," *expansion and manifestation, giving and receiving:*
"I create total abundance -- I see my life as limitless."

Now add "W" to "U" (as in 'who') -- "ooowoo,woo,woo,woow,woooooooo."
"U" *and* **"W,"** *mean expansion and enthusiasm:*
"I live each moment to the fullest -- I encourage you to do the same!"

Now add "Y" to "U" (as in 'you') -- "Yoo, yoo,yoo, yoo,yoo, yooooooooo."
"U" *and* **"W"***bring sovereignty, generosity, enthusiasm:*
"I see the adventure and challenge of life, and we're here to enable each other to fly!!"

5..... YOUR NAME - HOW TO UNDERSTAND & ANALYZE IT

(This information is my expansion of the original research on names by Shirlee Kilee & Rochelle Gordon.)[1]

From the voice and its expression, we move to your name, the sound pattern for your life. Many ask me - "How can my name be important if I didn't even choose it?" No choice exists. You are a specific sound-print and couldn't be named anything else! You embody your name as an aspect of the total Sound Body. Within the womb, every cell resonates with your frequency, even the DNA spirals sing your song! And through some mysterious soul-to-soul process, your unique and special "sound" comes into the mind of someone (often your mother) who then names you with it. When I tell this to people, I receive a barrage of questions including the following:

"My name was changed after being adopted, what does that mean?"
"They named me after my grandfather, does that make me the same as him?"
"After my divorce I wanted a new identity, so instead of returning to my maiden name, I chose three completely new names. Don't they cancel out my original name?"
"I detest my name. It reminds me of being screamed at as a child, that's why I'm changing it.....and you're telling me it contains my personality and my *destiny*?"

These and other questions will be explained as we proceed. We all have an intense interest in names, but the idea that they could hold any special or redeeming qualities never occurs to us, particularly if we happen to dislike our own. Part of my research has been to demonstrate the validity and importance of all our given names. An interesting example of this occurred several years ago. An elderly man came to me for name analysis at the urging of his son - a previous recipient of my research. They had decided to give me a name challenge based on the father's unusual situation. As a youth, the father, together with his parents, had escaped to England from Germany during the political rise of the Nazis. Being Germans in a country that ended up desperately fighting Hitler during World War 2, they put origins behind them by changing their names - and this gentleman had not used his birth name in 50 years. During our time together, I compared his German and English names in detail. The information astonished him, especially the depth of relevant meaning in his forgotten, unused name. I explained that succeeding changes act as filters for the original name (as for instance, when women drop their maiden names at marriage). In this man's case, the discarded birth name took on the function of a middle name, becoming a reservoir for deeper, more hidden elements within the personality. *It doesn't matter how many names are subtracted or added, the one on the birth certificate will always filter through the new ones. We never really lose or nullify that original name; its energy-influence always prevails, even if remaining in the background.*

Terms Used in Connection with Names:

Given name - the one on your Birth Certificate.
Christian name - your first name.
Maiden name - another word for a woman's last or original family name.
Family name - the last name regardless of gender.
Surname - another term for the Family or last name.
Legal name - this *could* be the one on your Birth Certificate, unless you have changed your name through marriage or naturalization. If you went through the Court system to change and re-register a new name, the most recent one becomes the new legal name. **However, the original, given name on the Birth Certificate contains the Master tape for your life - *not* the changed name!** A new legal name creates a fresh 'experience-filter' for the original one and can become an energy extension, an evolutionary progression for the initial birth name.

Most of us have two or three names - first and last - or first, middle and last, and married women commonly have a first, middle *and* a married name (their maiden name hiding in the wings). Unusual as it sounds, occasionally a man will take on his wife's last name by adding a hyphen between his own and hers creating a new legal double-name for himself. It's traditional in Western cultures for

---

[1] See "Personal Power is in Your Name" by Shirlee Kiley and Rochelle Gordon. A Dell Book.

the lady to drop her last name and assume her husband's - the old idea of the blood line passing through the man with the woman just being his channel (and chattel!). Now, with more equality a woman will frequently keep her maiden name at marriage, or will add a hyphen - retaining her own as well as gaining his. Such a novel arrangement often makes for extremely interesting partnerships! The mutual and individual energies change according to the letter combinations in the new joint name. Sounds complicated?.....it used to be all so simple!

Very occasionally, you will meet someone with an unbelievably long name. A possible example: a first name followed by two or even three middle ones, as well as a hyphenated last name. Likewise, if you have the usual two or three names, but they add up to being exceptionally long, for instance: many lettered names like Geraldine Camperdini; Zachariah Sylvester Schulyer, or Bernadine Maria Kopalowski--then they would share similar challenges to those with multi or hyphenated names. In the scheme of understanding names....what exactly does this mean?

Long and multiple names *present a serious energy challenge. Usually, the longer the name, the more diverse and fractionalized the energy:*

You may give others the impression that you're scattered and unfocused, with a wealth of interests pulling you in many directions - often all at once! Such diversity and lack of purpose can be confusing and creates the need for self discipline and narrowing down your interest spectrum. Then again, some of you handle this heightened energy without stress. You thrive on intense activity and enjoy the excitement of trying many different things - often to the chagrin of friends and relatives who wish you would settle into a solid occupation instead of being the dilettante.

Another group of **long-namers** *embraces the other extreme:*

In spite of sometimes overwhelming difficulties, you seem to be born with a built-in "radar" tracking down and locking on to your chosen path. You also emerge graced with the power to handle chaos and overload and follow your purpose *without* being moved - but **you** are one of the rare ones!

Short and compact names *usually hold a keenly focused energy with less inclination for distraction. The more concise the name, the more centered and concentrated the life:*

When disciplined or inspired, you direct your energy like a laser, cutting through doubts and fears, incinerating obstacles and invariably inspiring others. You too involve yourself in a multitude of interests, but underlying the apparent diversity burns the flame of a single passion - a special goal or pursuit that eventually becomes your driving force.

This explains why some people attract nicknames; subconsciously they want to simplify an unacceptably overwhelming name energy. Have you met a person who has been nicknamed from birth and *never* been called by their real name? It happens occasionally - and stranger still, have you heard of a person whose nickname has no similarity to their actual name at all?

Are You a Nicknamed Person? If so, remember that this shortened version (or substitution), has its genesis on your birth certificate where your **longer** original name awaits your understanding, re-assessment and possible reclamation....if you want to participate in all of your potential.

"But I never **use** that name, no one's called me that since I was a tiny child"!

Protest you might, but the unused name contains part of the energy pattern from your essential sound-print, and warrants inspection even if just to discover what you have been avoiding by using a shorter version. Think of the people you know with long first names, who do *not* allow others to shorten them and feel uncomfortable when it happens; I remember a **Barbara** (in my home land of Australia), who would never let anyone condense her name to **"Babs"** or **"Barby"** - some instinct in her felt the importance of keeping her name intact!

In spite of my seeming disapproval of nicknames, there are certain exceptions ***when it could be beneficial, or to your advantage,*** *for instance:* if you attract an abbreviated name, not because of avoidance, but because you've made a subconscious choice to concentrate on the energy in the shortened version - as if the rest of the name would be a distraction from the **real** lessons you came to learn. To illustrate, we'll use the name **PAT** (short for Patricia). The **"P"** energy naturally tends to retreat into a core of peacefulness or has the knack of smoothing the agitated feathers of the less-than-peaceful people surrounding them--unless of course it's unbalanced, then it becomes the "Disturber of the Peace"........and delights in stirring up strife and controversy wherever it goes!

To attract a **PAT** nickname, maybe the person wants to understand or *use* more personal power (power comes from the letter **"A,"** with its egocentric and natural leadership qualities) and in using the nickname Pat, all of a sudden the **"A"** energy takes center-stage in the middle of the name saying, **"Here I am! Get your ego on line, you can now be strong......you can now be a leader!!"** Mind you, such ideas aren't always to the liking of some "peace-at-any-price" **"P's."** But observe the letter on the other side of the power-loving (or power-fearing) **"A"** in Pat - the intuitive, spiritual, nervously sensitive, even psychic, letter **"T."**

Now let's arrive at a possible meaning for **PAT**. **"P"** in the front and **"T"** at the back could modify the **"A"** ego along the lines of peacefulness and self-containment; with a more sensitive and compassionate reaction to power and anger situations....that's of course, if you're a 'positive' Pat!! The 'negative' Pats get power-high on staging as much disharmony as they can. *So depending on how one chooses to use the energy, you can have several versions of "Pat."*

<u>The Different Parts of a Full Name.</u>

<u>**First name**</u>: (Christian name) reflects your outer personality, who **you** think you are and how, for the most part, you appear to other people....who **they** think you are!

<u>**Second name:**</u> (middle name) hides the more private aspects of your personality; it's from a deeper, almost subconscious level (perhaps not fully realized even by yourself) and sometimes contains unrealized gifts and abilities. If you believe you have lived before and bring in the energy of past lives, this second name (or names) reveals tendencies from those lives. By sounding or meditating on the letters of the middle name, you can often release these hidden strengths to benefit your outer life.

But what if you don't have a second name? In that event, your first name carries loaded information conveying a surface as well as an ulterior meaning. Certain letters in the name will magnify this 'hidden' disposition especially **"K's, T's, P's** and **W's."** Do others think of you as hard to get close to, enigmatic, puzzling? With only two names you may have an outer manner, a facade, that obscures and protects who you really are--even from yourself!

<u>**Last name:**</u> (the surname, maiden or family name) discloses the specific family atmosphere, the emotional, mental and physical milieu you found yourself born into. In addition, this name relates directly to the outer environment and governs specifically your life path. After growing up, leaving home and venturing out into the world, your last name continues to attract the opportunities needed to fulfill that life path, part of which includes your occupation, how you'll earn your living and support yourself and others in the environment.

<u>The Key Letters of Your Name.</u>

There are certain "key" letters in your name that give special emphasis to your life's direction. And every step along the way, you constantly have to choose between a positive or negative alignment with this key energy. Each letter in your name tells a story but certain letters have greater importance, these are the **first**, **last** and **middle** letters, or the middle <u>**two**</u> **letters**, if the name has an *equal* number of letters.

<u>The First Letter</u> -- THE DRIVE:

The energy you lead with, how you 'drive' your life, how you *appear* in the world.

1) The first letter of your **first** name....the persona, your personality mask, how you primarily impress or affect others. Sometimes, it's what you'd *like* others to think you are!

2) The first letter of your **second** name (or names)....the active force of your inner nature, the mostly hidden "stuff" relating to the sub-self personalities you were born with.

3) The first letter of your **last** name (or names)....the driving force in response to your environment, your relationship with your family, your work and how you face the outer world.

<u>Drive letter Examples</u>:
Let's take a look at the name of a rather notorious and famous figure: ex-football hero and accused murderer (of his wife and her male companion), **O. J. Simpson**. The Drive letter energy of his Christian names is so dominant, that hardly anyone in the general public even knows what those two initials stand for - he's always referred to in the media as **"O. J"** and *only* that. In effect, he has attracted a nickname created from the Drive letters of his actual names....thus drawing attention to how and for what, he will be the most recognized.
*Anyone else who initializes (rather than uses) their first names might also be saying "This is **<u>only</u>** what I want to project - I don't care to deal with any more of my personal identity; the first letter (or letters) is enough - that's **all** I want to be known as!"*

In relationship to **O. J. Simpson** and his both fortunate and unfortunate life, the revelation in these linked Drive letters astounds one!! Of course, being tried for a horrible crime and acquitted in a criminal court, then being re-tried and found responsible in a civil court, has totally polarized the energy of the accused! We have been forced to look at the dark side and the bright side of this man.

Therefore, I present to you the effect of **O.J. Simpson's** polarized Drive letters and keeping in mind the countless newspaper and magazine articles and the months of TV coverage of the murder events and the subsequent trials, you will note that both sides (given below) of letters **"O" "J"** and **"S"** from O.J. Simpson's now very famous name have been shown up for public scrutiny.

Consider:
<u>Letter "O" positive (constructive):</u> nurturing, caring, compassionate, loving, supportive, considerate, charming, open, gentle and above all--emotionally balanced.
or.....
<u>Letter "O" negative (destructive):</u> emotionally manipulative, dominating, controlling, self-indulgent, demanding, threatened and threat<u>ening</u>. (Of course, *every* word following "manipulative" must also be prefaced by "emotionally.") With **"O"** as the Drive letter of the first name, you can be a master of emotional manipulation and others will only know you through the particular emotional-mask you happen to be projecting onto them. The 'mask' changes constantly as you either respond or try and control, depending on what feelings others reveal. In whatever way the **"O"** projects itself, emotions direct the energy, and whether through weakness or strength, cruelty or compassion, the lesson remains the same--you have come to understand and master the power of emotions.

<u>Letter "J"</u> <u>positive (constructive)</u>: upholding justice and the law, the defender and supporter of just causes, a spokesperson against private and social injustices.
or.....
<u>Letter "J"</u> <u>negative (destructive):</u> perpetrating injustices while claiming innocence, attracting trouble, accidents, false or real accusations, or openly bent on mischief.

<u>Letter "S"</u> <u>positive (constructive)</u>: ethical, a positive public role model, setting an example through honesty, uprightness, trustworthiness and good deeds, upholding constructive and wholesome traditions.
or.....
<u>Letter "S"</u> <u>negative (destructive)</u>: unethical, presenting a false front to the community, society, the world, often behind an admirable public image eschewing the traditions and morals of upright society.
(The above are the two polarities of the three Drive letters in the name of O.J. Simpson.)

<u>Interpreting the Drive Letters:</u> *Turn to Chapters 6 and 8 in reference to the first letters of your first, middle and last names and discover the energy in your own personal "drives." All the letters following the first, express themselves through, or in relationship to, that initial Drive letter.*

The Middle Letter(s) -- THE FOCUS-CHALLENGE:

The energy of greatest challenge and ultimate victory, that which you were born to gain mastery over. Also, how you challenge (or aggravate) other people and the way in which you assist others to focus on things they need to pay attention to.

I'll give you a personal example: Over the years, an old Yoga student of mine would periodically visit me en route between Canada and Mexico. She always made me feel nervous, on my guard and somewhat aggravated, but It wasn't until her most recent visit that I realized where the challenge was coming from. It was the two letters in the middle of her last name, letters **"I" and "S."** (*I decline to supply the entire last name to protect the innocent!*) In less than 8 hours, her traveling companion, a large dog (part wolf, part malamute), proceeded to tear up an 8x6 ft. blind slung on my back porch and dug up part of my prized circular maze garden (twice) to deposit its excrement. Furthermore, against my friend's entreaties, I refused to let the dog sleep overnight **inside** my mobile home! The prospect of extra fleas and possible ticks depositing themselves plus the feared desecration of my humble treasures --not to mention my Persian cat--quite alarmed me!! In the face of my shattered peace (including sleeplessness), I began to mentally scrutinize her name letters and (as mentioned) found the answer sitting discomfortingly in the middle of her last name. During her visit (primarily through her dog), she succeeded in drawing attention (letter **"I"**), to my attachment to my 'stuff'- my possessions (letter **"S"** can include one's worldly goods). My sense of security through home and surroundings felt threatened by her/their presence! Interesting!! So next time an acquaintance upsets *your* composure, analyze the Focus in their last name. Also, not only look at what your middle letters challenge **you** to focus on, but study what potential effect those same letters may have on those around you.....it may not always be comfortable--for yourself or for them!

1) The Middle letter(s) in your **first** name show your biggest and most pressing personality challenge.
2) The Middle letter(s) in your **second** name(s) show your private, more hidden, possibly karmic personality challenges and potential.
3) The Middle letter(s) in your **last** name(s) show your work, family and environment tasks and challenges.

These Focus-Challenge letters stop us in our tracks and mark the line we won't go past, or fear to go past. (Some of us fear success more than anything!) They show us our blockages and defeats, what we would like to ignore, where we feel the most hopeless, foolish, helpless and humiliated. They're also called **Focus** letters because **If** we focus on their challenge **our lives will attain their greatest fulfillment and purpose.** The challenge always presents a superb opportunity, the choice between staying put or entering into the excitement and adventure of becoming a Master! You can either look at these central letters and say, "Yes, it's true, that's where I 'm always stuck," or "Wow, so that's how I'm going to change and get things moving!" Occasionally you will encounter an exceptional person, a person of enormous determination (or grace) who sweeps through life unfazed and undiscouraged by any kind of difficulty, who recognized in training-pants that being alive was the greatest challenge of all! Talk to them and you will hear the same story, at a key moment in their lives they made a simple decision, **"This is what I want to do!"** And they set out and did it--usually superbly!

How to *find* the Middle Letters.

If you have a name like JANET or BRUCE, names with an *uneven* number of letters, the **Focus** letter would be the one in the middle, the **"n"** in Janet and the **"u"** in Bruce. This changes when there is an *even* number of letters, as in GORDON or MARGARET. Gordon's **Focus** letters are the middle **two** letters, **"rd"** and Margaret's are **"ga."**

Interpreting the Focus-Challenge letter(s): *Consult* Chapters 6 and 8 ("The Secret Meaning of Vowels and Consonants" and "More Letter Meanings A to Z") *and read the meanings for your name's particular Focus letters. Also read the definitions for the letters immediately adjacent to (the left and right of) the Focus; they will help you comprehend the nature of your challenge.*

The Last Letter of your Name -- THE AIM :
The energy of final attainment or resolution, what you're aiming to fulfill and complete this lifetime.

1) The Aim letter of your **first** name...............what your outer personality needs to develop the most.
2) The Aim letter of your **middle** name(s)......what you need to release and develop from your hidden, more karmic potential.
3) The Aim letter of your **last** name(s)............what you want to achieve or resolve in your family, your work and the world.

Interpreting the Aim letters: *Look up all of the last letters in your names and try and decide what are your true objectives for being alive....remember, you have the choice of making the energy constructive or otherwise!*

Some names have extra sounds.

Extra letters appear in some names that are 'voiced' but not spelled, for example the **"J"** *sound* in the name ROGER. This means that all Rogers actually have *two* Focus-Challenge letters rather than one, **"G"** *and* **"J."** The spelled yet silent **"G"** represents a work Focus: you either have great pride in your work and become a happy workhorse -- or you want to avoid effort and toil like the plague. The **"J"** *sound* however, gives a completely different twist to the work challenge of letter **"G."** For the name Roger, this **"J"** energy predisposes them to a mini-holiday-mentality, they're able to open an escape valve from intense job-related stress--or else you get a counter-productive personality that avoids becoming work-responsible! And, some **"J"** people attract trouble like bees around a honey pot; they love the thick of a fight, be it verbal or fisticuffs. When negative, they choose trouble and when positive, they're uniquely gifted in trouble-shooting and solving problems.

One Roger I knew had all the qualities of a fine and dedicated worker, but his delight in wild trouble making, especially in his youth, had me puzzled until I remembered the *sound* of the "J" in Roger. "Piggyback" letters like these in a name have symbiotic functions--they appear to be unlike in form and function, yet each mutually nourishes the other in some way. The hard working Rogers *need* to have their wild side! A less rambunctious outlet is their love of travel and the outdoors (from the "J" sound). On the highest level, the Mastery of **"GJ"** would be to bring beauty, harmony and joy into troubled or unjust situations, and accepting what "is" rather than judging, condemning and stirring up dissent.

More Silent Letter Examples:

The "E" sound for the "Y" letter. A very common occurrence is a **"Y"** for the last letter (the Aim), as in RICKY, MARY and many other names. Here the **"Y"** is silent and an **"E"** is *heard* instead.....giving a **"Y"** ending two Aims instead of one. This means all **"Y"** Aim people are 'aiming' to speak their power (either verbally or through creativity), they're under pressure to *really* communicate because **"E"** is the dominant final sound. The **"Y"** remains a silent agenda beneath the **"E"** *sound* .....**making it crucial** that they learn to assert themselves in their own way! **"Y"** like **"A,"** needs to be independent and free.
On the transcendent level, *the mental will power of the* **"Y"** *surrenders to the higher will power of Spirit - and that changes how you communicate and express yourself (the* **"E"***)!*

The "V" sound instead of "PH" as in **STEPHEN** - the letter **"V"** brings the challenge to serve the world or communities through one's explorations of balance and harmony (**"P"**) and to bring it to public attention (**"H"**). With a silent **"H"** one might try to avoid fame, or one gains attention *mainly* within ones chosen field of expertise. Apply this to wheelchair-bound **Stephen Hawking,** one of the world's greatest physicists, but also bear in mind, the central Challenge letter of **Stephen**--the silent **"P."** *It brings the focus of inner serenity in the face of supreme outer problems....which pale in the light of his brilliant and luminous mind.*

The "F" sound instead of "PH" as in PHILLIP and PHYLLIS. ("**P**" for balance and harmony, "**H**" for vision and success)...as in the enormously successful, 16th Century High Renaissance, Italian artist **Raphael,** who was known and honored as a master of composition and harmony. The "**F**" sound can bring the added dimension of pride and prominence along with success.

Here are some for *you* to ponder: when "**I**" sounds like "**E**" as in **Heidi,** when "C" sounds like "**SH**" as in **Patricia.** *In these cases, you'll need to look up the meanings of the extra sounds as well as the letters that are written but* **not** *sounded.*

Consider also the *ignored* letters, like the "**E**" at the beginning of **Eugene** and **Eunice**. Then you really have two Drives, a silent one ("**E**") and the spoken one ("**U**") which stresses all the things that "**U**" means and with all the qualities of silent "**E**" being retained as a foundation.

And three totally unique sound-letter combinations occurring in names: - "CH," "SH" **and** "TH." *These sounds cannot be categorized* (broken down into couplings of other distinct alphabetical sounds), and represent a unique dynamism in the language of names. Remember that "**H**" generates ambition, vision and self-discipline or the exact opposite--procrastination, dullness and self-indulgence. Those few "**H's**" who knuckle down with a plan and a purpose can realize their dreams and become enormously successful, even famous.

Combination "CH," When "**H**" sits next to "**C**" curiosity and creative skillfulness prod ambition and help manifest money. A weak "**C**" impels the person to develop some specific skills or they'll spin their wheels and moan, "I just can't find what it is I'm supposed to do!!" On another level, many "**CH**" people go into the visionary aspect of the "**H**" and yearn to help their fellow man in some personal way...and often do! Like successful actor (and practicing Buddhist), **Richard Gere** who is passionately committed to the plight of the Tibetan people; actor **Arnold Schwarzenegger**, who works with inner city children to curb drugs and voilence; early 20th century brilliant musicologist **Albert Schweitzer**, who backed away from his glittering gifts and devoted his life to others as a medical missionary in Africa; and also **Winston Churchill**, Prime Minister and outstanding statesman during Britain's darkest hour in World War 2. The "**CH**" energy also involves itself with helpful research and specialized knowledge set to benefit others. **Examples: Rachel Carson** ("**CH**" middle Focus letters), concerned pioneer on the harmful effects of man on the environment; her controversial and crusading books written in the 50's and 60's ("The Sea Around Us," "The Edge of the Sea," and "Silent Spring") were harbingers of our now seriously threatened eco-structure. And real-life superman, actor-director **Christopher Reeve**, who even before his paraplegia, had devoted his life to health and environmental causes.

Combination "SH," this strong combination fits together perfectly for money, fame, a public image and social standing; it pulls dreams down into the practical world and compels the world to sit up and take notice. **Shirley Temple** was a wildly successful child star at the age of 5; her charm and grace cheered millions during the economic collapse of the 30's and her early black-and-white films still delight a host of fans today. Both "**H**" and "**S**" share the energy of ambition, incentive and the drive for recognition--with money inevitably following in the wings! "**H**" however, includes the aspects of willpower, self discipline and hard work to achieve its goals and where they also hold fast to a Grand Vision, staying-power mixed with patience is necessary--and results can be more delayed.

On the transcendent level, "**SH**" *bridges the veil between the mundane and the mystical. It holds the power to bring the esoteric before the public.* As with **Shirley MacLaine,** accomplished actress and writer of several mystical and self-improvement books including "Going Within, a Guide for Inner Transformation." *Also, it can make practical an enlightened vision.* Example: selfless, dedicated and practical visionary **General George Marshall,** the unsung organizational genius and hero from World War 2, who amongst his many military accomplishments, authored and orchestrated the Marshall Plan that rebuilt and healed war-torn Western Europe. (Notice the "**SH**" as the compelling Focus in the center of his environment name.)

Comment: In both **"CH"** and **"SH."** I find more than twice the number of male names over female names beginning with these letters. The reason could lie in the old tradition of men being the ambitious, money making heads-of-the-family preparing for the future; while women were supposed to stay at home with the children and not push themselves into public life. While researching, I discovered the **"SH"** *sound* sometimes occurring instead of **"CH,"** but only in female names (CHARLENE, CHARLOTTE, CHARMAINE, CHERIE, CHERYL), verifying that their skills **("C")** *could* be directed towards public and community concerns with subsequent recognition and honor. A different use of this could be an intense interest and curiosity (a factor of "C") in *other* people--who happened to already be public figures, in other words, they enjoy the energy vicariously!

A couple of intriguing male names CHRISTIAN and CHRISTOPHER have the **"CH"** but with with a substituted **"K"** sound. In these cases, the sexual, creative force invariably provides the dynamic energy *behind* the skills and ambition of **"CH."** Here, the underlying sexuality might be obvious and part of the person's charisma, or sublimated into a driving ambition or passionate interest. I also found three female names (not counting spelling variations) with the same **"K"** substitution for **"CH,"** CHRISTABELE, CHLOE and CHRISTINE. One immediately thinks of sexual challenges, *but for more insights, people of both sexes with this interesting **"K" instead of "CH" sound,** should study the relevant text in* Chapters 6 *and* 8, *and also the affirmation for* **"K"** in Chapter 7.

Combination "TH," names with the **"TH"** commencement present a very different kind of energy and in this case, I found an almost equal number of **"TH"** names for men and women. Here you have (in the **"T"**), the sensitive, mystical and religious....or their skeptical opposites. **"T"** as the first letter 'drives' the personality but is immediately linked to the ambitious, worldly, hard-working **"H"**....an interesting energy combination! In a few of the names, THERESA, THOMASINA, THORA for girls and THOMAS, and THOR for boys (you may know other names), only the **"T"** is sounded with a silent **"H."** In these names, the **"T"** would dominate as the Drive for the personality, while the silent **"H"** would bring in the need to develop practical forsight, self discipline and willpower.

Of Final Interest: the curious combination of **"ST."** With this, the potential for practical mysticism takes a curious turn, one that enters the realm of altered states of consciousness and interdimensional realities. I know several (legal) hallucinogenic plant and mushroom researchers and growers, also some intuitive healers, psychics and shamans with **"ST"** in their names....other **"ST's"** remain adamantly skeptical!

As you see, your name contains much more than the spelling; how it sounds when it's spoken, also makes a difference. Check your name. Has it any unspelled or unsounded letters--there are many more than I've mentioned? If so, look up their meanings and you may want to practice sounding them also to tap into that part of your energy.

Doubled letters.

Many names have doubled letters, such as Wa**rr**en, Ru**ss**el and Phili**pp**a. When a letter becomes doubled, you have to deal with a double-dose of the energy; it presents a special challenge, even if it isn't always in the middle of a name. Rather than analyze these name examples in detail, we'll concentrate instead on the tendencies of the doubled letters they contain. It's also important to consider the letters *each* side of the doubled ones - **"A"** and **"E"** for Warren, **"U"** and **"E"** for Russel and **"I"** and **"A"** for Philippa; these give you the most important modifying influences connected to the doubled letters.

Double "R." A fierce almost crushing mental force and at times, a great deal of anger; tremendous power for mental aggression; an intense interior world of ideas, ideas that can be immovable and narrow-minded or open and free ranging, depending on whether the person is balanced or unbalanced. There is always some kind of "conversation" taking place inside the head. **Note:** **"R's"** (and **"D's"**) give a distinct advantage in the legal profession (like **Gerry Spence** the famous defense lawyer--and a very good speaker!).

Double "S." Very responsible, dependable, upstanding. Has to keep a good public image. However, hidden underneath could be seething sensuality, that may or may not be acknowledged and satisfied! The opposite picture shows the sensual, unpredictable, social rebel; the late Greek multimillionaire and shipping magnate, **Aristotle Onasses** (who married Jackie Kennedy after **JF** was assassinated) provides a perfect example (four **"S's"** including one doubled!).

Double "P." Often attracts enormous problems that challenge the ability to be peaceful. When handled constructively, the person can learn great forgiveness, acceptance and peace. For instance, one such **"P"** person--who was shot and left for dead--later forgave the assailant! Then again, the double **"P"** energy can *cause* mayhem for others.

Some Notable Double-lettered People:
The enormously successful T.V. evangelist **Jim Bakker**, who fell from grace through a sexual scandal. **Bill Gates** (called "The most famous businessman in the world" by Time Magazine), has affected the lives of millions by dominating the revolution in personal computing. **Ted Koppel**, outstanding T.V. interviewer and host. **Truman Henry Safford**, brilliant turn of the century astronomer, mathematician and also famous for an encyclopedic memory. **Andrew Lloyd Webber**, composer of theatrical hits including "Phantom of the Opera," "Cats" and "Evita." Unusually talented and hard working song writer, singer and author, **Jimmy Buffett.** Religious authority **Mary Baker Eddy**, founder of Christian Science.
When you analyze doubled letters in names, always keep in mind the intensification of the energy - for good or bad.

HowTo Analyze a Name in Full.

To receive a fully rounded-out look at another person's life, you must of course consider every letter contained in all their names *and how these letters modify and relate to each other.* Begin with the key letters--the first, middle and last (Drive, Focus/Challenge and Aim), then study all of the remaining letters plus any *extras* in the form of those sounded but not written...such as the **"E"** *sound* at the end of **Ricky**. Observe how family members who share identical last names express themselves similarily (or differently) with the same energy. Notice the changes in people as the result of gaining a married name, returning to a maiden name after a divorce or taking on a complete name change. The full effect of the new name usually takes about two years. *These changes can be directly related to the new names.*
The Letter explanations given in Chapters 6 and 8, "The Secret Meaning of Vowels and Consonants" and "More Letter Meanings A to Z" are your general reference guides.

Name Analysis Problems.

You're looking to understand and analyze a particular name, but it doesn't quite make sense. The person may have a strong ability, tendency, gift or fault--but you can't fathom why from looking up the meanings of the letters in their name. See if you can track down their middle names, or check biographies to find out if a different one was on their birth certificate. Many famous people, particularly actors, actresses and musicians change their names for professional reasons. Authors also have a fondness for pseudonyms.

In the event of the above, here's a trouble-shooting check list:
Look for:

1) Hidden letters, that are not actually written in the name, but their *sound is present..*
2) Middle names that are not given out to the public (libraries can often locate them if the person is a public figure, also, biography software now exists for P.C's).
3) Check the maiden name of a married woman.
4) See if the person has an assumed name, or had their names legally changed in the past.
5) If the person is using a nick-name.

The Releasing Sounds from Chapter 4 are the five vowels of our language **A, E, I, O,** and **U**. And the most important and personally empowering ones will come from your own name. Vowels show how Spirit tries to express wholeness in a human form (mentally, emotionally, physically and transcendentally) - ***as you!*** They call you to reclaim your total Self through the unique sound signature of your name. The Vowels also intimate the primary method of your awakening into the expanded (transcendent) state of non-duality.[1]

Letter **A** *resonates* power and freedom.
Letter **E** *speaks* self expression.
Letter **I** *sings* inspired creativity.
Letter **O** *whispers* compassionate nurturing.
Letter **U** *shouts* expansion and generosity.

I hope you have been inspired to try some daily vowel sounding. Not only does this loosen up your speaking and singing voice, but it will also begin to activate the latent power of Spirit in your life. Read the following definitions for your **own** name vowels, then 'voice' them with new understanding. This will further vitalize the particular way your personal Spirit defines itself as **you**!

The alphabet also contains **21** other letters called consonants. In names, they supply the structure or *form* for Spirit's expression. As most of us are not integrated with our Spiritual Selves, the function of consonants becomes more guileful. They act as lesson bringers and limiters; in other words, 'cattle prods' to nudge and poke us towards reunion.

The combination of vowels and consonants in a personal name reveals the unique song or 'tone' of that life and displays on a higher level, the sound map of our deepest self-awakening and physical transformation. After you have read your name's vowel meanings, follow up by studying the consonants and get an overview of your personal name energy.

Although I discuss some of the letter energies under *balanced* and *unbalanced*, it's never really quite that black and white. Some of us reveal the weaker aspects of a letter, having attracted the energy to make us strong, while others appear naturally strong and balanced using the *same* energy.Then there are those who decide to express the dark side by being overpowering and destructive--the truly unbalanced! Generally, we sway a little between both sides, being weak or destructive in some areas, strong and constructive in others. I present the following information to help you realize where you are and where you are *not* - within the letter energy of your name, thereby giving you the opportunity to bring yourself into balance...should you choose to do so.

This Chapter contains only brief introductory meanings for the vowels and consonants; additional and more detailed information (with some name examples of real people), follows in Chapter 8, "More Letter Meanings **A** to **Z**."

---

1 Refer to Chapter 21, "The Sacred Symbols."

THE VOWELS IN THE NAME

A -- houses the ego, basic identity, body, sense of self-worth--the "I AM" factor.

One powerful "**A**" person I know, refers to himself as - "An independent S.O.B.!" Reactions to life occur in the face, particularly the eyes, which can *refuse* to 'see' or see very clearly indeed! "**A**" exerts control over the body through the head. The physical energy can be weak or strong, but in the long haul, it always overcomes. "**A**" delivers initiative for mastering obstacles (*and* getting ahead); rouses stamina for staying healthy (or reclaiming bad health) and establishing personal power.

"**A**" empowers and liberates by fortifying self-will. **Balanced "A" becomes unselfconsciously powerful--the epitome of 'effortless being.'**

In the expression of personal power and freedom, you know you belong to yourself and you're not bound or controlled by anyone. Yet you admire and enjoy other puissant people--you're already self-contained, so no one out there can threaten you. Difficult circumstances and people never really limit, they just provide you with stimulating challenges! A strong will and daring spirit guarantee you'll have many adventures! For those unbalanced in the energy, weak and insecure "**A's**" constantly need to prove themselves to others (even strangers); they feel compelled to impress the world at large with who they are and what they have done--or intend to do. A boastful person hides an insecure inner child. Neglected (unused) "**A**" energy can make them too scared to take charge of their life, or to stand their ground when facing overbearing people. *Take courage!* However, the energy can go to the other extreme with angry "**A's**" who throw their weight around aggressively and arrogantly. Their lesson would be: *Cool off and Back off, try respect and compassion for a change!* **"A" brings challenges and lessons in personal power.**

"A" -- Spirit as physical energy, self awareness and freedom--the Joy of Personal Autonomy.

Sound "**A**" when you want to reconnect with your true identity.

E -- contains the intellect; basic intelligence; communication; free expression--the "I SPEAK" factor.

"**E**" presents to the world: mental vitality, bubbling curiosity and a love of verbal expression. Some "**E's**" develop a unique rapport with the mental states of others and possess a special knack (through empathy and understanding), of putting people at their ease, always managing to say the 'right word.' They usually pursue multilevel mental interests and while a few might entertain a narrower focus, it's either because of deliberate choice or under-developed or neglected mental talents. Some prefer to be "Jack of all trades and masters of none" and the most inappropriate "**E's**" become superficial, insecure and disconnected from their purpose. **Balanced "E" empowers and liberates by sharpening the mind.**

You could be a great talker, an avid reader--or both! You may want to speak, write, research, teach and even get into music, art and theater! With your sparkling mind, you love a mental challenge and you'll never be at a loss for something to interest you...or expound upon! When unbalanced, "**E's**" curiosity or current intellectual passion carries them away to the point of being tactless or even boring. They tend to deteriorate into incessant "talk, talk, talk," draining the energy of others and wasting their own mental force. When really nasty, they become famous for diatribe. **"E" brings challenges in self-expression and communication.**

"E" -- Spirit as mental energy, intelligence, curiousity and speech--the Joy of Communication.

Sound "**E**" when you want to find and express your true 'voice.'

I -- inspires, skillfully creates and loves to perform--the "LOOK AT ME" factor.

When **"I"** triggers inspiration, creative ideas stream through the mind; those in this magical 'flow' delight to share their magic with others; this energy produces **performers** (dancers, jugglers, singers, musicians, conductors, composers); **performers-of-words** (actors, orators, comics, writers, poets, News Casters, Talk-Show Hosts, seminar-presenters) and the **performers-of-form** (artists, sculptors, designers, landscapers, architects, and craft-persons........does that include plastic surgeons??). Non-creative **"I's"** love and support the arts, others draw public attention to important issues. **Balanced "I" empowers and liberates through creativity.**

You are open to living your life creatively through mastering an art; this compels you to share, perform or communicate it in some way to the rest of the world. Then does your heart sing....."I feel so fulfilled, so alive, this has to be why I was born!" The closed down **"I,"** keeps the energy unbalanced; they remain defeated, frustrated and suffering from excuses. If letter **"I"** in a name points to *blocked* abilities, it also means the power exists to *release* those abilities. *Perhaps your natural gifts were squashed in childhood, but regardless of the past, you can still shout down those old discouraging memories and declare,* **"You were wrong--I AM supposed to be doing this!!"** *Next, you must reclaim your dreams from where they were smothered or misdirected; begin to pursue what brings you delight. Age is no excuse! (To quote Joseph Campbell, the Master of Myth, "Follow your bliss!".)* **"I" brings challenges in allowing yourself to be creative.**

"I" -- Spirit, as inspired creativity, playfulness, flexibility and talent--the Joy of Performing or drawing attention.

Sound **"I"** when you want to reach for the stars!

O -- *needs* nurturing, or *gives* sympathetic caring--the "EMOTIONAL" factor.

"O" contains all of our sorrows and cries of pain, our unspoken griefs and unspeakable neglects. It also reflects our wonder and joy, our caring connection with each other and all of life. It's the "Mother" in us all. **Balanced "O" becomes compassion without judgement, caring without an agenda.**

You embody compassion, emotional understanding, physical security and abundance. Your presence in a room, the words you speak radiate love and caring. For unbalanced **"O,"** life begins hopefully but instead of a caring family, the childhood environment can only be called a disaster! Not withstanding, **"O"** still demands eventual emotional maturity; this sometimes happens in a supportive surrogate family (friends and associates substitute for unfeeling, dysfunctional relatives)! *You need caring, safety, support and shelter, food for the body and security for the soul's unfolding. All of this points you directly to the inner child and your own mother and whether that relationship was supportive or not. "O" challenges and develops your deepest feelings, making you (eventually), physically and emotionally self-sufficient. You* ***will*** *stop expecting some one else to complete you. You* ***will*** *cease demanding constant approval. You* ***will*** *learn to supply your own needs and grow up emotionally!* **The presence of "O" also connects to the power of the Earth-Mother-Goddess, demanding responsibility for planetary stewardship.**

"O" -- Spirit as loving, nurturing energy--the Joy of Belonging.

Sound **"O"** when you're feeling neglected, abandoned, sorry for yourself; when you're eating to compensate--when you've forgotten to gaze at the stars and wonder! .

U-- ventures into the world, exploring, discovering and experiencing. "Life is magnificent!"-- the "EXPANSION" factor.
"U" presents a challenge to the heart. *Be open and generous!* In that mode, receiving is part of giving and giving becomes receiving. **An expanded, balanced "U" radiates Universal Abundance.**

Initially, you decide to master the mental laws of manifestation until eventually your thoughts and life reflect nothing but total abundance. Finally you realize that no matter what you do or where you go, how much you spend, or how little you appear to have--there will ***always*** *be more than enough for yourself and everyone around you!*

When held back and unbalanced, "U" becomes the epitome of paranoia! Fear and indecision rule every thought and commandeers the life: fear of not having enough or of losing what little one thinks one has; fear of future hunger, of homelessness, of possible accidents--fear of just about everything! The result: pernicious apprehension stifles movement while impending catastrophe lurks in every shadow! *The choice of contracting or expanding is always yours!* "U" **brings the challenge of generosity and receiving, expansion and exploration.**

"U"-- Spirit as abundant, limitless, expanding energy--the Joy of Cosmic Supply.

Sound "U" when you want to go beyond your boundaries and limitations.

THE CONSONANTS IN THE NAME.

While the vowels propel us into the environment to face the outer world, the consonants force us to look within and work on the lessons and challenges we were born to deal with--*all the things that eventually make us strong when we master them!*

B -- the five senses; the throat/voice; physical and emotional responses (sometimes food[2] and sex hang-ups). The "B" energy either *needs* sensual gratification, *fears* sensual gratification, or knows how to satisfy all the senses and **enjoys** life thoroughly! There's often an appreciation of beauty with a profound connection to nature.

TO BALANCE THE "B" ENERGY:

Embrace a new activity. Try gardening, or nature walks! Then again, working with **any** kind of creative interest will divert the energy normally wasted on compulsive addictions. Take charge of your body *and it will love you!* For dealing with your emotional reactions, see section **3** of Chapter 17, the "Disidentifying Technique."

A New Awareness for "B" comes through 'practicing' the five senses, touching and tasting, smelling, seeing and listening. **A transforming meditative practice:** Take each of the senses in turn, spend a day (or a week) with one and for that selected time, be aware of *tasting*--eat your food as a contemplation, experience everything as nourishment; next, try *looking* at the colors and forms around you; *listening* to the delicate patter of rain--*really* hear the birds, crickets and frogs; receive all the *smells* of your everyday life (pungent or sweet), and learn to *touch* everything with awareness. Give and receive a massage; in that event however, training in the art of enjoyment might be necessary....if pleasure makes you guilty! *Sound* **"B"** *and breakthrough to delight!* Delight and wonder lead to enlightenment, or at least to lightening up! (See Chapter 16, section **5.**)

---

[2] For food addictions and eating disorders, see Appendix 4, "Food Meditation."

C -- skills and curiosity, cleverness, intellectual pursuits. **The "C" energy** feeds on mental stimulation and devours information. **"C's"** passionate pursuit is *collecting* knowledge (but not necessarily *using* it); they tend to buy more books than they read. Some develop into seminar-junkies attending limitless lectures, amassing certificates or gaining College degrees. The really skillful read and research incessantly, then *write* the books and *give* the lectures! Most **"C's"** make Incorrigibly curious, investigators and some (in their intense and earnest desire to learn) unwittingly intimidate (even total strangers), by asking too many point-blank, penetrating questions! Others possess a tactless, childlike persistence inappropriately pushing through other people's boundaries and violating treasured possessions and privacy. They tend to drive their friends crazy! *The weak* **"C's,"** *retreat into sluggish states of mind, refusing to nourish their starved mental capacity!* Practically ALL **"C's"** **hate** to be misunderstood or misquoted.

TO BALANCE THE "C" ENERGY:

If your voracious mind is crammed full of facts and figures, it may exclude even the *possibility* of intuitive knowledge. *"Intuitive knowledge ! -- what's* ***that?****"* Learn to 'listen' before you leap into nosy action or dialogue. And you super-clever ones - there's nothing at all the matter with a well honed intellect, but you should get to know the part of your mind they didn't tell you about in school; you **do** have a superconscious higher Mind!. As for the neglectful and sluggish **"C's,"** they might become so intrigued, they could decide to be clever after all! *Sound* **"C"** *and develop curiosity!*

A New Awareness for "C" comes from relaxing the busy surface thoughts and opening the inner pathway to higher Mind and Spirit. **Suggested practices:** "Invoking the Stillness and The Nostril Breath" from Chapter 16 - also, "Accessing Instant Energy" from section **5** in Chapter 17, to experience some non-mental energy and expand your self-awareness.

D-- personal authority, all authority figures (Dad in particular), teachers, God, the Government, the Law. **The "D" energy** operates comfortably from its own authority, or needs to *develop* personal authority--or it provokes, fears and *resists* authority. *If you insist on taking certain authorities to task--it's an external reflection of what you need to take-to-task within yourself.*

TO BALANCE THE "D" ENERGY:

Do you have a history of heavy issues with authority figures and is your own self-command seriously lacking? Then Dad may have been a problem when you were growing up. Acceptance and forgiveness could be an issue here. Take time to review your relationship with *all* the power figures in your life (male or female). Sometimes a *lack* of Dad can cause problems if you didn't have an acceptable male prototype for the masculine, warrior-part of yourself! *Gals and guys, you're both in the same boat here, and wimps or ogres for care-givers aren't easy authority models to follow!* Reconciling these, if only mentally, and following firmly your *own* interests (regardless of criticism), will strengthen your confidence and personal authority.[3] Also, look up the sound-releasing suggestions for letter **"D"** in Chapter 9, "Sounding for Specific Needs."

A New Awareness for "D" comes through determined action on your part *for yourself,* and from knowing that in the long run, there's no one but **you** to answer to!
(Find letter "E" at the front of the Chapter under Vowels in the Name.)

---

[3] See "Emotional Healing Meditations" (Version Two) on page 145.

F-- pride and ambition, issues with fame, competition and one-up-manship; ostentation or the 'shrinking violet!' **The "F" energy** sometimes thrives on flamboyance, drama, self-comparison and competition, or it needs to *become* proud of itself, daring and accomplished. When unbalanced it breeds the excessive risk taker and compulsive gambler....particularly when the "**F**" is doubled ("**FF**").

TO BALANCE THE "F" ENERGY:

It's true! You've achieved (or inherited) more than most and you're justifiably proud of that, but does make you intrinsically **better?** And it's not absolutely necessary for you to prove yourself to the world....or are you really trying to prove yourself *to yourself?* Each of us has at least one strong ability or one incredible idea, and we could distinguish ourselves if given the right encouragement. **You have activated yours!** Sometimes you super-achievers can become the super-motivators for the rest of us. So don't feel alone or threatened. Share the glory with us lesser mortals! And for all those reticent and defeated--"What's the use of trying"--under-achievers, you attracted that "**F**" in your name to give you a jump start out of self-denigration.

A New Awareness for "F" comes when you accept that it's O.K. to attract fame, success and money--but it's your decision how you handle the consequences! You know you **have** got what it takes, so start believing in yourself; then you can appreciate and encourage others who might become the worthy assistants to your own saga. Read "**F**" in Chapter 9, "Sounding for Specific Needs." *Sound* "**F**" *for successful effort.*

G-- work oriented and work driven, pride and perfection in one's craft--or the opposite! **The "G" energy** often equates identity with work, or lack of. The extreme expression creates the compulsive workaholic--who judges self and others on work performance. Very rarely does it indicate the contrary--sloth, torpor and antipathy towards work of any kind, but once in a long while, it can! Also in some instances, the person may experience a variety of work related problems and challenges and when forced to support themselves--become mental and emotional wrecks. ("**G's**" may also relax by playing *too* hard, then they become heavy drinkers and womanizers.)

TO BALANCE THE "G" ENERGY:

We know you love your job, but there **are** more things to life--getting enough sleep, for one thing, and having some honest-to-goodness, time-wasting relaxation. Also, you might consider backing off from all that unpaid overtime and getting to know the spouse, the kids, the neighbors......yourself! Read Chapters 16, "Special Meditations" and 17, "Energy Exercises," and select some new experiences for yourself from those techniques. Regularly take your eyes off work and open them to the marvels of the world and who *you* really are. *Sound* "**G**" *to find your inner child.* Also, read "Time Shifting" (Creating More Time to Enjoy Your Life), by Stephan Rechtschaffen, M.D. *And for those who resist and even fear work try the affirmation: "I am well paid and recognized, by what I love to do." Then list the things you love doing, or do well.*

A New Awareness for G comes when you direct some of your intense work-related energy into being still and/or cultivating completely different interests. If you haven't a family, adopt a furry animal and start a relationship with another creature. Look at nature. Float a flower in a bowl of water and contemplate beauty--or roll in the grass, shuffle through the leaves, walk in gentle rain without an umbrella. Play! Look at yourself and realize how beautiful you are.....yes, you men, **you** are beautiful!

H -- dreams and goals, discipline and hard work, fame, leadership and money.

The "H" energy triggers tremendous desire and motivation for recognition and success. It polarizes between outstanding achievers and resentful failures. The achievers plan, dream and work very hard, never giving up--they know it's up to them to make it all happen. The failures make excuses, moan, wring their hands, blame and "drop the bundle" at the first sign of struggle; they were born with a fear of success and an equally strong fear of failing. It's called "Hanging on the Horns of a Dilemma."

TO BALANCE THE "H" ENERGY:

Contrary to mainstream beliefs, money and success do not result in great happiness; the richest, most famous people can be the most miserable, lost and even drug-addicted. So keep your goals in perspective, you achievers. *Take Five!* You've done all this stuff, made all this money....ever thought there might be another agenda, a 'Higher Plan' waiting in the wings, eager for an opportunity to attract your attention? **"H"** *does however, own an opposite face, one that needs encouraging!* Sometimes that scheme, that secret ambition seems just too impossible, too crazy; so you throw in the towel without giving yourself a chance. It often needs tremendous personal effort, self-discipline and vision to make a dream come true. **Motivate and discipline yourself.** Read and practice Anthony Robbin's dynamic book "Awakening the Giant Within;" or use the ideas in Stuart Wilde's powerful little book called "Miracles" and there's the delightful "Dare to Win" by Jack Canfield and Mark Victor Hansen.

A New Awareness for "H" comes when you choose higher vision goals, enabling you to advantage others as well as yourself; and for the failed **"H's"** -- when you believe in yourself enough to **realize** your dreams, *sound* **"Hah"** *and learn to laugh again.* See letter **"H"** in Chapters 8 and 9.
(Find letter "I" at the front of the Chapter under Vowels in the Name.)

J -- justice and trouble shooting - or injustice and trouble making, loving trouble!

On the "trouble" issue, **the "J" energy** falls into four categories:

1) Relishes trouble and finds it frankly stimulating.
2) Becomes an activist and takes on 'causes' for the good of others.
3) Inadvertently attracts strife, bumbles constantly into the rough end of the stick and tends to be accident-prone.
4) Fears and retreats from any kind of confrontation.

With many **"J's"** *in a name, you may cross-mix from all four of the above!* You're also physically oriented (sports, hiking, etc.), an outdoors person and love nature--or when unbalanced, you tend to neglect your health and console yourself with nature and animals. *(For* **"J"** *sounding instructions, See* Chapter 9.*)*

TO BALANCE THE "J" ENERGY:

You really get charged up and energized with a heated argument or fisticuffs and your eyes sparkle with pleasure when you talk about it later, but there's just as much excitement and joy in helping others as in battling them. And if, in the other extreme, accidents, misfortune and injustice sticks to you like glue, take responsibility for your life and stop blaming and judging others. You only attract what you need to experience. When you've learnt the lesson you keep pulling into your life, change the scenario! See yourself as worthy, be your own advocate and give yourself the best...also, be sure you keep your body exercised and healthy!

New awareness for "J" comes when your change your attitude. Give up judging yourself and others; place a smile within your heart. Your inner song: **"I live my life with great freedom and joy."**

K -- sexuality (or fear of), will-power, secrecy and moodiness, intense (mostly veiled emotions), creative power, vitality and health, or health issues and challenges. **The "K" energy** *compounds life with often overwhelming moods.* You have a much richer connection to the depth consciousness than most, which can be quite disconcerting, so you usually keep your real thoughts and feelings to yourself. **Sexuality is frequently an issue.** Unless you pretend, others might think of you as aloof, rude or proud. *To discharge emotional energy,* **"K"** *children will engage regularly in frenetic activities that culminate in happy, giggling hysterics. Once in a while, they laugh until they cry--which they find utterly puzzling....."Why am I crying when this is so funny?!"* Unfortunately we frown upon such behavior in **"K"** adults. Pity! It's such a marvelous release and tone-up to the nervous system; instead, they bottle up their feelings in scowling moodiness--**this is the unexpressed energy of powerful creativity.**

TO BALANCE THE "K" ENERGY:
Accept your uniqueness. In time, you'll find others out there who think and feel like you do. And you **do** come up with the most amazing insights and occasionally share them directly with someone you trust, but mostly we receive them through your creative genius. *Sound* **"Ka"** *to release your inner bliss. Channel the unresolved intensity into lightness and joy; once in a while surrender yourself to laughter. Watch a hysterically funny film..often!*

New Awareness for "K" comes when you take responsibility for your feelings. In addition to 'laughter therapy,' your mood swings will benefit greatly from a serenity type meditation.[4] You should possess phenomenal will power (or you need to *develop* it), but please use it constructively; the more creative you can be, the more fulfilled you will feel.

L -- Diplomacy, social expertise, loves or hates self and people; people pleasers or party poopers. The **"L's"** needs social contact to reassure their personal identity--they *must* be where the crowds are for their sense of self-worth comes from interaction with the public. The completely inferior-feeling **"L's"** get stuck in overcompensation and crave the crowd (or the group's) approval for their importance or competency. Balanced **"L"** remains up front and confident, really loving the "out there" milieu where they can practice their diplomatic charm. *The other extreme shuns public exposure and essentially dislikes or fears people.*

TO BALANCE THE "L" ENERGY:
As most of **"L's"** problems stem from lack of self-worth, you need to focus on **YOU** for a change, not on what others think of you! Spend time alone admiring, enjoying and affirming yourself, instead of expecting people out there to pump you up. Stop being a reflection of someone else's approval. **Approve of yourself--regardless!** You're O.K and what anyone else thinks of you is their problem! My favorite source for developing self-love is Louise Hay's book, "You Can Heal Your Life." Take her crash course to transformation!

A New Awareness for "L" comes when you love and accept yourself without fear or guilt. *Look in the mirror, smile deep inside and sound* **"L"**[5] *to start the process.*

---

[4]Check out Chapter 16, "Special Meditations."

[5] See Letter "L" in Chapter 9.

M -- emotionally nurturing or emotionally draining; mother, the Goddess, the ideal mate, preoccupied busyness; work for, or <u>from</u> the home. **The "M" energy** describes the nesting, mating, nurturing instinct in males and females. *(It shares some of the qualities of letter "O.")* **"M"** is productive, devoted, supportive and basically caring. Off center, it's emotionally suffocating, draining, demanding and at times, childish. (Some **"M"** occupations: catering, food and restaurant industries, home building & repairs, architectural, interior design.)

TO BALANCE THE "M" ENERGY:
As the **"M"** energy connects to your own mother and your good or bad childhood, you have the challenge of forgiving any past shortcomings on her part and going forward into self-nurturing and abundance. If you were more fortunate and had an absolutely marvelous Mom, the inclination changes; you often choose to remain connected and even provide some kind of meaningful support for her (should she need it), whether emotional or financial particularly in her old age. If you do *not* resolve any short-fall mothering needs, you tend to unconsciously demand that others complete your emotional insufficiencies; some of you close off these unrequited needs entirely and end up shy and withdrawn (or taciturn) emotional shut-downs. **The unresolved energies often discharge through compulsive busyness and workaholic habits** (*in this case, follow some of the suggestions for letter* **"G"***).* Practice the **"Mmmmm-ma,ma,ma"** resonator from Chapter 4, "Releasing the Voice," and also section 3 from Chapter 16 called "Finding the Power of the Goddess." And for that excessive busyness, read "Time Shifting."[6]

A New Awareness for "M" comes when you become self-nurturing and connect with your own feminine (Goddess) power.....not quite so easy for males! Sometimes, you may just have to 'grow-up,' break free from suffocating original-family restrictions and stop being overwhelmed by their demands. Each must resolve what a true family means for them--and then try and create their own!

N -- Smart, analytical, critical, sticklers for logic and intellect, yo-yo moods; the martyr complex. **The "N" energy** can be uppity, habitually negative and nit-picking, or suffering from inferiority in the "set-to-please" victim mode--pleasing everyone but themselves! The first kind has to learn dispassion and non-judgment; the second, "right service" and be able to say (without rancor), "NO! - I don't *have* to any more; **you** do it!"

TO BALANCE THE "N" ENERGY:
Take a look at the way you feel compelled to serve others; is it out of fear or out of love? Ask yourself--what are your *real* responsibilities? Do you control other people by making them dependent on you, weakening instead of strengthening them? Are your bitter complaints hiding the fact that you enjoy a sense of power by remaining in a situation as a thankless caregiver or provider? **"N"** often feels like the abandoned child, ignored and unappreciated. For some life-lesson reason, you decided to program this experience, but it doesn't mean you have to abnegate yourself forever. Develop that sharp and clever intellect, empower yourself and in so doing, you'll lift up those around you. *Sound* **"N"** *to enable yourself.* (Also, read **"N"** Resonator in Chapter 4.) *Balance excessive thoughts by physically activity.*
A New Awareness for "N" comes from staying centered in your own peace and balancing the forces that seem to pull you in every direction. Take a hard look at all your assumed (or thrust upon) responsibilities and place *your* needs first. The old injunction "Love your neighbor as yourself" - means loving yourself first!
<u>(Find letter "O" at the front of the Chapter under Vowels in the Name.)</u>

---

6 "Time Shifting" Creating More Time to Enjoy Your Life, by Stephan Rechtschaffen, M.D.

P-- private, peace seeking, mediating; challenging or destroying peace.

The "P" energy retreats from the 'madding crowd' and contemplates or vegetates--or it functions in the world as the serene center of the cyclone, unruffled--mediating in the midst of strife, calming all around him or her. Another kind of **"P"** unconsciously 'teaches' in the negative mode, deliberately stirring up hornet's nests, while challenging others to find their own centers-in order to handle confrontation and change! Letter **"P"** also contains a cruelty aspect; with such, you either perpetrate cruelty onto others, or attract it into your own life to learn how to transform the energy. Take note of the Peter, Paul, Penelope and Paula's in your life and observe how they manage their peace factor!

TO BALANCE THE "P" ENERGY:

"P" demands you understand the meaning of peace in your life. Can you boldly face the world and determine your own fate in a constructive manner, or do you retreat and follow the line of least resistance (which sometimes attracts an illness--then used as an excuse for not getting out of a bad situation)? As inspiration, motivation and (when necessary), for a good kick in the pants--every day read a little "Chicken Soup for the Soul." [7] *Also, Sound* **"P"** *and release your peeves!* Whenever I, or anyone else I know, suffers from a sudden bladder infection (it hurts to pee!), I always ask "Who are you pissed at?" To acknowledge the peeve will usually cure the painful urination!

A New Awareness for "P" comes from allowing the world out there to be part of the peace within you.

Q-- quintessentially quizzical, mentally focused, dynamic, and usually clever, energetic, expansive, enthusiastic.

The "Q" energy tends to be *quite* unique. I mean, how many people do you know who have the letter **"Q"** in their names? Most **"Q"** people appear as rare and unusual beings in this society; their mental intensity, energy and curiosity range beyond most of us. Perhaps they've landed from another planet and are here to learn, learn, learn--and get things done in spite of our resistence! Thrill-seeking often appears on the **"Q"** agenda and ranges from wholesome adventure to the criminal pursuits of theft and assault; though not usually both seen in the same person--this *has* been known to happen!

TO BALANCE THE "Q" ENERGY

Such intensity of soul and hunger for experience may result in compulsive behavior, such as gambling, impulse buying and excessive risk taking. What sends you overboard? Investigate your name for clues in the *other* letters surrounding **"QU"** (**"U"** mostly follows **"Q"** and means expansion), then study those and their balancing factors, applying them to your own case. Develop moderation. Take some of your thrills vicariously, watch films instead of laying your life on the line; reverence your body vehicle, it's all you've got to house the Spirit for its journey as you.

A New Awareness for "Q" comes when you redirect the passionate outer quest to a passionate inner quest; discover your potential magnificence as Spirit. See Chapters 14, 16, 17 and 21.

---

[7] 101 Stories to Open The Heart And Rekindle The Spirit, written and compiled by Jack Canfield & Mark Victor Hansen.

R -- mentally powerful and/or aggressive; superb orators or lousy speakers, deep, ruminative thinkers, embracers of diversity or the fixed, bigoted, restricters and controllers of others. The "R" energy covers the greatest intensity of mental force, there's a constant internal dialogue happening most of the time! When unbalanced, they equate their personal ideas with their identity and should you challenge or threaten these ideas, **"R's"** will turn verbally aggressive and abusive! Yet, when open and receptive to other opinions, they become expansive and tenacious researchers and/or leaders with innovative and empowering concepts.

TO BALANCE THE "R" ENERGY:

Relax control and delegate some authority. Keep a loose rein and let people make mistakes without coming down on them like a ton of bricks! Guide kindly. Allow yourself to be wrong, just once in a while.....you won't dissolve into a pile of tiger-butter! Listen to other people's opinions and ideas without throwing your own in as superior. There are other good minds out there! Suggest, rather than dictate. Don't be so intense and serious, relax and smile. And to the *faint-hearted* **"R's,"** who habitually attract the *overbearing* **"R's"** into their lives--why do you think you do that, since they give you such a hard time? It's to teach you to face the mental power that you fear so much, and become stronger. Like **"A,"** letter **"R"** also governs anger and rage; *Sound* **"Ra,ra,ra"** *to release yours or to connect with your own mental power.* For those with an overdose of power, practice the Heart Meditations from Chapter 16 and the Galactic Breath from Chapter 4.

A New Awareness for "R" comes with practicing compassion and taking the courage to change. Sound **"R"** like a resonator described in Chapter 18, "Power Tools for the Brain."

S -- public status-seeking (social/political), money-making; solid, down-to-earth practicality, level headedness, nest-feathering; concealed or secret sensuality - also, the jaundiced cynic, and the social rebel defying convention! The "S" energy usually settles itself comfortably into the workaday world of commerce and respectability. **"S"** people know how to get work whenever they want it, regardless of economic perimeters. *Good work-karma!* When philosophical, they *observe* life and society--often getting involved with clubs and organizations. Can be proud of their provider-skills and/or ambitious status-seekers. Also known for dogged, steady persistence and never giving up till they succeed! Occasionally, the **"S"** polarizes to practical ineptitude--the social drop-out, cadging a living off others, unable or unwilling to find work, harboring paranoias about possessions, other people's motives, the future - or taking on political extremism. In most **"S's"** there lurks a closet sensuality, sometimes acknowledged, sometimes suppressed..or it just hides under prudery.

TO BALANCE THE "S" ENERGY:

The **"S"** often attracts financial stability through easy work opportunities (if it's your birth name) and through endowments, or by marrying into an **"S"** name which enables the freedom to take up previously unexplored interests. Resist the temptation to get caught up in social 'back-scratching,' fear of the future and other rat-race paranoias, instead, develop social and monetary responsibility. Use your abilities and take advantage of opportunities, but also connect to the Earth Mother (Goddess) as your underlying support.[8] A disadvantaged **"S,"** or a deliberate social drop-out, may 'coast' for a number of years (building experience and gaining knowledge) before entering mainstream society, receiving recognition and making a positive contribution.

A New Awareness for "S" comes from community interaction, responsible self-support and in allowing yourself to do what you love--and get well paid for it!

---

[8] See Chapter 17, section 3, "Finding the Power of the Goddess."

T -- sensitive, nervous, idealistic, escapist; psychic, spiritual, religious; gullible, or fearful; skeptical debunker...or a sensitivity polarized to the gross and bizarre. **The "T" energy** can want to escape the outer reality by living in a constant day-dream world (you look at them--and they're miles away!). With its connection to the psychic senses, the energy may bring nervous overload, distress, confusion, fear of things supernatural--plus, avoidance. The avoidance sometimes takes the form of absentmindedness and/or blocking out the intuitive impressions with substance abuse--drinking, drugs and even overeating--it's called: *"Running from who you really are."* Fearless **"T's"** seek out the mysterious, they're fascinated by the unexplainable, the psychic, occult, mystical or religious and have a magical sense of the insubstantial and "otherworldly." **"T's"** who push away this side of themselves by ridiculing the psychic senses, still can't avoid their inner "hunches" - hunches that generally prove right. Some remain absorbed in their own interior world - others share it through creativity. **"T"** encompasses man's highest awareness--the mystic saint, to man's lowest--the enraged, irrational beast (particularly when incensed by injustice).

TO BALANCE THE "T" ENERGY:

All extremes of **"T"** need to accept their inherent psychic sensitivity. See it as an advantage and not a "curse" or something to be feared and ridiculed. Begin by sounding the identity-empowering vowels,[9] and ground yourself in the Earth Mother-Goddess (see section 3 of Chapter 17). One of the problems with oversensitive **"T"** - *too much activity in the head centers!* The remedy: try suggestions for an over-stimulated Crown and 3rd Eye under "Grounding Techniques" on page 110 and do the "Tranquillity Meditations" from Chapter 16. Finally, understand and sound the key letters from your own names and accept your potential. For all who denigrate their psychic and mystical tendencies, the choice remains the same - you can stay ignorant, or study to expand your awareness and claim your interdimensional skills. Why remain in fear and confusion? Wake up from day-dreaming--you're supposed to master the outer illusion.

A New Awareness for "T" comes from accepting, stabilizing and making your superconscious insights available to help yourself and others. Practice discernment so you're no longer easily deceived. **(Find letter "U" at the front of the Chapter under Vowels in the Name.)**

V -- visionary, perfectionist, political and social idealist or radical - or a pessimist; unconventional or clinging to conventions. **The "V" energy** gears its vision to the outer world and whether it likes or hates what it sees, it cannot remain unmoved or uninvolved. **"V"** people often have strong social/political opinions and can be active as a negative or positive influence--from futuristic utopianism to social revolt, destruction and mayhem. They either retreat into helpless or hopeless pessimism (as to the state of society, the government, the world in general), or maintain a visionary purpose to find ways to help, serve, and make positive contributions to others. *(**Unbalanced "V"** has vision that is destructive or defeated, rather than constructive.)*

TO BALANCE THE "V" ENERGY:

So you lack a personal purpose, a vision for your life; you can find no meaning in the senseless state of affairs and *your* life in particular! Take note of the letters in your name following or surrounding the **"V,"** they show the areas that reveal your hidden talents and mission in life; for inspiration, sound both the **"V"** *and* the adjacent letters.

A New Awareness for "V" comes when you connect with your special world mission, you are here to make a difference, so get going -- we need you too!

---

[9] See Chapter 4.

W-- impressive, confident, outstanding, motivating, bold - or willful, arrogant, boastful, brash, opportunist, standoffish. **The "W" energy** can be compelling, controlling and overwhelming, or warmly enthusiastic and friendly. They tend towards competitiveness with a natural sense of their "place" and importance in public situations; if someone threatens their (considered) rightful place in line for a bus, a plane, a table at a restaurant, etc., they usually get rankled. They also react if they're not acknowledged or given credit for something they've done (or think they've done!). Natural leaders, **"W's"** fall into three types:

1) Positive and uplifting.
2) Negative and self-aggrandizing (often pride hiding weakness).
3) Avoiding leadership; the permanently discouraged; very poor self-image and lacking courage to take charge and change things. These last attract the name energy in order to learn lessons in courage and self-pride.

TO BALANCE THE "W" ENERGY:

You sometimes feel quite insecure and *pretend* to know more than you do, just to impress people! A part of you feels you're supposed to shine at *something,* so you do your best, not always understanding why you *have* to come on so strong! Look at the following (or surrounding) letters to the **"W"** in your name; they will show you where you can place your powerful energies and develop yourself with confidence. **"W"** is a difficult letter to sound (look it up in Chapter 9, "Sounding for Specific Needs"); as you well know--it's also a difficult energy to come to grips with!

A new awareness for "W" arrives when you acknowledge your vulnerability and allow those that love and care about you to get close. Accept help once in a while and learn about true intimacy. *It doesn't matter if people see you with your 'perfection' guard down!* And for the restricted and restrained **"W's"** with limiting ideas of self-worth, stop feeling fearful and timid (seeing only 'impossibilities') and find the courage to believe in yourself.

X - INTENSITY! - mental, emotional and physical intensity, focused, brilliant, gifted, productive and powerful - or hyperactive, hypersensitive, confused and extremely scattered. **The "X" energy** is also relatively rare in Western culture, so when it occurs you can expect a *unique person,* either on the downside or the upside of the energy. Even the weak-willed and scattered **"X's"** are capable of phenomenal struggles to adjust and balance their emotional and mental extremes. Mostly, they tend to run around in circles, repeating the same old fear and depression patterns with their compulsive thoughts and activities; yet, the intensity of thought *can* periodically break through with incredible clarity allowing for life-changing action.

TO BALANCE THE "X" ENERGY:

Periods of over-excitement and turmoil frequently downside into depression and helplessness; and while some form of vigorous physical activity often produces a marvelous balancing effect--even this release may end up becoming compulsive. The person's natural balance for internal intensity will occur in the letters immediately following or surrounding the **"X"** in the name. Study those letters and see how their meaning applies to your own situation; also refer to Chapter 9, "Sounding for Specific Needs," and sound the **"X"** energy.

A New Awareness for "X" comes when you take that incredible fervor and focus it upon the *aim* of your life; for that, look at the last letters in all of your names. *This is what you came to achieve!*

Y - individualistic, charismatic leadership, self-contained, inspiring, persistent--or relentless, controlling, willful, commanding and demanding--or frustrated and intimidated. **The "Y" energy** when unbalanced causes trouble for everyone in sight--when it doesn't get its own way. Soliciting followers and surrounding themselves with "yes-men," they're selfishly insensitive to others.....you 'cross swords' with them at your peril! The other extreme lacks self-respect and will-power and often suffer lives of suppression and bitter frustration. When balanced, they inspire and lead with passionate commitment and make brilliant organizers in challenging situations, particularly in large scale visionary undertakings. From a very early age, strong "Y" children consider themselves equal with adults. They confront visitors with self-composure and gaze up into the faces of these "large" people - uttering wise remarks, quite oblivious to any differences in size, age or intellectual capacity. Occasionally, some adults respond with awe - and certainly with recognition - that here is a "person" of some power and substance--not just a tiny child! Years ago, a "Y" three year old (with some suprise) observed his mother (me) incapacitated in bed with the flu; after a brief survey at the foot of the bed, he announced magnanimously: "Today Mummy - you don't have to do what I say - I'll do what *you* say!!"

TO BALANCE THE "Y" ENERGY:

Try not to fly into a rage at the slightest provocation (no one is threatening your territory), you've established your power and domain! Rest in your own inviolability and from that foundation encourage those around you to discover *their* strengths. Furthermore, there *are* other ways of doing things, rather than dictate, be prepared to learn from others for a change....and occasionally, let some one else show you *their* way. When you're too angry, try discharging the anger by sounding **"Ah,rah,rah,rah;"**[10] when you need to be compassionate sound the last suggestion for letter **"Y"** in Chapter 9. For the weak **"Y's,"** prone to intimidation, you can also discharge your suppressed rage by sounding **"Ah,rah,rah,"** and do the **first** suggestion for **"Y"** in Chapter 9.

A New Awareness for "Y" comes from understanding the *constructive* use of personal power.

Z -- productive defiance, challenging destiny, changing one's fate - or being crushed and passively resigned to fate. **The "Z" energy** tends to observe destiny in a detached way, like the non-involved 'watcher' of the passing show. At other times they're in active confrontation ("I am the Master of my Fate; what I decide, I do") and sometimes engage in excessive risk-taking. They bring to full circle the progression of experience from letters **A** to **Z**. In many ways **"Z"** is similar to the empowered letter **"A,"** except that *balanced* **"Z"** has cultivated more wisdom. The weak and helpless (unbalanced) **"Z's"** are challenged to develop power over their surroundings--as well as detached awareness.

TO BALANCE THE "Z" ENERGY:

Look at what you think of as "fate." Are you blaming blind circumstances and unjust people for your woes? Do you feel helpless to control the events around you--as though swept up in them unwillingly? Accept that you attract or create what *a part of you* has decided to experience. Take responsibility and recreate, re-calibrate and restructure your life. Some of the knots you have tied yourself into can't always be easily undone, for *those* restraints, you need patience, persistence and a plan. Certainly, sound the **"Z,"** as described in Chapter 9, "Sounding for Specific Needs," and try taking one spoonful daily of "Chicken Soup for the Soul, 101 Stories To Open the Heart And Rekindle The Spirit" written and compiled by Jack Canfield and Mark Victor Hansen (these stories are so inspiring that several further "Helpings" have also been published).

A New Awareness for "Z" comes from accepting your own adventure with heart, courage and anticipation.

---

[10] See "Rah" bottom of page 11 and top of page 12.

7..... AFFIRMATIONS for the LETTERS in YOUR NAME

Now that you've seen a brief description of the vowels and consonants, here are some simplified (and even fun) ideas and affirmations to practice with your key letters - the Drives, Aims and Focus-Challenges in your name.

A

is looking at myself in the mirror and saying "You're the **Greatest,** you can **do** anything and **be** anything you want!"

"I **am** the Master of my fate,
I do what I **decide** to do."

B

is eating ice cream and chocolate cake - having a good massage, or sex, or something just as delectable, without feeling guilty.

"I **marvel** at the magic of life,
I dance, I play, I taste, I enjoy."

C

is going to seminars and classes, asking millions and millions of questions, or reading books for years and years - like Joseph Campbell, who then wrote:

"The Hero With a Thousand Faces."

"Everything I need to know -- a part of me **already** knows;
I open the door to my Infinite Knowing."

D

is holding back, I'm a tad reserved, but I really **do** know my stuff and if you touch upon my field with any intelligence, I'll **really** open up!

"I am my own authority--I'm completely self assured."

E is bewitched by **words**....written words, spoken words; *writing words, speaking words,* understanding other minds.

"I 'listen' to my inner voice--to understand how **others** think,
It whispers to me the *perfect* words,
The words that others are **able** to hear."

F is knowing without a doubt....I have **every** right to be proud of myself!

"I'm always the best that I can be--and you can be the same;
Please shine your gifts for us to see, don't hide your Light away!

G is working very hard and loving every minute, then knowing when to stop and rushing off to PLAY!!!

"Work, work, work--the day is just too short!
Remind me to relax, and go and smell the flowers."

H is saying with shining eyes, "I am **totally** committed, **totally** determined, and **absolutely** certain of fortune, fame, success!"

"I dream my dreams, I see my future,
I **patiently** work, it will **all** come true!!

I is loving the footlights, the fans, the acclaim, the unutterable joy of performing again!

"I need your attention, please look at me now;
I have something to share, to impart and to show."

J is "jousting at windmills" and planning to save humanity....but meanwhile, that trip out of town (out of state, overseas), looks ***pretty*** enticing!

"Wherever I am, Justice moves me and calls me,
But only in Joy, will my actions bear fruit."

K is never being able to hide from my sexual energy--that radiant, vibrant charisma! I love it and I hate it! My inner Phoenix **has** to fly!

"My strength of will shall **never** fail,
I forge through life with fearless passion."

L is loving the party, the people, the crowd and **best** of all, loving **myself!**

"I'm tactful, I'm charming, I work with the people,
They teach me my lessons--*they* show me the way.

M is keeping extra busy, but always thinking how **good** it would be to build that snug nest and my own family!

"The perfect love and home are always on my mind,
But first I need to find **myself** and then the rest I'll find."

N is declaring "No more, no way, no way! I **won't** be used and criticized, I **like** the way I am!!"

"When I say 'No,' that's **exactly** what I mean,
And I'm **not** the service doormat, that up 'til now you've seen."

O is sitting on the bed and holding my stuffed animal Care Bear and knowing I am hugging myself!

"I am **complete within myself**,
I love and take care of *me*."

P is keeping serene and together, when the rest of the world has gone mad!

"At peace within when the outer tempest rages,
I serenely watch the storm."

Q is outsmarting, out-thinking and outmaneuvering everyone, because I'm so darned curious and clever--and ***besides***, they just can't keep up with my pace!

"Life is my conquest my **daring** encounter,
And all of its answers are mine to discover!"

R is remaining in my own mental world. There's so much going on in my head I'm **never** really lonely, but watch out.....I'll argue if you challenge my ideas!

"I no longer have to be 'always right,'
I open my mind for a **wider** opinion."

S is success - with my feet on the ground and working each day; yet sometimes I know I'm incredibly **sensual** (but no one suspects), my public image is so impeccable!

"I am well paid and recognized, for the work I love to do,
And my inner sensuality empowers me through and through.

T is having too much sensitivity for my own comfort. Whether I like it or not I seem to be this sponge for other people's thoughts and emotions.

"My intuitive knowings and feelings,
Bring insights to help those around me."

U is opening my arms to the whole wide world and wishing I could give everyone exactly what they wanted to make them happy!

"I need to give and help, to get the action going,
And as I open up, my universe starts flowing."

V is having my vision for changing the world and knowing I was born for a **very** special task!

"In spite of the overwhelming chaos in the world,
I will **keep my vision,** I will do my work."

W is rushing energetically, showing off dramatically, being shameless, proud and pushy! I'm sunny and warm on the outside, but inside, I carry a secret part.

"I wear a mask of pride my fearful child to hide;
I must dare to feel the pain, and face my vulnerable side."

X is having a million interests and not enough hours in the day to keep up with them all!

"I discipline my thoughts and focus on my purpose;
My mind in perfect balance, all frantic-ness at rest."

Y is needing to do things exactly **my** own way. Just once in a while I'll step back and let some one else do it **their** way--but do I *have* to?

"I follow the beat of a different drum,
I work the best when I'm in charge,
But it's time for me, to relax my stand,
And allow my views to be enlarged."

Z is taking responsibility for everything happening in my life. When Fate opens the door, I walk right in and say "Thank you, Me!" When Fate shuts the door I say, "Obviously I have decided on something **better**!"

"My life's an adventure, a glorious game,
And my name contains the master key."

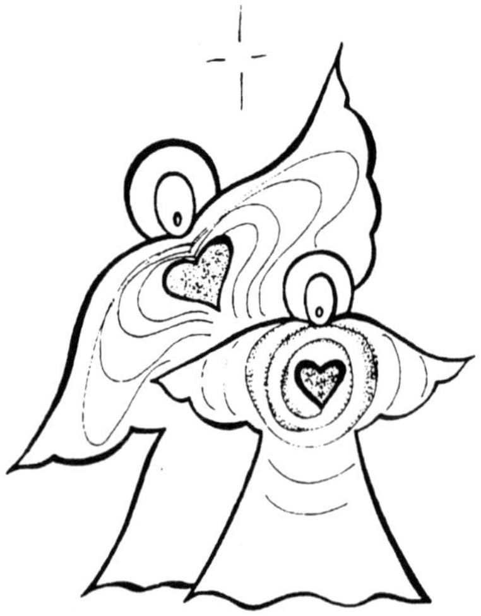

8..... MORE LETTER MEANINGS A to Z

LETTER A.

(For a list of famous **"A"** *names, see* **Appendix 5.***)*

Identity, ego, willpower, independence, self-mastery, self-empowerment, freedom, adventure. The physical body, strength, energy. **"A's"** outstanding quality might best be expressed as "presence"....*the presence of Spirit as physical power and freedom.* The more **"A's"** in a name, the greater the sense of power and presence. I once met an awesome, totally impressive man from the island of Samoa who had a total of ***eight*** **"A's"** in his name!! *Polynesian languages showcase the vowels.* In their power, **"A's"** live fully and fearlessly, expressing a strong need for personal freedom. Under privation, their life-force drive brings great courage, excellent survival skills and a knack for taking charge in group situations. Yes, they're natural born leaders and expect as much of themselves as anyone else. Their self discipline can be daunting, especially when mastering physical skills to gain goals. Ambition *does* come into it--so don't try and get in their way--you'll come off second best and find them quite uncompromising in the pursuit of those goals. *Of course the converse is also true* - there are flaky, gutless and weak willed ones! *Every letter has its polar opposite.* In these sorry cases, the presence of **"A"** in a name acts like a cattle-prod, to painfully challenge flagging courage and jump-start self love. Severe personal weakness *can* be overcome--*if* the person wants to summon up the will and determination. However, **"A's"** most uncomfortable quality is ANGER! Usually misinterpreted, anger shows a part of personal power that needs acceptance and understanding (especially in children). As a rule, once the **"A's"** have blown their top, their ire dissipates quickly and seems forgotten--except for the traumatized few in the direct line of fire--who tend to remember!! *"For God's sake, try not to make them **angry!!**"* Many flare-up's in the adult **"A"** stem from childhood memories of forbidden emotions and happen during extreme frustration; other hidden triggers are *fear* of powerlessness and the sudden loss of control over events and people. *For a balanced* **"A,"** *no one is in the line of fire.* They are singularly unblaming and take responsibility for their reactions; any bursts of anger, though intense, rarely get directed at anyone in particular...*they are simply anger reactions being released!* Observers of these outbursts (trembling in their boots on the sidelines and astonished that *they* are not being attacked) marvel at the pure and simple release of raw anger from someone with the skill to free it with such integrity. **So much for "A's" and anger!** Additionally, **"A"** means resolving to "take charge" of the physical body and maintain its health and strength. After all, we only have the one container and there's a saying "What you don't use--you lose!" Some **"A's"** attract physical challenges anyway--as part of their lessons in self-mastery. Two or more **"A's"** in the name mean you work with self-control, understanding power - and will-power in particular.

<u>Balanced "A:"</u> one who respects and is not threatened by, the power of others; power in action, a natural leader, self possessed, confident, daring, passionately excited with life and armed with a purposeful strength of will--a strength that motivates and empowers all who know them!

<u>Unbalanced "A:"</u> problems with personal power; egos frozen in the need to feel important; destructive and unpleasant; egomaniacs; operating from overweening strength and temper. **<u>Weak "A:"</u>** suppressing anger; wearing the mask of detachment, leaving unresolved rage seething inside; can't handle confrontation; hate playing the game of "sweetness-and-light." All their held-back energy builds internally causing sporadic blasts of anger--followed by even more determined efforts to push the feelings back down. Sometimes, the inner rage goes to the gums and erupts through abscessed teeth! They either possess too much or too little power and tend to fluctuate between the extremes, being weak one moment and overpowering the next--a part of them frantically craves attention, recognition, reassurance and praise. Weak **"A's"** when children, were never given a sense of self worth, so they frequently attract the opposite--humiliation and shame! When they express too *much* power, others find them (at best), overwhelming or awesome and at worst, imperious or intimidating. In either extreme, unbalanced **"A's"** secretly *fear* power!

When "A" is in YOUR NAME: *it's how you use or misuse your personal power and how you exert your power over others and the environment.*

<u>SUMMARY:</u> physical; daring, powerful, initiating, brave; the strength of the ego and personal identity; the capability to manifest and create one's own reality.

LETTER B. *(For a list of famous* **"B"** *names, see* **Appendix 5.***)*

The body, the senses, the psychic senses; pleasure, enjoyment, wonder; overindulgence, serious excesses - or *fear* of pleasure--especially sex and food. Money issues.

"B" has two extremes: the mystical (religious, healing, empathetic) and the hedonistic (enjoyment, pleasuring-seeking, sense-indulgence). Beneath them both rests the foundation of the sensing apparatus of the body--how we see, taste, smell, touch, and hear; these reflect our original child-like wonder at life and all its beauty. We perceive and enjoy everything through this sensory mechanism and that alone connects us to a 'probable' external reality. An initial curiosity about this sensory input can expand into a desire to extend life, to transform the species--even to becoming immortal! And because the outer senses connect through to the expanded psychic senses, there often arises a fascination with a number of esoteric practices and interests such as: interdimensional realms, religious mysticism, out-of-body travel, remote viewing, the feasibility of life after death, reincarnation, near death experiences...or instead, you have the skeptical **"B's"** who fear and reject such things! Along with heightened emotional responses, some own greatly expanded *physical* senses augmenting the normal sight, touch, taste, hearing and smell. These, the "empaths," are mostly *unwittingly* sensitive to the feelings and physical overloads of other people. First, they notice just certain persons who always produce uncomfortable effects on them--then they realize larger gatherings make them feel even worse! Many **"B"** sensitives end up shunning crowds simply out of self-protection. However, knowing *exactly* how others feel emotionally and *exactly* where they hurt physically can begin as a curse, but end up as a gift--a gift and a 'calling.' These empathetic **"B's"** eventually balance their people-discomfort by becoming healers, counselors and psychic advisers; the formerly unwanted sensory input is simply 'information' which vanishes as soon as acted upon (with healing thoughts and actions). Usually, *all* **"B's"** are *strongly* physical *and strongly* emotional with several levels and combinations of the two. The happiest ones remain naturally grounded, direct, practical, "earthy," and often bullishly stubborn; they show a guilt-less delight in the pleasures of the senses, with a joyous, natural lust for life! (The owners of a successful gourmet chocolate company in our town have *five* **"B's"** in their combined names!!) **"B"** *also has a connection with the voice and throat--the part of us that opens to receive and give nourishment. Some* **"B's"** *are good singers and speakers and others create or appreciate art and music.* The energy in names, usually indicates physical and sensual lessons and the challenge to develop the unrealized super-sensory and mental capacity latent within the human species. However, when a name contains more than one **"B"** *(and the person is inclined towards the mystical),* they no longer see themselves and others as isolated; their own sense of personal embodiment expands into a World-Body awareness and they inspire others with a vision of universal consciousness that springs from a greater "Cosmic Body of Mankind."

Balanced "B's:" know they are part of all the life on this planet and feel a need to maintain its fragile equipoise. They cherish the earth and delight in the family of mankind - like charismatic speaker and author on love and human connectedness, **Leo Buscaglia** (famous for hugging his entire audience after each lecture!). They also know that money is nothing more than energy, which needs to be skillfully used and enjoyed--rather than hoarded or feared.

Unbalanced "B's" *biggest bugaboos are food, sex and money.* The overindulgent ones love decadence and lack responsibility for the effect their lifestyle has on mind and body. **Example:** the late, talented British actor **Sir Richard Burton**, who had a serious drinking problem--and also really loved the ladies! Those in the opposite extreme (who fear pleasure), escape by retreating into self-denial or ascetic practices. **Weak "B's"** passively or stubbornly embrace defeat (give up too easily) and remain at the mercy of their fluctuating emotional and physical states and cravings; mentally they tend to jump-to-conclusions (habitually assuming), instead of waiting for all of the facts. *Very often suffer from throat blocks.*

When "B" is in YOUR NAME: *it's how you allow and experience personal pleasure - how you sensually receive, reject or ignore the world around you.*

SUMMARY: empathy with the physical, mental and emotional states of others; sensual wonder, pleasure and delight versus guilt, compulsion and addiction; expansion of the senses into psychic, mystical and spiritual awareness.

LETTER C. *(For a list of famous* **"C"** *names, see* **Appendix 5.***)*

The curious, collecting, clever quality of mind, clarity of thought, love of knowledge, innovative mental skills; skillful in a general way; hidden currents of passion! An intense curiosity characterizes the **"C"** energy and for some, anything that interrupts their wide-eyed and well-meaning interrogations upsets them and erodes their confidence. Beings of constant and rapid change, they vacillate between the blackness of doubt and the brilliance of certainty; there's no greater torment than a **"C"** in the depths of doubt!! Their energy can be described as "jumpy," with a tendency to scatter their interests, so they must learn to focus--and when they do, their curiosity becomes disciplined and they begin to *efficiently* gather information..like the good "fact-finders" they really are! Focused **"C's"** make incredible researchers, often making important discoveries (look up **Copernicus**, the father of modern astronomy). When skimming the intellectual surface, **"C's"** tend to ignore emotions, but as mentioned elsewhere, certain letters in name combinations sound like *other* letters. Most **"C"** letters in personal names, sound like **"K's"** (an intense, sexual and creative force). These two energies appear antithetical--moody and passionate **"K's"** want to protect themselves by being secretive, whereas curious, mentally oriented **"C's,"** love digging for information and giving it out as fast as they can get it. When **"C"** *sounds* the same as **"K,"** you have the calculating mind, inexorably joined to creative passion--which explains their drive to 'know, know, know!' Gathering skills for single or multiple purposes and always wanting to become the expert at what ever fascinates and compels them, they frequently work to uncover the hidden, the veiled and sometimes, the mysterious. (Like 19th Century Egyptologist **Jean-Francois Champollion**, whose burning curiosity enabled him to translated the hieroglyphics on the Rosetta stone and "unlock the door to the glorious past of ancient Egypt."[1]) They draw from the polarized **"K"** energy bringing its intensity into their up-front, unquitting curiosity; forever looking and *connecting,* researching and *correlating,* reading, listening and *weaving* the threads of knowledge for their own research and satisfaction. Some write, some teach, some are technicians and artisans; most love books. You could call them insufferable, nosy pests, or "Eternal Scholars," like **Joseph Campbell**, prolific researcher and writer on mythology. **"C's"** engage themselves primarily with the surface-mind through the eyes and ears; for them, these senses supply the food that titillates and feeds their intellectual appetites and satisfies their underlying quest for knowledge. *In one sense, letter "C" represents mental skills--set to serve (or deceive) the eyes and ears of the outer world, as in journalism or the legal profession.... or to provide an exclusive milieu for the "C" individual!*

Balanced "C:" conducts discussions in the manner of one who knows the (martial) art of Akido, yielding yet aware, aligning with the prevailing energy--not fighting it; then (contained in such flow), clearly seeing the openings in dialogue where they can present a point to the advantage of both. *When in the attack-defense mode of dialogue, the inner force that links us to the higher group-consciousness cannot function; (you also block what Spirit teaches or informs you through the vehicle of other minds). Remember, conversation is a mutual journey!*

Unbalanced "C:" carefully calculated responses; tightly controlled and circumspect; can seem unfeeling; regard their own skills and knowledge as superior. **Strong, negative "C's**," may cut others off--whom they consider intellectually threatening or mentally beneath them; cold and skillful, they always cleverly justify every suspicious action. **Weak "C's"** keep running old habitual mental patterns; like wheels stuck deeply in a rut....it's easier to stay in the old groove, than get out! Emotions throw them in a tailspin, they may have unresolved sexual hang-ups, which rather than face directly, they view vicariously through books and films! Weak **"C's"** argue defensively out of fear; strong, negative **"C's"** debate combatantly out of supercilious knowledge, education, or claimed elitist "connections."

When "C" is in YOUR NAME: *it's how you follow and satisfy your own curiosity and develop your mental skills - how you extract information and expertise out of others.*

SUMMARY: mental, clever, curious, skillful, inventive, intellectual; oscillating mental states; hungry for knowledge (facts, figures, details); creative; loves mental challenges. (When **"C"** *sounds* like **"S"** as in **Cecil** and **Cynthia**, they often possess social and success skills.)

---

[1] page 514 from "The People's Almanac" (1975) by David Wallechinsky and Irving Wallace.

LETTER D. *(For a list of famous* "D" *names, see* **Appendix 5.***)*

Dignity, authority, integrity, loyalty; Warrior-Self; the father; the family and community social structure; laws, regulations, governing institutions, authority figures. With our language based on a Patriarchy, society's behavioral boundaries are patterned within the family unit by the 'head of the house'- usually the Father. Just as the connection to Mom (Letters **"O"** and **"M"**) establishes emotional security, so the relationship with Dad (or a similar father figure), establishes confidence in the wider social boundaries of 'the tribe.' At home, we learn (in miniature), the behavior of the larger community--its work ethic, laws, social institutions, rules, regulations and government--with Dad as the good or bad measuring rod for how the society works. We also receive our *personal authority* imprint from our primary authority figure, regardless of that figure's gender. Generally, *how* the father projects his leadership within the home and *whether* he accepts or denigrates civic laws and public leaders, will either inspire a child to be constructive and confident in society or (with a negative father example) become a misfit or social rebel. If the father, as archetypal model, applies his own Warrior-self with distinction, his sons and daughters will take on the world with equal strength and confidence. An almost unnatural trait found in *some* serious-minded **"D's"** is an occasional and somewhat jolting wit; they laugh at life through different eyes--with clever drollness or sharp comment, leaving their listeners startled or pleasantly suprised! In another vein comes the **"D"** who habitually assails the unwary with insulting and non-stop glibness, like clever caustic comedian **Don Rickles**. On the other extreme sit the seldom-speaking, retreating, and very shy **"D's."**
Whenever **"D"** *appears in the name, the letters that follow or stand next to the* **"D"** *indicate the type of expertise that might be mastered.....or resisted (when* **"D"** *is unbalanced); there is usually a strong positive relationship with the father*--**or a strong negative one**...*either one spills over into the societal attitude.* The nature of negative **"D"** is dictatorial, from the word "dictator!" And both balanced and unbalanced **"D's"** share the characteristic of determination--for good or ill. *Try giving advice to a* **"D"** *person who is determined to fail!*

Balanced "D:" loyal and realistic; moving decisively forward in life; inspiring and encouraging others. Their motto: **"do it--do it now!"** They act with confidence, authority, integrity and dignity. Through their example, others find motivation to develop personal authority. **"D's"** often perform as community "Fathers" or looked-up-to leaders in a nation (like **Princess Diana** of Britain); most stand out as people who have become authorities in a chosen field.

Unbalanced "D:" Controlling or controlled; defensive; overly cautious, defeated by life; vulnerable with unsolved male parent issues; desperately searching for "Daddy;" want males and authority figures in general to empower, encourage and approve of them; tend to be very blaming and victim-oriented. The strong ones hide their feelings, *hate* being directed, resist or defy authority, make their own rules, appear emotionless, guarded, brusque, impenetrable, dour and retreative. Some antisocial **"D's"** take the law into their own hands and choose lives of crime. The serious **"D"** deviants become cruel, heartless and sadistic. A sadist is one who enjoys inflicting pain on other people and other life forms; (taken from the name of the infamous and depraved **Marquis de Sade**). Having lost touch with their feminine nature, their masculine side has become unfeeling and cruel. Sadism is an unbalanced and extreme characteristic of both **"D's** and **"S's."** *Great cruelty also marked the rule of Joseph Stalin in Soviet Russia* - **Stalin's** *real* name was **Djugashvili**. Also, there are those **"D's"** who suffer cruelty at the hands of their fathers, like gifted pianist **David Helfgott,** whose life was portrayed in the film "Shine."

When "D" is in YOUR NAME: *it's how you use and demonstrate your personal authority, and execute authority over others -it's how you honor and encourage others to exercise their personal authority.*

SUMMARY: good or bad relationship with Dad & authority, finding one's own authority in life; an expert (authority) in some field; a negative or positive search for the "Warrior-Self;" self-sufficient, realistic, competent or at times shy, non-communicative, dour, withdrawn; for some--the rebel against all authority figures.

LETTER E. *(For a list of famous* **"E"** *names, see* **Appendix 5.***)*

The Power of Speech, the physical voice; sound, words and language; self expression, intellect. Curious, clever, changeable, creative and gregarious, **"E's"** enjoy learning and expressing themselves in the company of others. *As the second vowel, it represents Spirit's need to freely (and audibly) communicate.* With **"E"** (or **"E's"**) in a name, you can bet on a lively mind, avid curiosity, sometimes a chatter-box - or - that a very specific *something* wants to be experienced and "voiced" in that person's life (the letters next to, or following the **"E"** will give a hint as to what the special something might be). Parents and educators (of **"E"** children) might carefully watch the child's interests, and rather than propel them into a "safe" or reasonable career, allow them the room and permission to investigate freely. When true interests are honored, the universe always opens a way for their expression. **"E"** may stay with the obvious idea of 'voice' and be primarily enchanted with speaking, writing, working in the media, or even studying languages - but there are other kinds of voices! *"A picture speaks a thousand words."* **"E"** artists, sculptors, painters, musicians and photographers speak to the world through their creations; dancers and even musicians talk with their bodies - who can forget the voice, songs, and gyrating hips of **Elvis Presley**? (Note the three **"E's"**!) With language in particular, **"E's"** (like **"C's"**), can't stand to be misquoted or misunderstood. Most speak fluently and always seem to find the right word or phrase, but weak **"E's"** need help in *developing* verbal skills. Again, some tend to talk too much rather than too well--and suffer from "diarrhea of the mouth." Think of the last time you were exhausted by someone's incessant and inane chattering! The exceptions: the magical, hypnotic storytellers, who charm us as they spin their yarns. My late husband had one such friend (an **"Eric"** I think), his non-stop talking bordered on the marathon! When this gentleman spun his fascinating yarns, he would hold forth without pause into the wee-hours of the morning--long past the time the rest of us needed to be asleep. In desperation, I would sneak away to bed leaving the men behind--my husband barely awake in his chair, helpless yet spellbound, with **Eric** striding around the kitchen, gesticulating (drink in hand) to make a point--and barely pausing between his words to sip his beer!

Balanced "E:" equally skilled in listening as well as talking; usually exhibit excellent negotiating skills; realize that most of us do not think alike. As masters in the art of true communication, their perceptions and insights entrain them directly with other minds. (*Mental entrainment:* ability to enter a similar mind-mode with someone else--even another life-form, and know exactly what they think--and why!). This requires inner-listening and receptivity to higher Mind, then it's possible (when appropriate) to link to the higher Mind of the *other* person; this ability can also be used to access the group-mind of larger audiences. Balanced **"E"** tunes into what someone else can comfortably receive--not what others assume they need to, or *should* hear! Such insights, the product of higher-Mind, bypass the conditioned, judgmental, outer intellect.

Unbalanced "E:" unable to understand other minds; can only think and communicate from their own limited standpoint; may remain aggravatingly fussy, mentally compulsive and locked into old thought patterns; find listening to others (instead of talking) difficult; often don't really 'hear' what's being said to them; will chatter out of insecurity (or just for the sake of hearing themselves talk). **Weak "E's"** hate being alone and frequently feed themselves on the captive energy of unwilling audiences! After intense mental stimulation, they find it impossible to turn-off their thoughts; can't unwind enough to fall asleep at night; need constant mental stimulation; being in their own company with no one to talk to terrifies them; you can't get them off the phone; the radio or the TV blares all night! Ineffectual **"E's"** neglect their mental potential and remain scattered and non-productive.

The more **"E's"** *you have, the more you are being called upon to truly understand how others think - try listening each time before you talk - and begin to pursue and freely express your creative talents.*

When "E" is in YOUR NAME: *it's how you use your voice, your curiosity and your self expression - it's how you listen to higher Mind and express yourself to others.*

SUMMARY: words, speech, "quicksilver" thoughts; higher Mind; need for constant mental stimulation; desire to express freely--especially verbally; media skills, (broadcasting, writing, interviewing); creative, curious, artistic, scattered, gregarious.

LETTER F. *(For a list of famous "F" names, see* **Appendix 5.***)*

Proud, dramatic, ostentatious, magnetic; born with "gambler's blood;" showy, brilliant, famous, attention-getting, daring, challenging, insistent, boastful...or shy, modest and retiring. The "F" energy acts as though Spirit wants to prod the rest of us out of our complacency. It often brings in a force to change the evolutionary flow--to "wake us up" with new activities, inventions, attitudes and ways of doing things, hopefully to make us think about our *own* lives - how we might make them more exciting, distinctive and productive. In the "F" ranks stand builders and changers of society, bringers of harmony, beauty, pleasure and invention, many of whom have forever changed the face of Western society and the world. From a long list of "F" luminaries, I mention only three: **Faraday** who created the electromagnet; **Ford** who gave us the first assembly line car and **Florence** (**Nightingale**), who pioneered nursing (on the front-line) during the Crimean War of 1853-6. Generally, "F's" have a reputation for being very friendly and likable, often displaying something for public scrutiny, such as a commodity they've personally created (in Australia, my cousin **Alec Fernie** became an engineer and built a spectacular bridge), or they attract attention with their sunny, ebullience (like the famous and unfortunate ex-Royal Duchess, **Fergie**...although she did end up creating a wonderful children's book!). "F's" tend to place themselves deliberately (or unintentionally) in the public - forcing a self-confrontation about their personal value. The more modest "F's" may play down their accomplishments, a part of them saying, *"Please don't notice me, I'm not sure I measure up to all this attention!"* (Note unassuming actor, **Harrison Ford**.) On the subject of displaying themselves, some drastic (over-or-under) dressers, tend to hold the world in contempt while using dress to accentuate their superiority! Then again, other "F's" really enjoy looking gorgeous and dressing outrageously--just for the fun of it! Add letter "B" and you get the beautiful bodied **Fabio**! Also, there's America's **Michael Flatley** - breathtaking Irish step-dancer of *Lord of the Dance* fame, and self-confessed "world's greatest living dancer" (and probably right)! When "F" combines with "R," there's either a negative or positive display of verbal skills bringing a curious mix of magnetic charm and powerful insistence--if they can't captivate you, they may end up shouting you down! Most "F's" love competition and want to be the "best of the best," often defining themselves by the dramas they create, *or they define society by creating dramas for the public.* **Example:** film director **Francis Ford Coppola**....and all the past and present actors and actresses with "F" in their names!

Balanced "F:" can appear both modest *and* justifiably proud of themselves; secure in their singularity, they bask in the visibility and hoopla without being egotistically attached to it; they also encourage motivation, pride and achievement in others. Some mystically inclined "F's" become spiritual teachers and exemplars, yet still retain an understanding of worldly ambitions and distractions, thus, instead of (permanently) retreating from the world, they teach us how to operate from the center of Spirit while remaining powerfully active in society. *Extra "F's" in a name increase the need to* ***dramatically*** *display something as well as be challenged by pride and fame. These additional "F's" stimulate ambition, without which, things of great importance (and usefulness to others) may never be developed. Some need courage to* **make** *themselves bring out the new and original, while others have all the drive in the world and* **want** *the glory of being the first!* "F's" *draw their ranks from the faint-hearted as well as the lion-hearted!*

Unbalanced "F:" may suffer from self-destructive arrogance; others, with a flair for risk-taking, become addicted to gambling. *And* there are those who enjoy being the center of *negative* attention. The ones who love to flaunt traditions often deteriorate into scathing smart-alecks. Cuttingly-witty, smug, shocking, and nonchalant, they nourish themselves (and even earn their living) from the public's reactions to their words and actions. **Weak "F's"** endure shyness, insecurity, shame and withdrawal; they desperately need encouragement to create a sense of pride in themselves. Sometimes, whether justified or not, the "F" lesson takes the form of public disgrace and humiliation!

When "F" is in YOUR NAME: *it's how you judge your personal achievements and strengths; how you compare your personal achievements and strengths with others.*

SUMMARY: often an irrational need to prove themselves, risk-taking; courageous, encouraging, serving others with innovative ideas; proud--or humble.

LETTER G. *(For a list of famous* **"G"** *names, see* **Appendix 5.***)*

Work-a-holic, loves work or lives to work, compulsive work habits; self-motivated, indefatigable; lazy or unable to work. **"G"** in the name creates the "Work-Perfectionist" or the idle sluggard. Mostly they're known as gluttons for work, energetic, persevering to a fault and driving others crazy with their obsessive work habits. My neighbor (a system's analyst), with **Giles** as a last name, says her best hours at the office are when everyone else has gone home for the day! Remember **George Burns**, the unstoppable geriatric actor-comedian? **"G's"** also want control over their efforts and bring high standards of personal achievement to their field. Some examples: Microsoft wizard and incessant work-a-holic **Bill Gates**; film maker **George Lucas** creator of the Star Wars Trilogy (and other marvels) and inexhaustible actress **"Whoopi" Goldberg** who prides herself on turning limitations into stepping stones - and advises, "Go with what you've got and make the most of it."[2] These and other high standards tend to bring 'performance-pressure' upon fellow-workers--or earn their admiration and respect. All of the go-getter **"G's"** still need to balance their intense labor habits with play and relaxation. If **"G"** **begins** a name, every letter in the *rest* of the name--has to be *worked with* and will also indicate the type of occupational energy. *For instance, my* **Giles** *neighbor "works" with aspects of letter* **"I,"** *finding intuitive and creative solutions to projects, and using tactful suggestions instead of mental manipulation when dealing with others; letter* **"L,"** *challenges her to be in a public occupation and work with people (she does!);* **"E"** *means communication skills and* **"S"** *at the end of* **Giles** *earns her respect and a good salary for her efforts.* **"G"** includes those who don't appear to be gainfully employed (such as habitually sick and disabled **"G's"**), also the able bodied slothful--working at being non-workers! - or deliberate drop-outs of mainstream commerce, who choose their own system of employment. All criminals with **"G's"** in their names have decided to work at crime--that's what they're doing this lifetime--unless they change their minds! *The challenge of gainful employment remains the same no matter what the extreme, it's only the lessons that vary.* Some **"G's"** know a more infrequent challenge; they possess either stunning beauty--or outstanding ugliness, which of course, affects their work! The beautiful are either unassuming and modest, carry a fixation about their appearance, or suffer their looks as a curse. Those branded with ugliness, sometimes transform it into a blessing and earn acceptance and love for exceptional inner-beauty. Handsome actor **Clark Gable** often felt saddled by his excessive good looks, whereas legendary actress **Greta Garbo** (equally famous for her sultry beauty), retreated totally from public view for the last few years of her life. Silent Movie heart-throb **Rudolph Valentino**, had a **"G"** Focus in the middle of his original name **Rodolpho d' Antonguolla**; women were so affected by his startling beauty they would either faint cold at the sight of him--or tear the clothes off his back! Another compellingly lovely actress **Ingrid Bergman**, also had the central **"G"** Focus in her name. **Special note:** when **"G"** *sounds* like **"J"** in names like Roger, George and Geraldine, the **"J"** energy sometimes overrides the **"G"** and they might enjoy (or attract) trouble and strife; creating injustices or battling injustices; others love to trouble-shoot and fix things. Controversial British playwright **George Bernard Shaw**, didn't exactly have it easy in his private life either! And 19th Century 'liberated' woman novelist **George Sand**, shocked fashionable European society by wearing male clothing, taking innumerable lovers (some female)--*and by being a successful female writer!!* She lived *way* before her time.

Balanced "G:" uncompetitive, dedicated, trustworthy, calm; standing alone as an example of reliable efficiency; rarely works to please anybody else--but essentially to please and satisfy themselves and their standards of a job well done; respects the efforts of others and with a quiet pride in their own achievements; skilled at keeping the balance between effort, play and relaxation.

Unbalanced "G:" In men, the lusty 'womanizer'..in women--definitely lusty! Also great workers, but with actions marked by negative pride, fear of competition and criticism of how *others* work. A weak type consists of those who have serious problems with being able to work and support themselves.

When "G" is in YOUR NAME: *it's how you motivate your self to work--or fear to work - it's how you measure yourself against (and judge) the work of others.*

SUMMARY: efficiency, endurance; lessons in work and play; beauty and ugliness.

---

[2] from an article by Mal Vincent who writes for the (Norfolk, Va.) Virginia-Pilot.

LETTER H. *(For a list of famous* **"H"** *names, see* **Appendix 5.***)*

Patience, vision, long-term goals, discipline, hard work, success, fame, public visibility (or the reclusive failure); the innovator; what you will be remembered for.

Although **"H's"** *can* polarize to extreme caution and paralysis, they're normally fearless risk-takers fired with determination and often the first to do something outstanding or unique. **Heinrich Hertz** (with three **"H's"**) discovered radio waves in 1886; **Sir Edmund Hilary** was the first man to climb Mt. Everest (tallest mountain in the world); American **Elias Howe** patented the sewing machine in 1896; **Hugh Maston Hefner's** "Playboy" magazine fueled the new sexual freedom after world war 2 and now at the end of that liberated era comes **Dr. David Ho**--revolutionary AIDS researcher! Money and fame may go together in the **"H"** energy; sometimes, they inherit it, as in the case of *young* **Howard Hughes** - who just went on to make more money, or they've a brilliant head for business and promotion like early skating star **Sonja Heini** from Norway. Combine the money aspect with **"H's"** futuristic energy and you get careers in projected trends and finance and occasionally, someone like **Barbara Marx Hubbard**, a leading social and spiritual visionary. Letter **"H"** governs concepts of time and all things connected to time management and efficiency - including the question of patience. *"How long will it take me to achieve this, what will I have to do to get from here to there??"* These time-scripts involve dreams, ambitions and plans for the future, with the determination, hard work and discipline needed to make them come true; it's also about learning and persisting through restrictions and limitations.
Note: talented singer-actress **Lena Horne** flourished during the turbulent years when black artists were struggling for and receiving very little recognition; now, several decades later and over 80, the self-affirmed "late-bloomer" is still beautiful, talented and successful! And consider another astonishing "late bloomer," the brilliant (and ill fated) concert pianist **David Helfgott**, whose life showcased in the film "Shine."[3] The **"H"** energy demands persistent willpower while you dare to own your wildest dreams - and even become famous for them. The *desire* for fame and fortune isn't enough--you also need a willingness to pay the price with dogged hard work. In the long haul, the hard fact remains - ***you* are responsible for your dreams, and only *you* can do the work!!**

Balanced "H:" positive willpower, mellowed by wisdom; patient striving--no matter how unusual or unlikely the goals; often has a strong business sense and the courage to take risks; an unwavering eye for the end result; a "success" consciousness. **Example:** the astonishing **Helen Keller**, who lived the "impossible dream," developing her talents for communication (four **"E's"**"), in a body that was blind, deaf and dumb; she became the inspiration of millions. (Letter **"K"** often means a physical challenge!)

Unbalanced "H:" craving for money fame and power; compulsion to succeed regardless of cost (to self or others); or the opposite--unpractical; undisciplined; a 'poverty consciousness' that avoids responsibility by non-action; an irrational dreamer who never amounts to anything; resentment over money--particularly if others have it and they don't! **Neurotic "H:"** epitomized by (the late in life), eccentric billionaire **Howard Hughes** (with three **"H's"**); initially, a wealthy, efficient businessman, aviator, visionary, successful film producer and handsome ladies-man; he spent his declining years as an obsessive-compulsive recluse in the world's luxury hotel suites. The fanatical **Adolf Hitler** took most of his life to become the supreme "Fuhrer" of World War 2's Germany; beginning in abject poverty with dreams and schemes that fell apart--and even within the political arena, it took him years of patient endeavor to rise to the strong heights of riches and infamy--with the megalomaniac power to enslave and destroy millions.

When "H" is in YOUR NAME: *it's how you deal with self discipline and delays - how (in a day to day practical way), you work and train yourself to fulfill your future plans .*

SUMMARY: restriction, delays, time and patience, distant goals; great fame and fortune (or infamy); leadership and success; foresight, tenacity, self motivation, self effort, rags to riches or riches to rags.

---

[3]See also "Love You to Bits and Pieces" by Gillian Helfgott with Alissa Tanskaya. Penguin Books.

LETTER I. *(For a list of famous* **"I"** *names, see* **Appendix 5.***)*

The "show-off;" joy & laughter; trying to please; mental manipulator; inspired artist; the Higher Spirit, the Breath of Life, Prana. ***The Zen of doing while Not-Doing.*** The last encompasses the mystical side of **"I"** which makes it possible to 'vanish' into the creative act. Such artists totally absorb themselves in their work (the ego ceases from "doing" and the sense of self fades into effortless-being). If a musician, they no longer "play" their instrument, the instrument plays *them*; the line between performer and performance melts away--they *become* the music! If a dancer, they dissolve into the choreography and the dance dances itself. If a painter, the painting paints itself--they merely facilitate the process and watch (with delight), the unfolding canvas! The same can be said for certain writers who have penetrated the superconscious mind. **Remarkable case in point:** I once knew a brilliant scholar (her first name contained two **"I's"**) who wrote her academic papers in "Higher-Mind-mode." First she did all her research, read the literature and took notes - then when she was ready to actually compose the paper or dissertation, she saw--as though on a screen in her head, everything she had already studied (along with her notes) laid out in the perfect order for presenting the material; then without further conscious thought or effort, she would sit down and write out the final, perfect draft! Another example of working through higher Mind came from **Tamegoro Ikii** (three **"I's"**), an ace Tokyo police Investigator, who enjoyed celebrity status for his deductive abilities. When polarized, **"I's"** fear to display their talent. Stage fright is an example. Brilliant singer, actress and director of films **Barbra Streisand** (letter **"I"** middle Focus in last name) has overcome this debility. And totally *without* stage-jitters (in fact, he loves to perform) is young Latin singing star **Enrique Iglesias** with an **"I"** Focus in his first name plus *two* **"I's"** in the second. For some, performing acts like food, it nourishes them *and* their audience--they only feel truly alive when "strutting their stuff!" **Note:** In Finland many personal names contain doubled **"I's"** and above all other peoples, the Finns take great national pride in creating and performing music and dance. *Physically, it can bring respiratory challenges;* also, many **"I"** people have researched and worked with breath and the Life Force; such as pioneer therapist **Wilhelm Reich** (two **"I's"** including a middle Focus in the last name), and with one **"I,"** modern 'breath-master,' **Gay Hendricks.**[4] *Letter "I" also lends itself to the mystical because it connects us (via the breath) to the life-force and Spirit.*[5] *The "I's" who use their gifts and abilities--challenge us to use our own and through creativity, to return to Spirit and share our inspiration with others.*

Balanced "I:" *positively* mesmeric and charismatic; loves life, gives out encouragement, joy, laughter; inspires others to their highest good through sharing their own talents.[6] Not every **"I"** wants to be artistic, but by means of their special charisma or through personal interest, become spokes-people and *draw public attention* to important issues that would otherwise be overlooked.

Unbalanced "I's:" very manipulative, calculated, mentally controlling; obsessed with what others might think of them; an almost compulsive need to be liked; always trying to say "the right thing;" terrified of showing themselves in a poor light. Weak **"I's"** play the buffoon (the habitual "show-off"), hogging center stage no matter where, desperately grabbing attention--always hoping for praise. Certain **"I"** performers (known for their emotional insecurity) become addicted to applause; they react to the audience's mood and suffer painful devastation when it's cool or critical; they display a childish need for attention--when children, they raged and pouted if they didn't get noticed on demand. Other **"I's"** alienate everyone with mocking put-downs and destructive displays--having frequent tantrums--regardless of their age!! *On a psychic level,* **"I's"** *can both give or rob energy through the 3rd eye.*

When "I" is in YOUR NAME: *it's how you draw attention to yourself and your creative abilities and how you present your creative gifts and interests to the world.*

SUMMARY: extroverted, attracts attention to self or important issues; encouraging (or mocking). Artists and artisans; the Life-force as creativity; Spirit--breath.

---

[4] "Conscious Breathing" by Gay Hendricks, Ph.D.

[5] See Appendix 1. "The Alphabet as a Ladder for Growth." All creativity begins and ends in Spirit.

[6] See Danny Kaye (David Daniel Kaminski), Chapter 19, "Name Examples."

LETTER J. *(For a list of famous* **"J"** *names, see* **Appendix 5.***)*

Controversy, judgment, justice and injustice; attracts/makes trouble or fixes/heals trouble. (***This also applies to letter*** **"G's"** ***that*** **sound** ***like*** **"J's"** ***as in "Roger" & "George."***) The letter focuses primarily on judgment and justice: justice for the individual, justice for communities and finally, justice for nature and the earth. It can pull in blame and accusation; **Janet Reno**, two term Attorney General, has had her fair share; singer **Michael Jackson** and his entire family have had theirs; retired Ohio autoworker **John Demjanjuk** found himself extradited to Israel and accused of Nazi war crimes (*three* **"J's"** in the name brought powerful issues with justice!)..and **O.J. Simpson** will always remain accused and guilty in the eyes of many. Letter **"J"** may attract unjust acts and situations; on that score, one might call **Jacqueline Bouvier Kennedy Onassis**, the First Lady of injustice! - and redoubtable comedienne **Joan Rivers** has bounced back after her "sea of troubles." Some **"J's"** choose political and social arenas and vary from being moderately involved to the out-and-out activist. In the name of social justice, early activist **"Mother Jones" Harris** instigated child labor reforms in the U.S. and became a champion for the poor; **Jacques-Yves Cousteau** ("The Jewel of the Sea") became the outstanding and outspoken advocate for the oceans, co-developer of the first aqua-lung and foremost exponent of marine conservation, he also fought the exploitation of our planet's dwindling resources. Generally speaking, most **"J's"** need a constant outlet for an excess of physical energy, many of them can't sit or stand still for long without wriggling or jiggling and most would rather be outdoors. They love to travel, or jog, do sports, race fast cars and boats, fly planes or engage in a passion for horses and other animals; some become daredevil adventurers with a wanderlust. The downside of **"J"** (similar to **"K"**): it may attract a severe physical challenge, often stemming from its tendency to be accident-prone......then the life reflects the lesson--in making the best (or worst) of an "unjust" situation! An accident-prone **"J"** child gets attention through trouble and catastrophe, they actually *need* extra attention and more acceptance, otherwise, later in life there's a struggle to find and keep employment, accompanied by a sense of being "put-upon" by others. The last physical aspect of letter **"J"** focuses on the health and fitness of the body; you develop a passion for keeping fit--or you even become a fitness guru, like **Jane Fonda** and the legendary health advocate **Jack Lalanne**. At a deeper level, some **"J's"** try to make sense out of life by taking it head-on and creating controversy--like provocative author **James Joyce**, whose writings were initially misunderstood, as was philosopher **Jean-Paul Sartre**--although Sartre also lent his energy and passion to revolutionary politics. Early psychiatrist **Carl Gustav Jung**, rebel and original thinker (from **"J"** *sounded* as **"Y"**), master of the unconscious, of symbols and dream interpretation and an investigator into the esoteric, was accused by his associates of abandoning medicine for mysticism; but he firmly maintained that psychiatry must reflect *all* of man's experiences! Finally, a more archetypal, mystical, heroine....**Saint Joan of Arc**, the martyred warrior-woman from fifteenth Century France, who listened to her "inner voices," rallied and successfully led her countrymen in battle--but was sold to her enemies for trial, torture and burning.

Balanced "J:" physical determination; persistence; reliability; accepting others without judgment; the capacity for joy and tranquillity in the face of trials and tribulations; an abiding inner faith in mankind and the spiritual forces within man and within all of nature; expert "trouble-shooters;" advocates for justice and just causes (like **Rev. Jesse Jackson**). **Note:** *where* **"J's** *sound like* **"Y,"** *refer to page* 69.

Unbalanced "J:" irresponsible, always in some kind of personal trouble; fear of being judged; projects trouble onto others--or personally takes *on* the troubles of others. Famous **"J"** perpetrators of injustice: Russia's "butcher" of millions **Joseph Stalin**; the **Rev. Jim Jones** (responsible for the mass suicide of his religious community in Guyana, West Africa); **Josef Mengele**, Nazi mass murderer; also, U.S. Senator **Joseph McCarthy,** who (all too quickly) judged and jumped to conclusions in his authorized communist witch-hunt after World War 2. **When weak**, they either deliberately avoid confrontations, or consistently attract trouble, especially when **"J"** begins the name...*but eventually, it makes them strong!*

When "J" is in YOUR NAME: *it's how you keep out of trouble or attract it - it's how you deal with injustice or physical challenges from others and your environment.*

SUMMARY: energetic, athletic; loves animals, sports, travel; dealing with justice, attracting or avoiding trouble, dare-devilish; mystical, interdimensional.

LETTER K. *(For a list of famous* **"K"** *names, see* **Appendix 5.***)*

The sexual force, sexual power transmuted into creativity; death or life; transformation; secrecy. The charismatic life force either as a sexual or creative catalyst - or both! Some **"K's"** attempt to disguise the energy with what appears to be a physically *unattractive* body, but it doesn't work--regardless of how they try to hide themselves, they still shine with libidinal charisma and can't understand why others find them sexually interesting! So **"K"** in a name may mean sexual and creative lesson-challenges...or you have a sex *researcher* - **Alfred Kinsey**! Turn this Life Force power outward towards nature and you find people devoting their lives to preserving endangered species or the seeds of plants, like botanist and molecular biologist **Alan Kapuler**, who started an organization called "Peace Seeds" in Corvallis, Oregon. Kapuler is part of a world network to save the seeds of hardy non-hybrid plants. Where **"K"** connects into death, there's both a positive and a negative fascination. The most famous person in this respect **Dr. Jack Kevorkian** (often referred to as "Dr. Death"- note the three **"K's"** in his name) feels his "duty as a doctor" should allow him to alleviate the suffering of the dying by helping them commit suicide. Other **"K's"** involved with the quality of death, devote themselves to hospice work like **Elizabeth Kubler Ross** and totally transformed, twice-back-from-the-dead, author and lecturer **Dannion Brinkley**. Some **"K's"** develop a passion for immortality and turn to the physics of cryogenics to preserve their bodies after death in the hope of later resuscitation; whereas others are more interested in the physical transformation of the *present* life and use rejuvenating breath-work, Yoga, Martial arts, diet supplements, etc. In the **"K"** criminal mind, the death interest becomes perverted; one convicted killer (whose name began with **"K"**) is on record as saying, "I love to kill." (Many people condemned to death have **"K"** in or at the ends of their names.) Some cultures favor death as a statement of personal or national honor; for instance, during World War 2, the Japanese used **Kamikaze** pilots from a suicidal branch of the Japanese air force to deliberately crash their planes (stocked with explosives) into American ships; and today, terrorists willingly die for their causes. The 'physical-connection' makes *most* **"K's"** robust and especially resilient to illness, but it sometimes brings temporary or permanent health challenges when it appears as the Focus (middle) letter of the last name. **Note: Stephen Hawking**, world renowned, brilliant astrophysicist suffers from life-threatening and debilitating Lou Gehrig's disease; yet inspite of years of almost total immobilization, his unfettered mind has "transformed our view of the universe."[7] The **"K"** Focus of his life has been to defy the dissolution of the physical--and soar to the heights of the mind! *The soul sometimes limits itself to develop special qualities and learn special lessons.* (**"K"** also means to uncover and bring forth deep and hidden things.) To sum up: **"K's"** have a reputation for being emotionally moody and secretive with (usually) strong sexual appetites and compelling willpower; some possess a singular and creative imagination and those interested in healthy lifestyles tend to advise or 'doctor' others.

<u>**Balanced "K:"**</u> inspires, charms and delights with unique creative abilities (like the inimitable and brilliant comic, **Danny Kaye**); self contained, charismatic and totally true to themselves, they disregard the opinions of others. *All artistic endeavor flows and energizes itself - from the sexual force.*

<u>**Unbalanced "K:"**</u> sexual excesses, or a distancing from others in an intense, antisocial reclusive world like accused Unabomber **Theodore Kaczynski** (two **"K's"**). Some have their inner intensity blocked and appear to be icy, emotionless, entirely without feeling and totally insensitive to others. This extreme category also includes the **"K"** neurotics and criminally insane. <u>**Example**</u>: famous cyanide killer **Stella Nickell** (**"K"** Focus letter in last name); cold and calculating, without remorse or conscience, she delighted in planning the deaths of others--here **"K"** means the *negative* power of death. Also ponder the **Ku Klux Klan**, which desires to cull "inferior" racial types from the face of the planet!

When "K" is in YOUR NAME: *it's how you accept or reject your sexuality -and how others respond to your use of the creative Life Force.*

<u>SUMMARY:</u> Sex, emotional intensity, moodiness, passionate creativity; secrets; hidden mysteries; death, execution; rebirth, immortality, life extension, health or illness.

---

[7] to quote from the dust jacket of his book, "A Brief HIstory of Time."

LETTER L. *(For a list of famous* **"L"** *names, see* **Appendix 5.***)*

Humanity, society; social skills, diplomacy; being in the public. **"L"** *reflects the energy of the people.* There are three levels: **1)** Self-love in relationship to other people. **2)** Sharing research, knowledge, and teaching about aspects of society and its viability. **3)** The culture *itself* and how leaders attempt to mold and change public opinion. **Example: Abraham Lincoln**,16th U.S. President; his self-identity remained colored by shame (at being illegitimate); he tried to compensate through tremendous personal effort to *be* the best. Lincoln also *did* his best to educate and change the people's attitude towards slavery--which shaped the America we know today. Other **"L"** leaders who have influenced their countries during times of crisis: **Charles De Gaulle**, (for France-World War 2); **Winston Churchill** (for England-World War 2) and **Nelson Rolihlahla Mandella**, with six **"L's"** in his name (for South Africa, to end apartheid). On a personal level, **"L"** presents lessons in self esteem through social interaction and adaptability; usually, if you dislike yourself, you'll dislike other people! **Louise L Hay** has written *the* definitive textbook on self-love,[8] it's now practically a classic. The **"L"** social energy thrives on networking, furnishing diplomatic skills to connect people in mutual endeavors or interests. Notice how the **"L"** members of the family keep track of where everyone wanders to (whether across the street or across the country); they organize great parties and facilitate family reunions. Profession-ally, **"L's"** gravitate to occupations in which they deal with, or are surrounded by, the public. Some **"L's"** have a special 'people-radar;' just by looking over a crowded room, they instantly know who they want to talk to and who they should avoid. The powerful ones can hold an audience spellbound, like the early jazz singer **Al Jolson**, and **Adolf Hitler**, with his almost hypnotic control over the masses. When **"L"** doubles in a name, it causes an intensification of the energy: to Australian **Bill Mollison**, it gives the vision of a sustainable future for lands and peoples in the earth-saving concept of "permaculture;" to the famous author, playwright and activist **Lillian Hillman**, it gave a strong social responsibility; to **Agatha Mary Clarissa Miller (Agatha Christie)**, it gave a fascination with how people interact, enabling her to delight millions with her timeless tales of mystery! There ARE **"L"** misanthropes--but apart from them, many great-hearted **"L's"** do very reclusive, private research gathering information in relative isolation and eventually presenting it in books and lecture tours. **Examples: William Sullivan**, who walked the wilderness alone for years remapping old hiking trails for the benefit of posterity--eventually returning to share his love of nature through lectures and slides; **Jane Goodall**, famous for her lifetime commit-ment to wild apes; natural historian **George Schaller**, who lived for considerable time in remote places studying rare animals and fighting to save them (his organization helped establish 50 nature reserves throughout the world); archaeologists **Louis** and **Mary Leakey** spent decades digging fossils in Africa to unravel man's ancient origins. Lastly, there are the world-visionaries like designer-inventor **Buckmins-ter Fuller** and Oregon's **Dr.Ralph Lewis**, preservationist, outspoken geology professor and watchdog for man's effect on the environment.

Balanced "L:" true humanist; lover of people and the human race; natural diplomat; very sensitive to the dynamics of social relationships (this tendency begins in early childhood); an affinity with nature and the earth; a conserver of that which is valuable, beautiful and of advantage to others such as Oregon's **Alan Kaupler,** who networks to save non-hybrid seeds; and in art, famous restorer **Lido Lippi.**

Unbalanced "L:" may be a social snob or racial bigot; dislikes people; suffers from insecurity, especially in public. (*Famous public* **"L"** *insecures:* actress **Liv Ullmann** and showman pianist **Liberace.**) The inner dialogue goes something like this: *"Is my hair OK, am I wearing the right clothes, what will they think of me??"* They have difficulty in making choices and struggle to find their identity through the reactions of others. **Extremely unbalanced** suffer from self hatred and hatred of life itself; can be fearful or repelled by others. Russian author **Leo Tolstoy** said: *"My life is some stupid and spiteful joke."* His books were miserable, life-defeating and depressing, yet filled with the power of his tortured soul.

When "L" is in YOUR NAME: *it's how you accept and love yourself - it's how you relate to a crowd and accept people generally.*

SUMMARY: people; love (or dislike) of humankind; social graces; harmony, public confidence; self love; beneficial research.

---

[8] called, "You Can Heal Your Life."

LETTER M. *(For a list of famous* **"M"** *names, see* **Appendix 5.***)*

Mother, house and home; family unit, the "nesting" urge, busyness; support, security; the Homeland; the Goddess. *Learning through close relationships, family and home.* Most **"M's"** search for the ideal mate in order to settle down and live happily ever after! These **"M's"** fall into four groups: eternal searchers; ideally mated; stoically mated (holding a home and a marriage together--but with things far from perfect) - and lastly, the *"I don't want to* ***ever*** *be mated!"* Most have strong family bonds and prefer to work in the home at a residence-based business. **"M's"** tend to chafe at inactivity and hate to waste time; they want to keep very busy and get miserable unless they're constantly working at something...(sound like **Martha Stewart** to you?) - or they put up with work they hate (fearing change) just to keep the home and family together. Many **"M's"** nurture themselves by nurturing others--this can be negative and controlling, or enabling and selfless. Like **"O,"** letter **"M"** has a food-thing lurking in the background and can also emotionally drain (and feed upon) the unsuspecting...it's called the "vampire" aspect! *Ever felt drained and exhausted after spending time with a needy* **"M"** *or* **"O"** *person??* Other **"M's"** feel more secure when they collect things--like money and possessions! Billionaire **Malcolm Forbes** understood the principles of collecting, but *unlike* most of the very rich, he also knew how to really enjoy his wealth! In a general sense, **"M"** represents the basic cultural unit of a society--the family, and how it sustains or destroys itself. **Karl Marx** with his radical philosophy of communism redefined the interactions of a culture and ultimately affected billions of families; early anthropologist **Margaret Mead's** interest in "the family unit" extended to the study of (the then) unspoiled Polynesian cultures; writer-columnist **Erma Bombeck** made us laugh at the funny side of family life and **Martha Stewart** presides in the media as the American Guru of housekeeping. *The presence of* **"M"** *in a name denotes a key interaction with the mother....*she may be a best friend--or a worst enemy! In either case, there are major lessons within the relationship. Occasionally an **"M"** child takes over the role of 'mothering' an elderly parent (most frequently the mother), to the extent of having the parent live-in with them indefinitely. For the balanced **"M,"** this live-in, caring service becomes a willing act of love, but when unbalanced, the same filial duty is highly resented and complained about! Sans an aged or ailing parent to care for (a natural part of family life in more 'primitive' cultures), **"M's"** tend to collect a menage of people not necessarily blood related--and/or animals, as part of their home or extended family. **Example:** actress **Mia Farrow** (the epitome of home and dedicated motherhood) cared for ten children, some her own, the rest adopted....and not all of her lessons in "mothering" have been easy ones!! Vulnerable **"M's"** need constant emotional support from a wide circle of friends.

Balanced "M:" emotionally self sufficient; efficient; very adaptable yet nurturing; love to make others feel comfortable and welcome; can easily *create* a home (or feel at home)....anywhere...regardless of what's going on; never bored, can always find something to interest, busy and absorb them.

Unbalanced "M:" emotionally needy; a compelling quest for the ideal love may suffocate and drive would-be mates away--especially if the searcher felt rejected or abandoned as a child (the search is *really* for the denied and unattainable perfect mother!).**Weak "M's:"** unwilling or incapable of providing their own 'nests;' they learn how to "camp" in other people's homes for free--where they keep very busy (like good **"M's"**) making themselves useful to the hosts, but essentially, they're only pervasive parasites! When the foundation of a loving mother and supportive childhood has been denied, **"M's"** reactions can become neurotic to sociopathic, in their rage, they turn against accepted family values and lay waste that which *they* never received. These misfits find their "clan" within the ranks of gangs, other criminals, or form their own destructive anti-social groups (the **Mafia**). They reverse the nurturing aspect of **"M "** by destroying members of family units, pillaging homes, targeting public institutions and committing antisocial acts against women in particular and society in general--it's their way of 'punishing' the aberrant **real** mother along with the rejected community. The personality types run the gamut of the emotionally needy to the psychopathically criminal--deviants because of their **"M"** problems. **Classic example:** **Charles Manson**, society-hating, Californian commune leader in the late 60's with a 'family' of devoted female followers who master-minded the Tate-LaBianca murders.

When "M" is in YOUR NAME: *it's how you relate(ed) to your mother - it's how you find the perfect mate and create your own ideal home/family/business.*

SUMMARY: mother, home, family, mate, the earth - or reviling and destroying same.

LETTER N. *(For a list of famous* "N" *names, see* **Appendix 5.***)*

Clever, analytical, critical; detailed work; integration & balance; service; the martyr. Perfectionists and obsessed by details, **"N's"** are the detail-junkies of the alphabet..if you're *not* - the **"N"** in your name might be there to help you *pay attention* to details! Or you might be orderly and systematic like the music of **Johann Sebastian Bach** (who had three **"N's"** in his name). Specifically, **"N"** is one of the 'inward-turning' letters--so a part of the personality tends to be reclusive and introverted. Usually much personal-work needs to be done as "N" necessitates reconciling compulsive extremes. First you bring yourself into balance, then you're fit to help others. Furthermore, it involves rendering *right* service--*not egotistical or martyred service.*

<u>The "N" extremes:</u> 1) Physical. Some **"N's"** fluctuate between neglecting or wrecking their bodily health; may compulsively over-exercise, yo-yo between junk-feeding and dieting, try periodic health food kicks, flip between living like a slob and rushing after every speck of dust - or from being lazy to a dynamo of energy and compulsive activity. **2) Mental.** Some swing from mental languishing to analytical cleverness and nit-picking perfectionism (also "second-guessing" everything and everyone)!

3) Emotional. Some polarize from helpless, self-pitying victim-pathos to attack-mode, criticizing and blaming everything in sight! *In each of these polarities, the middle road must be discovered.* Because **"N"** *goes* to extremes, it has the power to *reconcile* extremes. When misunderstood, **"N's"** often become enraged, they generally go to great pains to clarify themselves. Many **"N's"** suffer from the "soft-touch," they're selfless to a fault and so compassionate (or striving to please), they can't say *"No"* when someone wants something. The healing aspect of **"N"** may be the challenge to heal yourself, like **Norman Cousins** (three **"N's"**) who healed himself of a lethal disease by developing "laughter therapy."[9] (Laughter releases healing chemicals in the brain.)

<u>Balanced "N:"</u> the Balancers; experts at self-management; people of great integrity, above reproach, high personal standards; will listen inwardly to higher Mind before speaking; frequently combine linear logical analysis with intuitive thinking; serve with compassionate awareness instead of willy-nilly "rescuing" or "helping" others. *Sometimes the most compassionate thing to do is nothing--the other person may need certain experiences for their own growth.* **<u>Serving-"N's"</u>** will observe in what ways humanity needs to come into balance--then gravitate to a particular aspect of service subsequently dedicating their lives to that endeavor. One who sought to bring a sense of balance to society through his art was famous illustrator **Norman Rockwell**; he painted only idealized details of American family life in 317 covers for "The Saturday Evening Post." A great servant of the people (especially children), who also healed with laughter was actor-comedian **Danny Kay**.[10] **Norman Vincent Peale** (four **"N's"**) began the public's fascination with self-improvement. And today, **Ralph Nader's** detailed analytical and critical research makes him the nation's foremost consumer advocate.

<u>Unbalanced "N:"</u> the Martyr; failures at self-management; suffer serious abandonment issues; frequently moody and depressed; super-critical perfectionists--yet cannot endure being the butt of criticism. When on the receiving end they immediately erect defensive walls, behind which they either whimper their weak excuses or vociferously protest their intellectual superiority. Ruled by compulsion, emotionally vulnerable weak **"N's"** frequently hide their real feelings; always taking offense, whining and complaining, attracting constant criticism and put-downs and lashing back with self-pitying diatribes. However, when roused, they can be powerful, **and furious** *"Oh-poor-me's,"* almost glorying in their misfortunes! Another version (determined to fail)--just give up--sinking into self-rejection and neuroses...the ultimate martyr!

When "N" is in YOUR NAME: *it's how you handle and deliver criticism, it's how you balance your polarities and use your brilliant mind.*

<u>SUMMARY:</u> the analytical perfectionist, critical, clever, balancing, compulsive; attentive to detail; service to others; healer; yo-yo moods; the martyr.

---

[9] See "Anatomy of an Illness" and "The Healing Heart," by Norman Cousins.

[10] See the Danny Kay entry in Chapter 19, "Name Examples with Analysis."

LETTER O. *(For a list of famous "O" names, see* **Appendix 5.***)*

The emotions, empathy; the breasts and belly; the mother and the wounded child; the Goddess; the magical, sacred Inner Child; wonder, delight and pleasure; food; birthing ideas. "**O**" shares similar energies with "**M**" as both relate to the mother and the Earth-Mother Goddess. Whereas "**M**" yearns to *create* the ideal family, "**O**" needs to have been *part of* an ideal family, to have had basic emotional needs satisfied--a factor vital to emotional health. This directly ties into eating habits developed from the way mothers use food to destructively control or positively nourish their offspring. *The* "**O**" *curriculum includes lessons in learning to be self-sufficient without expecting or demanding that others supply your emotional needs.* An Oedipus complex develops when mothers turn their sons into substitute husbands (from the Greek myth of **Oedipus Rex** who unwittingly killed his father and married his mother). It's interesting to note how many early ex-Presidents of the US had several or doubled "**O's**" in their names....and to study the weak or strong emotional reactions they showed--plus their responses to food! In passing: **Herbert Clark Hoover**, the 31st President was famous as a humanitarian and food-relief administrator. **The Food Issue**: *If you are deprived of unconditional, self enhancing love as a child, you never completely mature emotionally and may turn to food for compensation. It's called "feeding the Hungry Ghosts" - the starving inner selves; yet when you nurture yourself (by doing what brings joy and wonder into your life), your body's metabolism changes radically, you respond differently to food; cravings vanish and you enter the realm of the magical, sacred self. Look to the letters each side of the* "**O's**" *in your names to find what brings you deeply into joy and wonder.* Some "**O's**" become amazing cooks - others just get involved with food and nourishing others. T.V. Talk show host **Oprah Winfrey** reveals her great and caring nature through her films and daily programs, including the heartwarming "Angel Network" (spare change to help others), but she also does constant battle with her inner "hungry ghosts." Also, buxom "**O**" T.V. host **Rosie O'Donnell** (with *three* "**O's**"!!); known for her caring, positive programs and fund raising.

Balanced "O:" Master of emotions; patience; understanding; wisdom; contentment; detached empathy; compassion; bringing 'nourishment' and healing through actions and words; loving role-model; moist and flowing rather than dried-up and arid; *secure in the ability to give and receive love;* self contained and self nurturing; reaching out to **give** instead of reaching out to take; appreciation of good food without guilt or addiction...and (regardless of gender), merging with the feminine principal (the inner Goddess), as well as the outer Goddess (the Earth Mother); sustaining the planet; maintaining an underlying oneness with all nature, peoples and creatures; concern for the suffering of others.

Unbalanced "O:" self-absorption, imagined insults, emotional demands, the wounded child; emotional manipulation or indulgence; hedonism. **Oscar Wilde**, brilliant, ostentatious ("**W**"), nineteenth century successful playwright and author; his one novel "The Picture of Dorian Grey" reflected his own self-indulgent downfall. Some manipulate by discerning the emotional vulnerabilities of others, then cleverly use the information against them - or they control their surroundings through unpleasant and unpredictable moods. **Weak "O's"** become the victims preyed upon by stronger emotional manipulators (including stronger "**O's**"). To *earn* love and acceptance, some become "responsibility sponges," running around trying to do the impossible and by sopping up other people's puddles of unhappiness. The converse: searching for sympathy, the *"Oh poor me"* syndrome!

Severely unbalanced, "O's" tend toward paranoia with many fears: loss of possessions, loss of food (fear of starvation and deprivation); loss of love-objects (fear of emotional deprivation).

Note: 16th century, Italian anatomist Gabriel Fall**o**pius (with the "**O**" as Focus-Challenge) was the first to dissect, study and name, the female parts of reproductive anatomy.

When "O" is in YOUR NAME: *it's how you nurture (or feed upon) yourself - it's how you nurture (or feed upon) others and how you relate to the inner and outer Goddess.*

SUMMARY:- gentle, caring, master of emotions; wonderment, pleasure, self-containment, self-nurturing, feeding others; sentimental or moody; accumulating, clinging to money and possessions; self-indulgent or abstemious.

LETTER P. *(For a list of famous* **"P"** *names, see* **Appendix 5.**)

Bringer of peace, tranquillity, balance and harmony - or the perpetrator of disharmony, disunity, strife and war. Very aesthetic, usually demands quality, beauty and harmony in surroundings; restores itself in aloneness and solitude; tends to avoid situations and people disturbing to their predetermined mind set; often attracts disharmony as a 'teaching mirror.' *The Lesson: instead of withdrawing they need to open to new insights and emotional experiences.* The **"P"** energy also dips into the unreal worlds of alternate realities--like computer-animator expert **Phil Tippett** (three **"P's"**), his work is the stuff that dreams are made of. He designed the marvelous dragon in the 1996 film "Dragon Heart." You'll find other **"P's"** drawn to occupations that harmonize, blend and synthesize and the obvious ones are music, art and choreography--the more intriguing are medical, industrial and food chemistry! From the latter came **Earl Tupper**, a Dupont Chemist who invented "Tupperware" (in the 40's), the versatile kitchen containers with their unique vacuum sealing system. Of even greater benefit to mankind was 19th Century French microbiologist and chemist **Louis Pasteur**, founder of modern microbiology, who developed several vaccines and the process of pasteurization; whereas **"P's"** with supersensory taste and smell may become tea and wine blenders, creative chefs and skilled perfumers. Certain **"P's,"** like British physicist **Edward V. Appleton**, look for underlying meaning and harmony in the world around us; his research into the upper atmosphere revealed what is now called the "Appleton" layer in the ionosphere, and German physicist **Max Plank** developed his theories to explain the nature of light. The obvious polarity of peace and harmony--brings us to war and violence, so you'll find specific **"P's"** attracted to professional soldiering, some with a primary desire to *keep* the peace and others who want to *make* war. Famous war strategists: **Napoleon Bonaparte** (two **"P's"**) and **General George S. Patton**. Even as I write, **O.J. Simpson** defends himself in Court for the wrongful death charge in the murder of his ex-wife and her companion. A glance at his last name reveals a central **"P"** as the Focus letter--it would appear his choices have **not** been in the direction of peace, balance and harmony!! Then there are those **"P's"** who deliberately or inadvertently challenge the status quo like Alabama's **Rosa Parks**, who in 1955 was too tired to give up her bus seat to a white man and her subsequent arrested triggered the great civil rights movement of the South; **Elvis Presley**, the 'times-changing' rock-and-roll legend whose sensuous hips and sultry voice drove the girls crazy--and their parents up the wall!...and artist **Pablo Picasso** who with his paintings became famous (or infamous) for dissolving solid form into dissected, two dimensional segments. **Note:** **"P"***concerns itself with consolation, relief from pain, solace for the soul--thus the words, "placebo," "pampered" and "panacea." When totally reversed,* **"P"** *brings pandemonium and panic.*

Balanced "P:" peace-loving; peace-inducing; introspective, private, self-contained, with often solitary pursuits - generally creative; realize what makes them happy and comfortable and absolutely *refuse* to remain in stressful or destructive relationships or situations; diplomatic and charming; naturally take the role of mediator. Unruffled in any crisis, they have a total sense of who they are. To quote my unfluffable neighbor Pat, **"I always carry my own space with me."**

Unbalanced "P:" self-punishing; some are known to *endure*--to stoically remain in stressful and painful situations even to the point of illness and death (like my old friend **Penelope**). And while the innocuous ones disturb the peace, create their diversions, and love practical jokes, the insidious remain contentious and cranky, needling and nasty, ruffling feathers and delighting in causing disharmony and havoc while getting high on other people's discomfiture. *The dark side of* **"P"** *is cruelty and punishment--even to the self!.* **Weak "P's"** become emotionally immobilized and can't (or won't) deal with people and the simple mechanics of living. They blame and constantly judge the disharmony of others. Another form of unbalanced **"P"** sells-out for "peace at any price" - as did **Marshall Philippe Petain** (four **"P's"** including one doubled), who took control of France in World War 2 and capitulated to the invading Germans.

When "P" is in YOUR NAME: - *it's how you bring peace or create havoc in your own life and in the lives of those around you.*

SUMMARY: The 'loner' instinct; serene, self contained and private; perfectionist; innovative researcher; loves or shuns people; keeps the peace, or destroys the peace.

LETTER Q. *(For a list of famous* **"Q"** *names, see* **Appendix 5.***)*

A unique (often brilliant) mind-set; freedom loving, daring, fearless, efficient, organized, energetic, restless, cunning - or mentally lazy, slothful, inept, wimpy.

The thrill-seekers! Often known for their enormous enthusiasm and overwhelming openness. *"Let's try it--let's do it now!* Frequently leaders in their chosen field, the **"Q"** factor often creates a mental-set so precise, organized and perfect (in a unique way) that others find it hard or difficult to match--or even to keep up with. They have the inventive power to master any challenging situation--preferably without interference from others. **"Q's"** tend to have their own reality, but not necessarily in line with the rest of the world and need to find their own niche in life where their unique mental brilliance can shine on others: like Grammy winner, TV, film producer and Jazz musician **Quincey Jones**; influential British fashion designer, **Mary Quant** and the "perfect performer," actor **Anthony Quinn**. When **"P's"** and **"Q"** combine (as for 17th Century **Philip Quarll**, who found himself castaway on a tropical island), you may find the resourceful, self-sufficient hermit, creating their own peace and tranquillity - Judging from his journal, Quarll aligned himself totally with his environment and was so content with his personal "kingdom", he refused to accept rescue when found 50 years later. **"Q's"** also make ingenious criminals like 19th Century **Francois Eugene Vidocq**, who began as a scoundrel, then a prison spy, then a brilliantly successful Paris Police detective. He founded the famous Surete, where ex-convicts were hired to *catch* criminals; Vidocq soon became the feared nemesis of the French underworld. **Note:** the **"Q"** at the end of his name *sounds* like a **"K"** and in addition to the sexual aspect (he was known as a womanizer in his youth), the **"K"** energy can be involved with secrets and spies, life and death...in Vidocq's case, with catching and sending criminals to the guillotine! Also using the **"K"** *sound* for **"Q"** (and allegedly involved with subterfuge and death through international terrorism) is Libyan ruler **Muammar el-Qaddafi (or "Gadafi"..or "Khadafy"!)** *The three* **"M's"** *produce a great nurturing and sense of family solidarity including love of children--within the context of his own people, but it's usually reversed in regards to non-Muslims (with some notable exceptions--American mothers visiting their children in Libya); plus his* **"D's"** *present him as a powerful father-figure--which all goes to highlight the outstanding uniqueness surrounding a strong* **"Q"** *energy.* The most commonly found letter combination: a **"Q"** followed by **"U"** often resulting in the challenge of expansion--the search for new worlds to conquer and discoveries to be made in whichever direction the **"QU"** person's passion lies. For some, adventure flows in their veins--not blood! Other **"Q's"** hunger for absolute truth. The search could be of a spiritual or mundane nature, but they want to know *for sure*--then they may force their beliefs upon others for "their own good!" And they want their questions answered 'in person' - *"Talk to me God!"*

Balanced "Q:" open-ended searching mind and spirit; very creative; singular attitude to life; accepts the fact that they will have few mental or visionary companions; content to follow their own perception of life without imposing it on others. Their questing minds often leave a beneficial legacy.

Unbalanced "Q:" tend to get into mischief or real trouble when bored; often lonely and misunderstood (few people comprehend the **"Q"** mental energy); can attempt to align or fit-in with others, but there's always a part of them that's out in left field, like **Raymond Queneau**, a 20th Century French novelist and poet whose "bizarre, erudite humor, full of puns and Surrealism, cloaked a profound pessimism."[11] And when the quest for danger-high's combines with "conquest" it often becomes criminal and turns to blood-lust as in the case of **William Clarke Quantrill**, known as "the bloodiest man in American history," who in the mid 1800's turned from teaching school to gun fighting and murder. Unbalanced **"Q's"** have "tunnel vision" and see only their own reality, which is sometimes shared by a few odd-balls but mostly makes them frustrated loners or overpowering leaders.

When "Q" is in YOUR NAME: - *it's how you allow your questing spirit to enrich your life and benefit others - or to feed a need for destructive danger.*

SUMMARY: a different mind-set; intensely curious, brilliant, uniquely creative and inventive; unstoppable, frenetic, uninhibited energy - or a wimpy, weak conformist.

---

11 from "The Reader's Digest Illustrated Encyclopedic Dictionary."

LETTER R. *(For a list of famous* **"R"** *names, see* **Appendix 5.***)*

Mental Power and push, persistence, cogitation, abstract thought, the ideas-person; Wisdom Mind. When I think of **"R,"** I mentally see **Rodin's** famous sculpture "The Thinker," chin in hand--lost in thought. It was my husband **Roger's** favorite stance. The thinking rarely stills, there's always internal dialogue; if it's not "self talk," they're rehearsing for impending conversations and most **"R's"** have a strong introverted side that keeps them deep in their own mental landscape. Although President **Ronald Reagan** was known as "The Great Communicator" and famous for loquacity (letter **"E"** in Reagan), **"R's"** mostly need silence, even solitude, to mull over their thoughts. The more articulate tend to be the friendliest, but the mentally aggressive ones love to silence others! Some weak **"R's"** suffer from verbal insufficiency, they struggle and stumble to find the right word, take instant offense (where none was intended) and on getting riled, lash out with verbal abuse--or they sulk, simmer and brood. The most aggravating **"R's"** don't like to make decisions *about anything*--from the little things like choosing an ice-cream flavor, deciding on a restaurant - to the big life-demanding issues. They will *beg* you for advice--which they instantly ignore! Finally, it hit me--they only need to *hear* advice, then what they ***really*** *want to do* clicks in!! For your sanity, resist the temptation to advise an indecisive **"R,"** instead, walk away and *force* them to make up their minds on their own!! Now consider a few interesting **"R"** people (some with multiple or doubled **"R's"**): **Gerry Spence**, famous defense lawyer and powerful speaker; **Garry Kasparov** (three **"R's"**), chess champion of the world; **Don Rickles**, well known sarcastic humorist; **Larry Flint,** outspoken publisher of Hustler magazine; misspoken novelist **Salman Rushdie**, under an Islamic death-threat for blasphemy; **Sally Jessy Ralphael**, TV talk show host and **Larry King**, skillful TV interviewer. *When letters* **"R"** *and* **"H"** *combine in a name it can result in a life of aggressive financial success or public fame; the* **"R"** *and* **"O"** *combination tends to manipulate (or heal) through emotions;* **"R"** *and* **"E"** *in a name may create a thinker-writer, or the articulate investigator.*

<u>**Balanced "R:"**</u> marriage of verbal skills and concepts; exceptional reasoning power plus innovative ideas (or able to expand, augment and honor *existing* ideas); not easily aroused to anger--takes responsibility to process anger without blame (as in balanced **"A"**); respects the opinions of others; selfcomplete and contented with a natural need to look for deeper meaning in everything; able to leave the outer intellect and expand into higher Mind; shares wisdom and insight with others.

<u>**Unbalanced "R:"**</u> instant rage; the mental control-freak; revengeful against "slights" (real or imagined); opinionated, disdainful, superior, critical, controlling, domineering and mentally overbearing; fixed, bigoted and irrational; not open to any viewpoint other than their own. Operating through mental aggression; masters of insult, demeaning put-downs and unassailable arguments (if it appears they might lose, they begin to shout and scream). There's an "Army" joke that fits them to perfection: An assistant is briefing a new member of the staff in the General's office - *"The General is always right--even when he's wrong...remember that!"* <u>**Vulnerable "R's"**</u> will identify their ideas and possessions with their ego (this stems from a hidden, insurmountable, insecurity); therefore, disagreeing (even mildly) with one of their opinions or even criticizing one of their *possessions* will immediately threaten their personal facade of reality--causing irrationality in the face of hard facts! I have witnessed such an **"R"** person tear a book in half and throw it away, rather than face documented data that would contradict (and illuminate) their closed opinions! They hear only what they want to hear, making it difficult if you happen to have said something *other* than what they remember--you are then accused of lying--witnesses notwithstanding! When linked with **"O"** they're possessive and smothering (often painful to have as family members or close companions). <u>**Weak "R:"**</u> very fragile ego (same for unbalanced), sense of well being topples with the slightest criticism; tendency to live in their own internal reality; fear of change, resistant to even smallest of changes; have to learn at their own rate, can't be pushed or pressured to try new procedures or they close down their minds; a profound fear of failure--so why bother to try!! Favorite phrase: **"I can't"** (meaning) **"I won't."**

When "R" is in YOUR NAME: *it's how you handle your mental power and how you interact with the mental power of others.*

<u>SUMMARY:</u> aggressive mental power; very persuasive; outspoken; in love with ideas; skilled speaker; open minded or bigoted; easily angered, intimidating, pig-headed.

LETTER S. *(For a list of famous* **"S"** *names, see* **Appendix 5.***)*

Respectable, practical; money and success oriented, providing for future needs; steady, solid, resilient; social activist; social visionary; closet sensualist or kinky-sex.

"S" *is the American Dream* - being immersed in traditional society, paying taxes, not 'making waves,' 'playing the game,' following tradition, living up to Mom and Dad's expectations, toeing the accepted line - expecting to succeed (make money, buy a house, marry and rear a brood, put down securities, enjoy a contented old age)!! At this moment in history, the previously solid social-ground has become a quickly disappearing mirage. Some socially minded and concerned **"S's"** who have woken up to the superficial and vapid nature of the old paradigm are pouring money into the world's crumbling facade. Billionaire American financier **George Soros** (in 1996 alone), gave away $360 million to ten European countries for social projects; he now intends pouring $5 billion into American areas where he feels change is needed....or you have the localized compassionate activism of **Bernard Glassman,** Zen monk, social entrepreneur and founder of the successful Yonkers Greystone Bakery, plus other inner city projects for AIDS and the homeless. Glassman and his New York Zen community are fully immersed in the problems of 20th Century urban life. Although **"S"** links to conventional society and success, it also polarizes to anti-money and anti-mainstream society ambitions and life styles. Early in the Century (1875-1965) you had **Albert Schweitzer**, brilliant musician, humanitarian and medical missionary who turned his back on the world and created his own idealized community in the jungles of East Africa. Those who want to maintain or patch-up the old life styles are usually at odds with those who want to change them radically or have a destructive elitist view, like the supremacist **"Skin Heads."** Notable amongst those **"S's"** who influence, entertain, palliate and sometimes re-educate the community mind-set is **Steven Spielberg**, prolific director, screen writer and sometime co-producer of films, - remembered from the 70's: *Jaws* and *Close Encounters of the Third Kind;* from the 80's: *Indiana Jones* movies; *E.T. The Extra-Terrestrial; Temple of the Sun, The Color Purple* and the 90's: *Hook; Jurassic Park, Schindler's List, Amistad...*to mention only a few! For most **"S's,"** a life commitment to social involvement cannot embrace the vast philanthropy of a **Soros**, the spiritual vision of a **Schweitzer**, a **Glassman**, or the inadvertent (or intentional) mind-manipulation of media moguls like **Spielberg**--it may be smaller, yet still important - an old friend of mine **James South**, a nutritionist, designs special herbal and vitamin formulas for the health and welfare of humanity. Whenever **"S"** begins or is **in** a name, there are money issues and challenges of basic survival, when these come into balance, you have the foundation for **"S's"** *real* purpose--the betterment of society. Your personal part in that will depend on the letters following or surrounding your **"S"**...look up their meanings and find your place in the world. *On the personal, practical level,* **"S"** *challenges you to represent, or to bring, credibility; to support yourself successfully, be recognized by others for what you really enjoy doing....and finally, there's this sensuality issue! No matter how conventional an* **"S"** *person appears on the surface, there usually lurks a unique set of underlying sensual needs below the facade of respectability; when* **"S"** *doubles or the name contains a multiple of* **"S's,"** *the tendency is magnified.*

Balanced "S:" being in the system, yet transforming the system; ability to move comfortably and non-judgmentally on all levels of society; business and money savvy; will always find something they love to do for a living--and then do it! Reminiscent of **Malcolm S. Forbes**, unabashed capitalist and founder of *Forbes* magazine, who was truly contented with his millions--he enjoyed lavishing them on himself and others and lacked the paranoia and guilt that's usually associated with great riches.

Unbalanced "S:" the puritanical, "What will others think?" versus *"To hell what others think!!"* - beating or breaking the system; social climbers; paranoidal anti-social terrorists; money issues; irrational needs for respectability, success and money; business guile; rough-shodding over people for personal gain; scam artists, the **"S"** con-men/women. Kinky sensuality may turn into ecstatic masochism or sado-masochism especially when combined with letter **"D"** - the late **Jean-Bedel Bokassa**, ex-self-proclaimed Emperor of Bangui in the 70's, considered one of Africa's most bizarre and brutal despots and **Saddam Hussein** (three **"S's"** and two **"D's"**) with his reputation for ruthless, cold and calculated cruelty.

When "S" is in YOUR NAME: *it's how you will interact with money, success, society.*

SUMMARY: The conformist, or the social rebel; money, success or money struggles; fear of success, distrust of money; acknowledged or latent sensuality, prudery.

LETTER T. *(For a list of famous* **"T"** *names, see* **Appendix 5.***)*

Idealistic, perceptive, empathetic, intuitive, psychic, mystical, religious; sensitive, nervously stressed. "T" represents the mystical part of the human bio-system that links into higher out-of-body energy centers. Some **"T's"** examine consciousness by pushing beyond normal boundaries within the nervous system, they expand awareness with breathing, energy and movement techniques; others rely on psychedelic substances like Harvard psychologist **Timothy Leary** whose 60's research involved psilocybin and LSD; and ethno-botanist **Terrence McKenna** (hallucinogenic mushroom researcher) who has been more motivated by the mystical and spiritual aspects of the expanded mind. *Letters* **"T"** *and* **"B,"** *share a similitude:* **"B"** *governs the outer five senses of sight, touch, taste, hearing and smell, by which we connect to outer reality;* **"T"** *expands these physical probes into the 68 psychic senses of mystical and interdimensional awareness.* Our material-based Western culture tends to put down and ridicule all those with developed psychic senses (the "Sensitives"), particularly children, who usually shut off their abilities--or suffer the secret fear that there must be something terribly wrong with them. *The intuition aspect of letter* **"T"** *doesn't only apply to the mystical and psychic.* I once knew an electrician in a large industrial Plant who loved to fix problems that stumped the other electricians - he could align his mind with the machines and always knew exactly where to find the breakdowns. His middle name Milton, contained the **"T"** (middle names often carry our more hidden talents). In the cut-throat commercial world, **"T"** in a name can give an edge, an uncanny instinct--the hunch that always pays off. Computer genius **Bill Gates** (with a **"T"** Focus in his "work" name), pictured the super Information Highway (Internet) and is now one of the richest men alive. **Donald Trump**, brilliant real estate entrepreneur who maintains his wealth in spite of financial challenges - says it's not the money that brings him personal fulfillment--it's the "Art of the Deal;" another enormously wealthy **"T"** person was billionaire **Jean Paul Getty** (with **"T"** doubled), who turned an inherited oil business into a giant financial empire. In the Arts, **"T"** functions as the envisioned dream that must be made practical--**Michael Flatley** creator and star of *Lord of the Dance* (with a **"T"** Focus letter), kept a precise mental picture of all the show's dance routines --long before he was able to recreate them on stage.

<u>Balanced "T:"</u> an empathy with nature; relates, interacts, unites and communicates with people and other life forms--even inanimate; bridges dimensions with awareness and understanding (like **Tom Brown Jr.,** renowned Tracker, Scout and author who teaches self-discovery through nature); chooses personal fulfillment instead of a high-stress life-style - **Dirk Douthitt,** (with three **"T's"**) gave up Silicon Valley computer engineering for the peaceful country life of breeding rare and exotic pheasants.

<u>Unbalanced "T:"</u> also high in empathy--they feel the emotional, mental states of others, receive psychic impressions, even interdimensional input--*but entirely without awareness*--causing nervous overload, confusion and eventual "shut-down." Some get easily distracted, thinking they've done something (turned off the stove or disconnected a switch, or paid a bill), but 'taint so!!--*must learn to focus on details and pay attention to their intuition.* Escapist dreamers fill themselves with irrational, impractical schemes, or blurr the lines between inner and outer reality (*always be in control of the vehicle!).* The overzealous mystic **"T's"** end up as religious fanatics or recluses, while the other extreme breeds psychic or religious skeptics and intolerant persecutors (often just a mask to hide their fear). Some deliberately exacerbate their over-sensitive nerves with drugs and drink like **Tanya Tucker**, country singer and tough "Wild Child." Underneath, they're often romantic, idealistic and unpractical--yearning for perfection in an imperfect world. Ex-heavyweight boxing champion **Mike Tyson** chewed a chunk out of an opponent's ear in the ring; his suppressed sensitivity hits the **"S"** Focus letter in his last name (he inflicts pain through boxing for prestige and money), on this occasion he flipped into **"S's"** aspect of cruelty and sadism! Filmaker, writer, actor **Quentin Tarantino** (three **"T's"**), sensitizes only the bizarre and macabre in his work, polarizing *away* from the mystical and spiritual.[12]

When "T" is in YOUR NAME: it's how you expand your inner awareness and respond to external input.

<u>SUMMARY:</u> impractical dreamer or hard-nosed hunch-follower; sensitive, romantic, intuitive; mystical; master of illusion or prone to deception; psychic or skeptical.

---

[12] See letter "T" on page 186, Chapter 21 "The Sacred Symbols."

LETTER U. *(For a list of famous* "U" *names, see* **Appendix 5.***)*

Generosity; giving and receiving; extravagance or stinginess; courageous expansion into life or pulling back (*at times, retreat can also be valid*). The "U" energy pulses with the ebb and flow of life - venturing forth, returning within, giving out and receiving back. It mirrors the balance of beginnings and endings. But what we receive inexorably reflects what first was given out--the old idea of reaping what we sow. With "U" in the name, this lesson is of prime importance. As Spirits (clothed in flesh), we are *supposed* to attract and receive all that we need and want to fully relish life and turn it into an adventure--and live harmlessly with the rest of creation. *The lack of this balance now pollutes the planet, depletes its natural resources, destroys flora and fauna and keeps us warring within our own species.* Letter **"U"** brings lessons in expansions and contractions, generosity and receiving. Note real estate mogul **Donald Trump**, (builder of skyscraper Trump Towers in New York city plus various glittering hotels and casinos around the country); he regards his business manipulations as a "game" while expanding and contracting his holdings (seemingly) without fear in the mega-buck world of high finance. (Trump also boasts a million dollar--expanded ego!!) *Christian scriptures state a puzzling Law of Abundance: "For he that hath, to him shall be given: and he that hath not, from him shall be taken even that which he hath."*[13] *Now does that sound fair?? Actually, it has nothing to do with fairness but everything to do with mental vibration. Put simply, if you are positive in your attitude to money, see the Universe as essentially abundant, give to yourself and others, you will develop an "abundance consciousness" and will always attract everything that you need--and more. If, however, your train of thought remains resentful about money and opportunities, this negative and doubting nature will keep you in a state of lack and despair. Habitual thoughts breed their equivalent situations, therefor change your thoughts!* Another vainglorious and brilliantly talented self-made man was artist, naturalist, ornithologist and writer **John James Audubon** (1785-1851), with two **"U's"** in his name, who expanded his love of birds into a massive book of stunning paintings and detailed notes.[14] Those who support *aggressive* expansion are the munitions makers and suppliers, a famous one was munitions genius **Dr. Gerald Bull** (with **"U"** in his "work" name), who designed a never-to-be-completed Super Gun called the Intercontinental Cannon. The lucrative pursuit of destruction focuses in Brussels, capital of Belgium and the European center for the world arms business (including illegal and smuggled arms).

Balanced "U:" the unconditional, generous humanitarian; follows the inner promptings of higher Spirit when relating to others, the world at large and the unfolding events surrounding them; becomes the channel for infinite abundance and generosity; helps others expand and open to life; a champion of the environment, like oceanographer **Jacques Yves Cousteau** (with three **"U's"** in his name), who dedicated his life to undersea exploration and drawing attention to the endangered state of the world's oceans.

Unbalanced "U:" conditional giving; creating obligations and debts by "buying" and controlling others through false generosity. *"I have done this for you - therefor you owe me that!" Not* giving for fear of scarcity; *not* receiving for fear of becoming indebted...or out of unworthiness--it's sometimes difficult to let yourself receive anything (from a compliment to a favor). Some **"U's"** deliberately withhold benefits, blame others for their own misfortunes and won't accept responsibility for attracting life-challenging events. *(Take responsibility, learn the lessons and the circumstances will change.)* **Despotic "U's"** remove the basic human rights of others--even their right to live! Consider the twisted life of serial murderer **Andrew Cunanan**, who in his 1997 rampage, brutally dispatched a stranger, ex-lovers and world famous Italian fashion designer Gianni Versache. And one always has to watch governments for suppression, as in the **"Huston"** Plan, suggested in 1970 by the Nixon administration, which would have enormously increased domestic spying, through opening private mail, burglarizing homes etc.

When "U" is in YOUR NAME: it's how generous you are to yourself; how you allow yourself to fearlessly expand and experience life - how you give and receive from others; how you encourage *their* expansion and exploration.

SUMMARY: generous or self-serving; indulgent; positive or destructive expansion.

---

[13] St. Mark 4.25. The Holy Bible, Authorized King James version.

[14] "The Birds of America" by John James Audubon, also "Viviparous Quadrupeds of North America" (mammals).

LETTER V. *(For a list of famous* **"V"** *names, see* **Appendix** *5.)*

Idealistic, world and social visionary; hopeful; community minded; breaking with tradition and convention; pessimistic. An externally directed personality, more concerned with group and community fulfillment than personal ambition; co-operates with others to benefit the many--they simply want a better world! Some envision national goals and carry world-wide interests or affiliations; some serve as leaders or organizers. *This name analysis system is not based on conventional numerology--although my discoveries relating to that science appear in Appendix 1 & 2. However,* **"V,"** *the 22nd letter of the alphabet, ranks as a Master Number in the "old science" and a comment must be made! Master numbers are not supposed to be added together (2+2=4), but I have always found that to be in error:* The highly visionary nature of **"V"** *and* 22, tends to remain in wishful thinking pipe dreams, unless brought down to earth and made practical. Two plus two *should* equal four--then the two arms of the **"V"** meet in a focusing point--four is the foundation number of practicality. In other words, *you get to make your 22-vision real!* I have met many **"V"** people who waste opportunities to positively impact the lives of others. Even those who *do* dedicate themselves to service, at times, the outcome may not always fit the intention: **Jeannie Van Velkinburg**, professional nursing assistant (note the two **"V's"** and four serving **"N's"**) was shot and paralyzed from the waist down while trying to help a hate-crime victim, yet her cheerful courage and loving attitude continue to inspire others. **"V's" don't always** receive a world-vision for making a difference, but develop a personal one that still impacts their immediate community; like **David Van Dorien** of Washington State (two **"V's"**); when over 80, he still rose daily at 4 a.m. to put in 8 hours of work shoveling live oysters at an oyster packing plant. His health, energy and purposeful living inspired the much younger men working around him. And versatile, cross-over black actor **Ving (Irving) Rhames**, brings a fresh, far-reaching vision to racial (not only black) issues. Other examples of social visionaries: **David Smith**, founded the Haight Ashbury Free Clinic in 1967; **Ellen Bravo**, 60's anti-war activist, organized a group called 9-to-5 to protect employee rights of women office workers. Quite a percentage of **"V's"** discount their dreams--they decide fulfilling them would be too difficult or impossible and rather than daring to put themselves "out there" with what their hearts demand, they settle for something more 'realistic' and practical. Some who do persist (and their vision demands country-wide, or world-wide coverage) become "the travelers," promoting their message with much of their time spent in transit. Some **"V's"** tout a perfectionist mentality, especially if their names contain **"N's"** and they're into the critical discernment aspect rather than service, then nothing is quite good enough--even their own efforts! **"V's"** can be super conservative, and look askance at all unconventionality while harboring a fascination for wild, showy and away-from-the-norm individuals. To others they say, "Heavens! Take a look...aren't they scary?! I'd never dare *look* like that, *speak* like that, or **do** anything like that!" Yet, another part of them *longs to!* While some **"V's"** openly embrace the odd and off-beat, others will *appear* conventional, yet have hidden quirks they display (with great delight) to the unwary!

Balanced "V:" an open being who brings fresh vision to potentials within the human race and society; who actively inspires others to change themselves in positive ways, and presents a socially encompassing picture of the future race.

Unbalanced "V:" those with myopic vision serving an isolationist view of society; like **Chevie Kehoe** in Little Rock, Ark. (with one **"V"**), who conspired with other white supremacists to overthrow the government and through polygamy, build an elitist republic; and **Joseph Visarionovitch Djugashvili (Stalin)** of the former Soviet Union (with three **"V's"**) who dictated the ruthless regime that changed the Imperial based society in Russia to a communist controlled regime. **Weaker "V's:"** socially distant, withdrawn, detached, fatalistic, cynical about society, locked into a private world; often have a vision, but fail or refuse to implement it; others are meddlesome, or critically observe certain local or world tendencies, but retreat into hopeless or angry pessimism.

When "V" is in YOUR NAME: - it's how you envision the perfect local or world society and how you place yourself in an active role to assist or bring about change.

SUMMARY: traditional, socially minded; untraditional, breakers of convention.

LETTER W. *(For a list of famous* **"W"** *names, see* **Appendix 5.***)*

Proud, flamboyant, sunny, warm, hearty, generous, Royal, motivating; boastful; control-freaks. **"W's"** feel compelled to promote the things that excite them, their high powered enthusiasm just *has* to be shared and the often showy ego masks a much more vulnerable and private side that they don't readily reveal. You'll find puzzled acquaintances, who, try as they might, just can't get close to the popular **"W"** life-of-the-party (or the office); when too insistent, they receive the inevitable cold shoulder....."Thanks, but no-thanks! See you around with the rest of the crowd." It's not that **"W's"** don't have any close friends, they do, but not as many as you might think--too few can be trusted to see a **"W"** up close and personal--sans all the public bravura! So yes, some **"W's"** love to come out and roar impressively to the world, but don't disturb them when they retreat into their dens, underneath, they're very self protective. Domestic guru and reputed control-freak **Martha** Ste<u>w</u>art (with a **"W"** Focus Letter), carefully protects her mystique. **Howard Stern**, the outrageous and infamous talk show host whose book "Private Parts" was made into a fan-popular film, has letters **"W"** and **"A"** forming a doubled Focus in Ho<u>wa</u>rd (his personality name); he's an egotistical braggart in public, but privately, he's more shy, insecure and sweet! Most people equate his attention getting flamboyance (**"W"**) with his actual identity (**"A"**)....but it would all appear to be part of a calculated front....and the real **Howard Stern** hides behind the facade! Again, when **"W"** is the Focus letter it may draw a person totally *into* themselves, as with an Australian Buddhist nun (formerly **Janie Stewart**), who began by wearing the glamorous and successful mask of an actress-producer in films, plays and TV then renounced it all to become a serene recluse, "free of ego concerns and the need to impress" - the polarity within the **"W.!!"** In the world, the astute **"W's"** penetrate the "masks" of others--while keeping their own intact!

<u>**Balanced "W's:"**</u> *People with heart who delight in encouraging others to find their place in life.* A famous **"W"** motivator often asks this question: "How much do you love what you're doing? - If you don't really love it, find something you can put your heart into." These **"W's"** are known for their unconditional warmth and generosity, they want to bring the best out in others and do it in respectful and non-invasive ways; they're modest and unassuming, yet confident and proud of their own achievements and see themselves as role models to encourage and inspire others.

<u>**Unbalanced "W's:"**</u> extremely competitive; always want to impress people with the right appearance, the right word; might go as far as pretending to be an authority on all subjects, embellishing the truth, exaggerating for personal attention or gain--or are downright congenital liars! Although egotistical and very self-absorbed on the surface, underneath it all--doubts gnaw at their innards. In order to push the self-doubt away, they constantly crave attention, praise and reassurance - to them, flattery becomes a food! <u>**Strong and controlling "W's"**</u> may display a calculated charisma drawing attention to themselves through their commanding appearance and scintillating manner; this makes *them* feel important (and possibly more real). Others (with charm, talent and knowledge), set themselves up as some kind of unique leader and spend their days inviting *or demanding* that the world 'play them court;' some of this ilk, carefully foster a dependent group following, thus ensuring a constant supply of ego-food in the form of captive admirers! **Werner Erhard** (Jack Rosenberg) the controversial founder of "est" comes off as a strong and controlling **"W"** - backed by the mentally dominating **"R's"** in his original name of <u>R</u>osenbe<u>r</u>g. <u>**Weaker "W's:"**</u> habitually discouraged and discouraging; tendency towards fear and paranoia; live in a torment of insecurity and self-recrimination (vacillating between attracting or running from attention) and frequently 'catch' themselves - *"Oh, darn, I've done it again! I only said that (or did that), to draw attention to myself! - why would a total stranger care what I said or did ?!!"* Most **"W's"** *want* to be admired, but the weak and fearful have attracted **"W's"** in their names to enable them to *develop* ego-strength, pride and courage in themselves. Also, when the **"W's"** childhood has been a constant put-down, they can't endure witnessing *other* people's loss of face through embarrassing situations--a reaction stemming from their own (unhealed) dis-empowerment.

When "W" is in YOUR NAME: *it's how you attract or discourage notice to yourself and how you empower, or control others.*

<u>**SUMMARY:-**</u> **public/ego: charismatic, inspirational, irrepressible, enthusiastic; controlling, overconfident, bombastic, officious, paranoid; lessons in pride and humility.**

LETTER X. *(For a list of famous* **"X"** *names, see* **Appendix 5.***)*

Intense, clever, highly focused, efficient, methodical or mentally scattered. "X" presents the focus point between extremes--between physical and mental polarities, such as psychic sensitivity and the mundane world, intensity and passion versus practical tasks. When spoken, the extremely mental **"X"** contains an **"S"** *sound* forcing it to get down to earth about money and self-support issues, or embrace a need for public acceptance, respect and social charisma--sometimes at any price (the downfall of ex-president **Richard Nixon**)!! The energy also polarizes (in some) to *denigrating* social values...*did Nixon also do that with Watergate?* As well, the underlying sexual issues inherent in **"S"** will surface in the **"X"** person. **"X's"** often remain stuck in compulsive mental patterns--mainly because of overwhelming input from the psychic as well as the ordinary senses. In a way, it's similar to **"T's"** nervous sensibility, the difference being, that **"X" has the power** to fully focus and understand from a multi-level mental input; and the more mystically inclined know how to bridge dimensions through expanded mental states. While **"T"** shows us the breadth of human consciousness--its range, **"X"** seeks to *understand* and even interpret that range. They should be our "way-showers;" their **ex**tra intelligence and supernormal sensing could solve the mystery of consciousness itself--but too many remain overly intense and scattered. Eminent British novelist and psychedelic experimenter **Aldous Huxley** investigated expanded mental states, describing his interest in the occult and his experiences with mescaline in three books;[15] these generated discussion on the relationship between drugs and mysticism and later fueled the early drug culture of the 60's and 70's. Huxley also experienced LSD and realized it would not bring liberation and understanding to everyone, he wrote of its dangers in his last book "Island." Whereas traditional shamans journey between dimensions with the aid of powerful hallucinogens, **"X's"** are the *natural* shamans; their sensibilities when focused and developed need no outside stimulants, they're often visionaries and see-ers of future events like (my daughter **Dixie**) and famous sensitive **Jeane Dixon**[16] who predicted president Kennedy's assassination. *How you express the complex power of* **"X"** *depends on its surrounding letters, which it will bring into intense focus, along with the rest of the letters in the name --**this can be both positive and negative.***

<u>**Balanced "X:"**</u> rare and complex individuals; highly perceptive with great clarity, brilliance and depth of spiritual insight; masters of their multi-level nervous systems; *bringing us intimations of the fully integrated superconscious being;* serving society and others with their gifts and abilities; skilled and sensitive to both inner and outer realms; forming a point of passage between dimensions; communicates constructively with nature Devas, discarnate entities, guides and angelic forces; can seemingly handle a multitude of activities simultaneously--yet remain focused and stable; mentally, physically and emotionally disciplined; the gift of stabilizing (mentally-scattered) people and situations; transforms through the power of the will; aware of all the options in worldly affairs and business - with the power to bring them into focus. *There are not be many of these beings around!!*

<u>**Unbalanced "X:"**</u> often suffer from misplaced or underrated brilliance; unable to make decisions easily; confused and unfocused; weak-willed; thinks compulsively in circles (or remains stuck in habitual or defeated thoughts); prone to intense depression; constantly fluctuating in up-and-down moods; over stimulates the mind causing frequent nervous collapse and exhaustion; will spread themselves thinly with too many interests; a *need to be selective or* becomes overwhelmed by certain tasks; retreats from obligations, prefers to live in an unpractical personal world; disorganized or the opposite--*excessively* thorough, *too* meticulous and driven; tricky and deceptive to attain own ends; needs stimulation most of the time or gets depressed; unstable and unsettling for other people; intense often tactless curiosity.

When "X" is in YOUR NAME: how you focus your personal energies without being scattered and how you interact with and balance outer distractions and interruptions.

<u>**SUMMARY:**</u> **hypersensitive, hyperactive, compulsive, undisciplined; befuddled, over-extended or focused; intelligent; deceiving, tricky; visionary, psychic, prophetic.**

---

15 "The Devils of Loudon," (1952), "The Doors of Perception" and "Heaven and Hell," written in 1954 and 1956.

16 Books on Jeane Dixon:"The Gift of Prophesy," Ruth Montgomery; "Jeane Dixon:The Wittnesses," Denis Brain.

LETTER Y. *(For a list of famous* **"Y"** *names, see* **Appendix 5.***)*

Unique, charismatic, grandiose; a natural leader, self-contained or offensively self-important; must be in charge to do it *their* way..or needs to *develop* "Y" qualities.

Practical visionaries--relentless, persistent, accepting no boundaries or limitations and often known for outspoken candor, **"Y's"** exude a passionate commitment. In their strength, they emerge with a "Grand Vision" and swiftly proceed to organize and complete it! In their weakness, they're dominating and reluctant to delegate authority demanding everything be done *their* way. Without a doubt, their ideas and methods often *are* the best and they do **not** work happily under direction--especially if **"Y"** begins or is exactly in the middle of their name. (Bosses will get the best out of their **"Y"** workers if they give them lots of slack--or put them in charge of special projects.) Unless evolved, **"Y's"** should learn to give the *appearance* of co-operation--or at least to *consider* a different point of view if they want to make friends instead of enemies! They're known for embracing causes and spending large amounts of time trying to convert others to their beliefs. Confrontational tactics and stand-offs mar many a passionate **"Y"** -- "Making people angry to make them think" was said by "homeless" activist **Mitch Snyder** (a **"Y"** Focus in his name). Those who lead by personal example, may bark orders like a taskmaster but still earn devotion and respect. In 73 A.D. revered **Eleazer Ben-Yair** led a party of Zealots (including women and children) who held out against the Roman Empire in the mountain fortress of Masada, choosing mass suicide rather than surrender. These strong **"Y's"** exude charisma and with their powerful organizing abilities (and often considerable talents) collect hordes of adoring followers to assist them with their projects. In 1963 archaeologist (and General) **Yigael Yadin** discovered the legendary Masada site in Israel; he then directed and inspired a large party of excavators for two difficult years at this inhospitable site. Today, there's **Yanni** (born **Yanni** Hrysomallis in Greece): brilliant creator of inspiring music for the masses; a musical prodigy with perfect pitch and his own method of notation who only hires the best musicians in the world to perform with him and engages thousands (even governments) to help prepare his lavish productions. His first on the "grand scale" was staged in Greece's famed Acropolis, the second after extensive planning and involving millions of dollars, occurred at India's Taj Mahal *and* China's Forbidden City. **Yanni's** own words entreat tolerance and brotherly love; his music uplifts the listener regardless of nationality. *The letter's formal sound "Wi-ee" asks the question "Why?" The lives of some* **"Y"** *bearers are characterized by questions--asked and answered for everyone...even if the answers bring despair and resignation.* Eleventh Century Persian poet and mathematician **Omah Khayyam** (although instrumental in reforming the Islamic calendar) shines brightly down the ages for his exquisite "Rubaiyat" - verses extolling the joys of wine and women, the insecurity of faith and the surety of death and decay.

Balanced "Y's:" know they have a special quest or questions to be answered and feel it their duty to find and share their discoveries to benefit others. **Jacques-Yves Cousteau** made his questing ground the oceans. Pioneering undersea exploration and research through his co-discovery of the Aqua-lung; he then became our conscience for polluting the earth's life-blood. **"Y's"** radiate a "presence" with a sense of tremendous force behind every word and action. Their will is essentially constructive, and personal needs are blended into whatever is appropriate for the moment. Grasping or self-denial do not exist for them. Moving with assurance in alignment with a greater universe, they know exactly what they want.

Unbalanced "Y:" difficulty in co-operating with others, often deliberately disruptive in order to keep control of a situation; a fear of failure and a compulsion to win (only enjoy playing games so long as they are winning); selfish, willful, insensitive; a contrary uniqueness alienates them from others; they don't care what they say or do--it's the only way they know to be themselves. Controversial and startling interactive artist **James Lee Byers** was quoted as saying "As soon as I open my mouth, I find myself in a state of alienation."[17]

When "Y" is in YOUR NAME: you stand accountable for the burning questions in your life - have you pursued them, and have you benefited others as well as your self?

SUMMARY: the Grand World Vision; questioning, visioning; original; headstrong; charismatic, inspiring, persevering, or alienating others with stubborn willfulness.

---

[17] TIME, June 9th, 1997.

LETTER Z. *(For a list of famous "Z" names, see* **Appendix 5.***)*

An instrument of Fate; fatalistic; marked by Destiny; sensual; fame and money issues.

"Z" sees the need for change--and tries to implement it. Mexican revolutionary **Emiliano Zapata** (1877-1919) led a revolt for agrarian reform--and here at Century's end, now inspires modern day Mexican **Zapatistas**, who struggle for the same reasons; whereas **Fang Lizhi** ("Z" Focus letter), China's well known dissident intellectual (given asylum in the U.S.) can only act by urging *other* governments to apply pressure on China. The "Z" energy brings things to a "head" through incidents occurring in the life, which (on the surface) appear to be random and almost out of one's control--yet a compelling pull inexorably moves us into them--and from that moment, life changes forever. Sometimes it's just a matter of being in the right place at the right time - or the wrong place! From a crowd-lined street in Dallas, Texas, Nov.22nd,1963, **Abraham Zapruder** filmed the fateful shooting of President Kennedy and with 15 seconds of movie, captured the crime of the century. That morning he had felt "compelled" to take his camera to film the motorcade, and as though some force in the universe demanded a record, fate placed him in the exact place at the precise time to present visual evidence of a possible second assassin[18] thus linking his action forever in history - and with the last few living breaths of President Kennedy. It may just be *one* fateful decision, *one* spur of the moment event that implodes the life, or begining more subtly, it sits in the consciousness like a nagging compulsion--until you actually DO something! In one such case, a "Z" man felt driven (because he'd reached the fateful age of 40), to make a drastic change; after months of dithering, and then planning, he finally went back to college--but in a foreign land. He took his family with him. Their lives were never the same again....partly because the discontented wife (under the "Z" name), found herself inwardly compelled to leave the marriage, but unable, until a fateful event gave her the courage to do so! You could describe the energy as a "door" - a door of opportunity, or a door closing in your face. For some **"Z's,"** only one fateful door opens in their entire lifetime, for others, many doors appear--seemingly miraculously and with the closing of one, another will open immediately--apparently from nowhere! You could also say "Z" is an **"S"** *with sound added*--bringing the **"S"** qualities of success, money, public prestige, along with sex and sensuality; but **"Z"** usually takes the sensuality out of the closet making it concrete and open--or in the other extreme--more desperately hidden! And when the **"Z"** softens and sounds more *like* an **"S,"** you have an intensification of sexual desires--as with 19th Century's flamboyant and sensual pianist-composer **Franz Liszt**, not only lauded for his pianoforte virtuosity (which sent men and woman into ecstasy), but well known for his prolific Don Juan appetites! Then long before the TV era, opportunist and impresario **Florenz Ziegfield** (two **"Z's"**) opened new doors in entertainment and for the first time on this continent, brought extravagant musicals filled with briefly-costumed, glamorous show girls - the sensational Ziegfield Follies. **Ziegfield** too was a famous womanizer and addicted to the high life with a compulsive passion for gambling--he more than tempted fate - and on a daily basis!!

Balanced "Z": the ability to flow with the changes; seeing the power of life as the power TO change; moving into new experiences quickly and without regrets; lusty and fearless; enjoying the adventure of being fully alive; aligning with nature, perceiving the oneness in all beings without judgment; initiating positive changes for themselves and others. **"Z"** says: It's time to change - to take the next step in human physical and spiritual evolution! **Question:** *are those nations whose peoples possess frequent* **"Z's"** *in their names, more fatalistic in temperament - more aligned with the natural flow of life??*

Unbalanced: violently polarized personality extremes (even schizophrenic and manic depressive); and (as in the case of **Franz Liszt**), creating part saint, part passionate sensualist; resignation and acceptance of doom, gloom, corruption and decay; a feeling of being pulled into a downward spiral that can't be stopped or changed; hopelessness and brooding, at the mercy of circumstances. The dark to despairing sexual, sado-masochistic side of **"Z"** expresses in the purely nightmarish, pain wracked music and lyrics of "shock rocker" **Trent Reznor**, lead singer, composer and creator of Nine Inch Nails.

When "Z" is in YOUR NAME: it's how you flow with opportunity and change; whether you feel helpless in the grip of Fate, or the orchestrator of your own joyous destiny.

SUMMARY: a life open to sudden changes - or resisting opportunity and change.

---

18 See page 794-5 "The People's Almanac #2" by David Wallechinsky and Irving Wallace. Bantam 1978.

Here's a wild thought for the karma-inclined! Your DNA cell patterning might result from your incarnating soul/Spirit and past-life subselves, collaborating to create a pre-programmed physical vehicle in the womb, embodying old problems and unfinished businesses. They could also predispose the uterus to certain histamine reactions (allergies), diseases and other anomalies linked to emotional and mental triggers from past-life events!

It would appear, that certain deliberate tones and sounds can shake loose these old patterns, particularly the letter sounds from your own name.....but not *only* those letters. Some letters augment or overlap each other in meaning; for example: "**A**," "**R**," "**H**" and "**Y**," which address different phases of personal power. Say for instance, your name contains only one, *or even none* of those letters--you could still sound *all* of them to enhance your own physical/mental, visionary strength and willpower. When people alter their names, they intuitively set out to improve their given sound pattern. So if you wish to change or enhance your life, sound the appropriate letters--even if they *aren't* in your birth certificate name, or as a final extreme....create yourself a new name!

Below follows a list of the letters of the alphabet, with ideas on why and how you might want to sound them. *For all these exercises, you can choose to speak or sing - whatever you feel like doing.* And you don't have to use the *exact* same number of syllable combinations, I'm just giving you an indication. Always sound as many or as little as you feel you want to--and if you'd rather scream, shout or let loose with total abandon (as I suggest in Chapter 4, "Releasing the Voice"), *please indulge.* It will free you! You'll notice for the most part, I only offer one or two series of sounds to cover several different problems; the key here is to focus on **your** particular need while you sing the suggested sounds. Don't be limited by my variations, feel free to add your own! And you'll gain a much better result if you incorporate the **Galactic Breath** into your efforts (refer back to Chapter 4).

Finally, the letter itself (its visual image) reflects the Sacred Form.[1]

How to combine Sound with Sight.

1) Decide which sound-combinations seems best suited to your needs.

2) Take a practice run with the sounds of your choice while viewing the instructions.

3) Now look at the letter that goes with the sounds, as though you are receiving it *into you* with your breath.

4) Then close your eyes and remain "seeing" the image in your head **as you sound it.** If you lose the image, repeat **3-4**, or "draw" the image in your head, as though on a chalkboard.

5) Finally, make the sounds while *looking* at the letter. *This is much easier.*

For the letter image: *use either the larger sized capitals given here, the even larger ones from* Chapter 7, *or the meditation sized ones from* Chapter 21.

A.... Higher Self, identity/ego, personal and physical power.

1) When you lack the courage for some endeavor;
When you're expected to lead, but deem yourself inadequate;
When you feel humiliated and powerless;
When you need to *let* yourself be powerful and important;
When you need to discharge anger and frustration.....

a) *Make the more open* "**Ah**" *sound; curl your lip and begin with the almost soundless, threatening, spitting, snarl of a large wild cat -* "**Aaaaahrr.**" *Try several of these and let your mouth stretch and your feelings of rage come into your teeth and lips. Then feel your teeth as your animal weapons and growl some final warning* "**Aaaaaaaahhrrrr's**" *deep in your throat! All this may stir up and loosen considerable*

---

[1] See Chapter 21, "The Sacred Symbols."

matter, if so, gently clear your throat, cough if necessary - swallow several times and take a few sips of cold water. Next, release any tension you may have built up in your neck and take some deep breaths, relaxing completly for a few moments.

b) *Now you're ready to sound forth your anger and frustrations with sung or shouted* **"Aaahh, rah,rah, rah,rah,rah,rah, raaaaaaaaaaaaaaah's."** *Vary the tone and the pitch according to your emotions. Feel and release the rage, then open wide and roar like a triumphant lion. These sounds will resonate the nasal septum and at times you'll seem to be singing from the corners of your eyes!*

2) When you reach a creative or activity hiatus;
When you're not projecting and expressing your identity and personal power....

Use **"A-e, aee,aee,aee,aee,aee,aee,aee,aaaaaaaaaaeeeei."** *(The* **'i'** *at the end is the 'short-sound' as in* the word **"it."**) *Do several* **"Ae<u>eei</u>, - ae<u>eei</u>, - ae<u>eei's</u>;"** *accenting the underlined letters and pushing each sound out of you with a contraction of the navel, singing them higher each time - finally, when you're ready, finish by swooping the tone down.*

3) When you want to be more in charge of your life;
When some executive or management problem arises;
When you just want to do something *your* way for a change.....

Use **"Aaay, yay,yay,yay,yay,yay, yaaaaaaaaaaaeeee,"** *or extend the* **"Ae"** *sound with* **"<u>Aaae</u>-yay, <u>aaae</u>-yay, <u>aaae</u>-yay."** *Take a breath and conract the navel with every* **"Aaae-yay."** *The* **"Aaa"** *sounds like* **"hay."**

4) To activate and strengthen the Power Chakra at the navel......

a) *Use short dissonant bursts of the same "a" sound as in* **"apple"** *or* **"at"** *- "Aa! aa! aa! aa! aa! aa!"*

b) *Then try <u>short bursts</u> of the same sound that's in* **"may"** *- "<u>Ay</u>! <u>ay</u>! <u>ay</u>! <u>ay</u>!" You can make the "Ay" quite piercing and high or low. Move the pitch around. Each time you voice one of these short sounds, push it out explosively by contracting your belly at the navel. Should you start to feel considerable heat or vibration building up in the spine (directly behind the belly-button), it's time to stop....you've built up enough energy for one session. This is also a good tummy toner, but watch out for tender muscles after the first few days of practice!*

B.... the five senses (sight, taste, hearing, touch and smell), also the psychic senses.

The challenge of a soul incarnating into solid form, i.e., our body, carries the serious danger of distraction and forgetfulness. Either due to religious manipulation or social conditioning, our senses tend to polarize us painfully between guilt and addiction! The solution lies in reconciling the five outer senses with our extended psychic/mystical senses. *(Also,* **"B"** *is one of the powerful brain-resonators and in my experience, when sounded as a resonator*[2] *has a more active vibratory effect on the front of the throat down as far as the thymus, than the soundings given below. Resonating on different tones and pitches changes and extends the vibratory effect in the body - which will vary with the particular timbre of the voice doing the resonating. I suggest you also experiment with the sounds given below.)*

1) When you're fearful or guilty about pleasure and enjoyment, particularly eating and sex;[3]
When you're afraid to expand into a new experience that might prove sensually pleasant and different, such as a massage or a Jacuzzi in the buff;
When you don't like your body and hate your appearance........

---

2 See Chapter 18, "Power Tools for the Brain."

3 For eating disorders, also use the Food Meditation and Disassociation exercise from Appendix 4.

a) *Speak or sing short bursts of* **"Buh! buh! buh! buh! buh!"** *and really push the sound out from the belly with a breath between each* **"Buh."** *Make the* **'u'** *sound as in* **"up."** *At the same time contract your perineum/yoni and allow yourself to feel a mild bliss. Finish with a long sustained* **"Baaaaaaaaaaaa aaaaaaaaaaah,"** *while you simultaneously practice the P/Y contraction.* (For information on the P/Y contraction see Chapter 17, "Energy Exercises.")

b) *Sing a rapid, continuous* **"Bub,bub,bub,bub,bub,bub,bub,"** *really feeling the relaxed sensuousness of your mouth each time you make the* **'b,'** *then do a long* **"Baaaaaaaaaaaaab"***at the end.*

c) *Then try the wonderful rolling sound of* **"Brrrrrrrrah, brrrrrrah, brrrrrrah, brrrrrraah;"** *you roll the* **"Br"** *through your lips* (instead of the usually rolled **'r'** with the tongue behind the teeth.). *To finish, clamp your teeth together and make a long sustained* **"Brrrrrrrrrrrrrrrrrrrrrrrrr."** *Your lips will rapidly vibrate--sometimes juicily--as the force of the air blows through them.....yes, it's exactly the sound you make when you're feeling suddenly chilled, or the cold is finally 'getting to you!'*

2) When you wish you could just be accepted for yourself;
When you want to express who you really are -
And do what you *really want to* with you life.....

Use **"Bee,bee,bee,bee,bee,bee,bee,bee,beeeeeeeeeeeeeeyuh"** *and claim for yourself what you want to be. Then try several* **"Beeeyuh, beeeyuh,beeeyuh,"** *singing the* **'yuh'** *part higher than the* **'beee.'**

3) When you have a throat block to singing, speaking and creative self-expression......
Work with all of the above "B" sounds.

C.... governs the passionately curious, skillful, clever parts of mind.

1) When you want to focus on mental skills, or skills for success....
Use **"See, see,see,see,see,see,see,see,seeeeeeeeeeeeeee"** *several times.*

2) When you want to study, read and learn more to power and inspire your vision...
Try **"Seee-aah, seee-aah, see-ah;"** *sometimes stressing the* **'seee'** *at other times, the* **'aah,'** *finishing up with a long powerful* **"Seeeeeeeeee-aaaaaaaaah."** *Look at letter* **"C"** *when you sound* **1)** and **2)** above.

2) When you're feeling mentally stale;
When you've lost your sense of passionate curiosity;
When the joy of discovery has vanished.......

Use **"Kuh,** *(as in* **"cup"**) **kuh, kuh, kuh,kuh,kuh,kuh,kuh,kuh,kuh,kuh, kaaaaaaaaaaaaaaaah."** *Pull your belly button in strongly with the first four or five* **'Kuh's.'** *Feel the sound explode out of the back of your throat in little bursts. Then swoop up in a series of rapid* **"kuh's"** *as you contract your perineum.*

3) When your mental self-discipline lags;
When you lack motivation;
When you've thrown away your vision of success
When you yearn to help, to be of some social use, but don't know how to begin.

Let yourself sound like an old fashioned steam train chugging with power, patience and determination up a steep grade: **"Chuh, chuh, chuh, chuh, - ch,ch,ch,ch, ch,ch,ch,ch,"-** *(then let off a burst of steam) -* **"Chhhhh chhhhhhh".** *Repeat until energized and delighted!* **"H"** *reactivates determination and vision.*

Remember to look at the letter while you're sounding it.

D.... the "Warrior Nature," authority figures and how we handle our own authority.

1) When you want to summon up your inner "Warrior;"
When you want to develop determination and strength;
When you feel intimidated by people in authority--and wish you didn't;
When you want more dignity and authority for yourself......

Speak or sing **"Deee, deee,deee,dee,dee,dee,dee,dee,dee, deeeeeeeeeeeeeeyuh;"** *also try* **"Deeeyuh, deeeyuh, deeeyuh, deeeyuh,"** *with a strong accent on the* **'dee'** *and contract against the power center (navel), as you sound.*

2) When you flaunt, or 'throw' your authority around;
When you come down too hard on others under your influence;
When you need to soften--instead of being so rigid and hidebound.......

Do the same **"Dee,dee,dee,dee,dee,"** *as above, but now cover your ears and sound it several times very softly and gently, even lovingly...a love for yourself as well as others. Then take it softly and gently up an arpeggio scale to "re-chord" the way you relate to yourself and people.*[4]

3) When you have problems with your Dad, or authority figures in general........

Slowly at first, speak **"Duh!-duh!-duh!-duh!"** *several times, with a navel contraction for each sound;* ***then*** *sing* **"Dah, dah,dah,dah,dah,dah,dah,daaaaaaaaaaahd."** *Vary the tones and their intensity while sounding the extended* **'aaaaaaaaaaaahd.'**

E.... communication, all mental processes, the fundamental Self-intelligence, the voice.

1) When you have creative blocks, with trouble releasing your gifts and abilities;
When others discourage you from expressing yourself.
When you have to speak in public, but you hate it!
When it's hard to get your words out...to even **find** the words you want to say;
When you want to communicate your ideas to others--but doubt yourself;

2) When you really want to write, but don't know how to start;
When you've hit a writer's block;
When you want to communicate something special through a creative skill.....

a) *For all of the above use* **"Eee, eeee, eeee, eeee, eeee, eeeeeeeeeeeeee;"** *then try* **"Ee-yah, ee-yah, ee-yah, ee-yah, ee-yah, eeyah,eeyah,eeyah,eeyah, eeeeeeeeyaaaaaaaaaaaaaaaah!"**
Then, **"Eey,yeey,yeey, yeey, yeeeeeeeeeeey;"** *now* ***very*** *rapidly--***"Eeyeeyeeyeeyeeyeeyeeyeey, yeeeee-eeeeeeeeeeee."** *The last extended* **'yeeee'** *always goes higher and higher -- and higher!*

b) *More slowly and deliberately, now use the same short* **"e"** *sound as in the word* **"yes"** *and make* **"Eh, eh, eh, eh, eh, eh,"** *pulling the navel in with each sound. Sound-wise this is not easy--but persevere! Finally release it explosively (yet lightly) with short bursts of breath while you rapidly contract your diaphragm. Finish with a long drawn out, almost silent* **"eeeehhh,"** *the same sound as in* **"air."**

3) **When you suddenly realize that you talk too much and need to listen more.....**

Do the same **"air"** *sound as above, but this time close your eyes--cover your ears and make several long extended sounds; tuning in to your higher Wisdom-Mind. Mentally ask to be reminded - not to jabber away incessently, but to "Listen, listen, listen," before you 'shoot' your mouth!*

---

[4] Read letter "K" in this Chapter for information on arpeggios and personal Chords.

F.... brings issues with pride, achievement and public self-worth.

1) When you feel like you're a failure with nothing to be proud of in your life;
When you need to encourage yourself to be the best that you can be.......

a) *Slowly speak* **"Eff, eff, eff, eff,"** *gradually making the* **'e'** *a longer sound (the same sound as in* **"air"** *but with a strongly formed* **"ff"** *at the end of it) --and at the same time, contract the navel while saying each syllable. Be certain to stress the soundless* **'ff'** *at the end of each syllable.* **This is NOT an easy exercise to practice--but then, having pride in oneself isn't always easy either!** *After developing some strength of tone with just speaking the* **'eff,"** *now try to sound it. Begin with a comfortable low note and sound it through an arpeggio.*[5] *When sung, the "e" of course, seems to be all you can hear next to the silent "f." The nature of the "e" however, enables the "f" energy to be released and expressed.*

b) *Now follow with a more rapid* **"Ef,fef,fef,fef,fef,fef,fef,fef"** *for as long as necessary.*

c) *Then sound an extended* **'ef,'** *(it's the same* **'eh'** *sound as in* **"air"** ***-- but with an 'f' on the end).*** *Do several long ones interspersed with the shorter* **'ef'** *sounds.*

Important Note: when you speak the letter **"F"** (as if you were formally reciting the alphabet), the actual sound you make is **'ef.'** Whenever the vowel sound **"E"** *precedes* the voicing of a consonant in this way (as also in letters **"L," "M," "N," "S" and "X"**), the energy becomes introverted and forces you to understand that particular consonent's lesson *in relationship to yourself* - before you can express it outwardly in a positive and constructive manner.

G.... the proper balance of work and play.

1) When you realize you're a workaholic and need to slack off for the sake of health and balance;

2) When you need to focus on your work - to do your very best.......
For both the above, first speak the short form of **"Guh! guh! guh! guh!"** *expelling the breath with the navel contraction; try it in different spoken pitches, then* ***sing*** *the longer form of* **"Gah, gah, gah, gah, gah, gah, gah, gah, gaaaaaaaaaaah."**

3) When you need to become the child again--and play!
Here you use the **'j'** *sound of letter* **"G"** (remember from Chapter 5, how some letters share the same sounds?), *use the playful sound of* **"Jee,jee,jee,jee,jee,jee, jeeeeeeeeeeh."**

4) When you want to find a better job, or improve your present situation.......
Use the **'j'** *sound of letter* **"G"** *with* **"Jay, jay, jay, jay, jay, jaaaaaaaaaaaaaaay,"** *also,* **"Jaa-ey, jaa-ey, jaa-ey, jaaaaaaaaaaaaaaaa-ey."**

H.... the energy of ambition, future goals, self-discipline and patience.

The two sounds of letter **"H"** are unusual in that one is incredibly complex, while the other is simplicity itself. The first one is **"Huh"** (or **"Hah"**) and relates to release-through-laughter, and the physical heart; the second **"Aeech"** (or **"Aich"**), is used when just saying the letter. Interestingly, the letters comprising the *sound* of **"H"....."Aech,"** *imply the solutions to all of the difficulties that* **"H"** *names are prone to!!* **"A"** means personal strength, power and courage - **"E"** endows self expression and communication - **"C"** brings skills and know-how, plus the **"H"** sound itself, which is goals and success that comes from hard work. *Very complex - but then* **"H"** *people don't come in simple packages either!*

---

[5] See instructions for sounding an arpeggio in Chapter 12, "Training the Outer Singing Voice."

1) When you want success, money and recognition;
When you must plan and work for future goals;
When you need more will power and self-discipline;

2) When you **fear** success and public recognition, and that fear prevents you from getting on with your life's work.......

Difficult as it may be - use **"Aaeech, aaeech, aaeech, aaeech."** *Speak and sing it slowly and mindfully. Try it in arpeggio form (see* **Chapter 12**). *You can say it faster later by running it all together, then it sounds like* **"Aaechaaechaaechaaechaaech!"**

3) When you're getting far too driven, intense and compulsive;
When you're **only** money and success oriented.....

You are too involved in the ambition and achievement aspect of the **"H"** *energy and must balance by remembering to 'soften' and rediscover your heart. For this, sound lots of* **"Huh, huh, huh, huh's."** *Burst them out of you with little tummy contractions, then widen into a laughing sound* **"Hah, hah, hah, hah, hah, haaaaaaauh"** *and see if a real laugh doesn't eventually come out of you. Flow with the laughter and the feeling of the laughter.* ***Very healing!***

I.... the breath--Spirit, creative power, inspiration/performance, showing-off, manipulation, drawing attention to issues.

1) When you've lost faith in your value as a performer;
When your creative fires have burnt low - or gone out;
When you've pointed out a problem, but no one takes any notice....

Sound **"iii...yie,yie,yie,yie,yie,yiiiiiiiieeee,"** *and claim the power to do it your way!*

2) When you've lost touch with the inner voice of Spirit;
When you desperately keep drawing attention by showing off;
When you keep trying to manipulate people to get your own way

a) *Use the same sound as in* **"sigh"** *and sing* **"iiiee, iiiee, iiiee, iiiee, iiiee"** *- pause, and take a deep breath and repeat several times with a breath-pause. Begin at a low note and after each breath-pause, take the tone up another note until you are singing as high as you can with power and clarity. Direct the attention and the feeling of the sound up high inside the head; eventually feel that the sounds are ascending to the Chakras above your head.*

b) *For a more advanced, meditative way, project the sound upward using the* **Galactic Breath**[6] *and in addition, try the sound with your hands over your ears to take the mind into your core-center.*

c) *Finally, sing the* **"iiiee,iiiee,iiiee"** *quite rapidly in a continuous flowing line, then finish up with a long* **"iiiiiiiiiiiiieeeeeeeee."** *Sing as many as you want to.*

3) When you have a throat block.....

Work with the letter **"B"** *soundings as well as the ones given above for letter* **"I."**

J.... the justice and passionate-concerns energy, physical health.

1) When injustice dogs you at every turn and everything seems wrong;
When you need to start accepting and stop judging;
When you need to stir up joy instead of strife;

---

6 Read instructions in Chapter 4, "Releasing the Voice."

2) When you think you've become accident-prone;

3) When you want to get more physical, improve your health, strengthen your body and get motivated to start an exercise program;

4) When you're supposed to travel more and you know it - but you'd rather stay at home and avoid the inconvenience........

a) *For all of the above - begin with short bursts of the more closed* **"Juh, juh, juh,"** *then try several of the more open* **"jaja-jaaaah, jaja-jaaaah"** *(as in* **"car"***).*

b) *Use the more 'flattened'* **'a'** *sound (as in* **"say"***) -* **"Jaaey, jaaey, jaaey, jaaaey."**

c) *Try Sounding not one tone--but two notes on* **"jaaey;"** *then sing it more quickly,* **"jayjayjayjayjay,"** followed by **"jaaaaaaaaaaaaaaaaaaaaaaaaey."**

d) *See* Chapter 18, *"Power Tools for the Brain" and sound* **"J"** *as a resonator.*

5) When your name is *spelled* with a **"J"** but a **"Y"** is said instead - and you feel powerless, defeated and discouraged by life.......

Sound **"Yah, yah, yah, yah, - ya,ya,ya,ya, - ya,ya,ya,ya, yaaaaaaaaaaaaaah"** *opening your mouth widely and stretching your chin and facial muscles as you sing - or shout!*

K.... physical challenges, creative, sexual energy, intensity of thought and mood.

As **K** is a primary letter for the physical life force (health, stamina and resilience), you should really tune your body daily into its chord harmonics. Some esoteric sound researchers decree that we're born with a one-and-only "key" note, and you need an expert with special gadgets to tell you exactly what that note is! Yes, our bodies do arrive at birth tuned to a specific tone (which you might regard as an underlying 'drone' supporting the life energy), but unlike certain fixed musical instruments that can only be played in one key, your body-instrument is not limited to its birth-tone. It varies from hour to hour and day to day at times, depending on the variables of your experiences and thoughts. Particular trials and illnesses also have their own singular key notes comprising the chords that will release and integrate these disharmonies. If you have no musical background, refer to Chapter 12, "Training the Outer Singing Voice" for instructions on how to sing the four main harmonic notes (called an arpeggio) in a chord. *When you've read the instructions, begin with a medium to low note, and whatever you happen to sing, will be the first note of the particular chord you need to work with that day (or hour) - it could change by tomorrow (or in the next hour), or it could be exactly the same! Sing all of the* **"Kay,kay,kay's"** *followed by the long drawn out* **"kaaaaaaey"** *on the initial note, then repeat it on the next highest interval note in the arpeggio triad and so on until you are singing an octave note above the first.*

1) When your physical challenges - or illnesses, get you down;
When it's time to stir up your survival instinct........

Use **"Kay! kay! kay! kay!"** *fairly slowly and with each* **"kay"** *contract at the navel power center. Now make it more rapid (while you hold firm at the navel center),* **"Kay,kay,kay, kay,kay,kay,kay,kay, kaaaaaaaaaaaaaaaaaaey."**

2) When you need to activate your creative abilities.......

Use a rapid **"Ki, ki, ki, ki, ki,"** *(sound the* **"I"** *as in* **"it"***), while at the same time you execute a gradual perineum/yoni contraction,*[7] *at the end it should be held in very tightly and strongly while you sound a final extended* **"Keeeeeeeeeeeeeeeeeeeeeeeeee."**

---

[7] See Chapter 17, "Energy Exercises" under section 1.

(You could argue that the "I" in "ki" sounds similar to the "E" in "eeeeee" and you're partially correct; however, the "I" sound is much shorter and it's also important to *focus* on the "I" energy. Remember to visualize (**or look at**) the letter and be aware of its meaning.)

3) When you need to overcome your sexual hangups.
When you want to conceive (both parties could sing the sounds)..just kidding!!
When you need an extra burst of energy - or you want to activate the Kundalini in the Root Chakra and send the bliss energy into the cells.......

a) *The sexual life force is most strongly felt in the sound* **"Kah,"** *so for needs listed under* **3)**, *use a slow and strongly held P/Y contraction at the same time as you rapidly sound (with an ascending note),* **"Kakakakakakakakakakakakakakaaaaaaaaaa."** *This sound begins quite gutterally at the back of the throat, and you sing up the scale with each* **"ka."** *At the completion of the long note, you should be singing close to the highest note of your range, as though it's coming out of the very top of your skull--while all the time contracting the perineum/yoni.* **Relax, and repeat several times ...and be aware of the bliss.**

b) *Last, and equally powerful, this one is highly reminiscent of the Australian Kookaburra's bird call:* **"Kookookookookookookook,"** *which ends in an extended* **"Kooooooooooooo."** *You can also alternate these two sounds in a call that is quite similar to a full throated Kookaburra laughing at the rest of the world --* **"Kookookookoo,kaakaakaakaa, kookookookoo,kaakaakaakaa."** *While singing this, you make a rapid P/Y contraction (up-down),[8] for each change in the sound pattern.*

L.... the social service and expertise energy, love of people and love of self.

1) When you need to accept, like and love yourself more;
When you need self-confidence to be in a crowd, or to work in a crowded place.
When you need to accept, like and love others more.......

For all of the above - press your tongue (inside the mouth) on the hard palate--slightly above your top front teeth, while you sound **"Lllll[9]ah, llllah, llllah, llllah,"** *- (of course, lift the tongue it up for the* **'ah.'**) *You will feel a strong vibration in the back of the throat that extends down into the thymus gland and sternum bone. Expand it further into* **"Llllah, lul,lul,lul,lul,lul,lul, laaaaaaaaaaaaah."**

2) When you're organizing or integrating a large number of people--anything from a large function, a business bash, a reunion or just a dinner party.

3) When you're the "one in the middle" and everyone is looking to you for advice and counsel--this is any situation in which you're handing more than a couple of people.....

For **2** *and* **3** *- use the same sound as in* **"tell:" "Ellll, ellll, ellll, elll"** *- again, press your tongue on the hard palate to resonate the* **"L,"** *gradually speed it up with* **"El, lel,lel,lel,lel, lellellellellell,"** *finishing with an extended* **"Eeeeeeeeeeeeellll."** *(The preceeding* **"Eeeeeee..."** *sounds the same as in* **"air."**)

As already noted for letter **"F"** - if, in speaking the letter by itself, an **"e"** vowel *sound* preceeds it, (in this case you have **"el"**), the energy becomes introverted to make you understand that *particular* consonant energy before you can express it efficiently. The following letters **"M"** and **"N"** also fit into this category, as do **"S"** and **"X,"** e.g..."**eM,**" "**eN,**" "**eS,**" "**eX**".

---

[8] Instructions in section 1 of Chapter 17, "Energy Exercises."

[9] I have obviously changed the font for lower case "L" because otherwise it tends to give the appearance of a series of "I's."

M.... the home, family, mate - and bustling busily on their behalf, nurturing issues.[10]

1) When you're getting far too busy and fussy about the wrong things, or about everything.
When you've become a work-compulsive, which is even worse than a workaholic.
When you need to relax and do something nice for yourself.......

a) *For the above - refer to* Chapter 4, "Releasing the Voice" *under the section called* **Resonators** *and follow those particular sounding instructions for letter* **"M."**

b) *Also, press the teeth together on the* **"Mmmm"** *and sound a series of* **"Mmmm-mah! mmmmm-ah! mmmmm-aaah"** *quite slowly and deliberately, opening the mouth for the* **"mah,"** *followed by:* **"Mma,-ma,ma,ma,ma,ma,ma,ma,ma......maaaaaaaaaaaaaaaah."**

2) When you're yearning for the perfect mate to build the perfect nest with......
Try slowly and emphatically, **"Emmm,emmm,emmm,emmm,"** *finishing with* **"Eeeeeeeeeeeeemmmm mmmmmmmmmmmmm"** *(make the* **'eee'** *sound, as in* **"Emmy"** **or** **"air"**).

N.... critical analysis, right meaning of 'service,' the discerning mental energy that brings balance;

1) When you're sick of being the martyr and need to say "NO" to things you really don't want to do.
When you need to stop being so critical of yourself and others.......
Use **"Nah, nah,nah,nah, nahnahnahnahnah, naaaaaaaaaaaaaaah."** *Lift your lips and snarl the* **"Nah!"** *Also look at the* **"N"** *section on the* **Resonators** *towards the end of* Chapter 4, "Releasing the Voice."

2) When you're in a mental rut and need to sharpen your mind, until you get that sparkling, clear and clever feeling again......
Use the same sound as in "end" - "En, en,en,,en, eeeeeeeeeee, **eennnnnnnnnn,"** *(the long* **'eee'** *sounds like* **"air"** *and for the* **'nnnn'** *at the end, the teeth are together with the sound resonating against them).*

3) When it's time to stop compulsive 'back and forth' behaviour from one extreme to the other, and balance yourself physically, emotionally and mentally;
When something (or **everything)** in your life needs balancing.......
Sound the **"N"** *as a simple resonator with the 'intention' of bringing about balance. The tongue presses behind the top front teeth and you'll be aware of a strong drone between the ears, as well as on the nasal septum and in the skull bones on the back of the head. Make the sound continuous for as long as the breath extends,* **"Nnnnnnnnnnnnnnnnnnnnnnnnnnnnnnnn."** *Take it through a series of arpeggios to re-chord yourself.*

O.... emotions! Emotional needs, manipulations, understanding. Food and Mother.

1) When you know you carry emotional pain that needs to be felt, released, healed;
When you have unsatisfied emotional needs and ....
When you know it's time to become emotionally un-dependent;
When you want to be more self-sufficient and self-nurturing;
When you have unresolved eating disorders;
When Mother is a problem;

---

10 For food compulsions, see the Food Meditations and Disassociation exercise from Appendix 4.

2) When you have fears about the present and future (how will you support yourself, will you always have a place to live, enough to eat??--all the basic necessities).....

In addition, you need to reconnect to the Earth Mother. Practice the exercise, **Finding the Power of the Goddess** from Chapter 17, "Energy Exercises."

3) When you need to start looking at things again through the eyes of your inner child--to wonder and marvel and take delight in the simple magic of life;

4) When your heart feels like a stone and you have forgotten how to be caring, compassionate and loving.......

For all of the "O" needs use the instructions for sounding "O" in Chapter 4, "Releasing the Voice." *You should also sound* **"O"** *to your inner chord (arpeggio) and establish a firm emotional base. (See letter* **"K"** *in this Chapter.)*

Special Note: (a) when your Mother (or surrogate caretaker) is, or was a problem, read the section on "relationships" under the "Emotional Healing Meditations" at the end of Chapter 16. **(b)** when eating disorders are a problem, refer to Appendix 4.

P.... issues about inner and outer peace.

1) When you have to *hang in there* and not be fazed by a difficult situation.......

a) *Make up your mind to calm yourself! Try and be alone, sit quietly for a moment and take some deep breaths (even if the only place you can escape to is the toilet)! Now discharge by gathering the energy and pushing out strongly from the diaphragm,* **"Puh! puh! puh! puh!"** *let there be a pause between* **"Puh's."** *Do several and focus on releasing all the stored emotions in your gut and expanding yourself outward into Peace. Then do them more gently and softly--it's happening--you're opening into Peace! Finally, establish the* **Galactic Breath** *rhythm (from* Chapter 4).

b) *Softly sing* **"Peee, peee, peee, peee, peeeeeeeeeeeee"** *and feel that you're expressing Peace outwardly to others.* Try also the **Disidentifying Technique** from Chapter 17, "Energy Exercises."

c) *If you're dealing head-on with a situation and can't back out of the room, immediately be aware of your breath and reverse its usual pattern by breathing in slowly and evenly to your belly and out through the top of your head. Each time you breathe in, mentally think "Loving;" each time you breathe out, think "Breath." You will imediately calm down - and possibly the situation also. When confronting others practice the* **Figure 8 Breath** (from section 4 of Chapter 17, "Energy Exercises.").

2) When you're spending too much time alone and need to let others come into your life.......

Read the ***immediately preceding*** *instructions for Sounding* **"Puh"** *-- but now sing it more evenly, less forcefully and more quickly,* **"Puh,puh,puh,puh,puh,puh,puh,puh, paaaaaaaaaaaaaa aaaaaaaaaaah."**

3) When you feel anything but peaceful!

a) *Use* ***all*** *of the instructions given for letter* **"P,"** *but sound* **"Peee, peee,"** *more deeply from the belly much more deliberately and with lower notes.*

b) *When possible, do the following silent Galactic Breath meditation with letter* **"P."** *Rest on your bed, visualize the letter in your chest as you breathe deeply into your belly, then as you breathe out and up to the Galactic Center of our universe, mentally repeat "Breath," or "Loving breath."* **"P"***--IN,* **"Loving breath"** *OUT....over and over with the golden light from the heart of our Milky Way galaxy, pouring in through the top of your head and filling your body with radiance. I assure you --* ***you will feel peaceful!***

Q.... very unique, unusually energetic, clever, forthright and curious.

1) When you're between achievements and questing for a fresh challenge.

2) When your drive for perfection is getting out of hand and you need to slow down.....

For both of the above--return to the wonder, amazement and delight of the "small one' inside you; stop being so driven and compulsive--relax and enjoy like a child! Try **"Quooo, quooo,"** *(same sound as in* **"queue"** *-- to wait in line),* **"Quoo,quoo,quoo, quoo,quoo, quooooooooooooo."**

3) When the adventure vanished along with your enthusiasm and life feels flat and stale.......

Try **"Qwah, qwah, qwah, qwah, qwaaaaaaaaaaaah, qwah, qwah, qwah, qwah, qwaaaaaaaaaaaaaaah, qwaqwaqwaqwaqwaqwaqwaqwa--qwaaaaaaaaaaaaaaaaaah!"** *Somewhat like the sound of a duck but with the* **'ah'** *rather than the* **'ack'** *sound. Anyway, who ever saw a discouraged duck! They're always waddling or swimming off very busily and purposefully and, of course, they're incredibly curious. So remember the marvelous fearless, unstoppable duck--and for fun--make the* **'ack'** *sound instead! Read the references to the* **"Q"** *energy in the other parts of the book and sail back off onto the pond again with your insatiable curiosity and zest for life!*

R....constant ideas, inner dialoge, mental force and persuasiveness.

1) When you need to be quiet, to think and be peaceful.

2) When you have trouble expressing your ideas.......

For both of the above - use **"Ree, ree, ree, ree, ree,ree,ree,ree, reeeeeeeeeeeeeeee"** *in several tones until you get a good rolling resonance in the upper sinuses and frontal skull bones; deeper tones will also resonate and vibrate the chest area and higher tones will stimutate the 3rd Eye and Crown Chakras. After you feel you've had enough resonance, close your eyes and breathe very softly, taking your awareness deeper inside you.* In addition, try the **Tranquility Meditations** from Chapter 16. and for problem **1)**, also follow the instructions for letter **"P."**

3) When you tend to get too angry;
When you always HAVE to be right.......even when you're wrong!
When you're too dominating and controlling

Use **"Ahrr, ahrr, ahrr, ahrr, ahrr, ahrrrrrrrrrrrrrrrr"** *and roll your* **"R"** *vigorously, letting the final roll come out in higher and higher tones--to feel and release the anger. Also, swoop the roll both up and down in pitch then try the "roaring and anger" release instructions from letter* **"A"** *in* Chapter 4, "Releasing the Voice," *then do the* **Disidentifying Technique** *from* Chapter 17. *(saying "Anger is present, I am not the anger"), and try the* **Tranquility Meditations** *from* Chapter 16.

4) When you want to get more speaking confidence, to expand your power of ideas, and strengthen your mental force.......

Use **"Rah,rah,rah,rah,rah,rah,rah,rah, raaaaaaaaaaaaaaaaaah,"** *repeat several times and as you gather force with each sounding find the most powerful tone and stay on it.*

S .... social acceptance, traditional values, success, self-support, money, sensuality.

1) When you need to become fiscally responsible and stop expecting other people to take up the slack--pay your bills and bail you out of trouble.......

Use **"Esss, esss, esss, esss, eesssssssssssssssssss."** *The* **"e"** *sounds the same as in* **"essence"** *For the* **"ssss,"** *really push it out of you forcibly, like a powerful hiss.*

2) When you want social acceptance and recognition for who you are and what you are doing;
When you're between jobs and anxious to find another one.......

Sound **"Saah, saah, saah, sssssssssaaaaaaaah - saah, saah, saah, ssaaaaaah,"** *then* **"Saah,saah,saah,saah--saah,saah,saah,saah, ssssssssssssssssssss-aaaaaaaaaaaaaaaah."**

3) When you need to allow yourself to be more sensual.......

Refer to letter **"K"** *and letter* **"X."**

T.... perceptive, intuitive sensitivity; the psychic senses and mysticism.

1) When you feel too sensitive and want to retreat from places, social situations and certain people because they seem to drain you or make you feel frayed out, strange or terrible.......

When face to face with difficult situations or trying people practice **The Figure 8 Breath** from section 4, Chapter 17 *and try the actual* **"T"** *soundings when alone.*

2) When you tend to feel exhausted most of the time;
When you've really overdone it and feel on the verge of collapse.......

a) *Explosively use* **"Tuh! tuh! tuh! tuh! tuh! tuh! tuh!"** *contracting your navel power center with each sounding. Start at your lowest most powerful note and gradually raise the tone with each* **'tuh.'**

b) *Next repeatedly sound* **"Tah,tah,tah tah, tah,tah,tah,tah, taaaaaaaaaaaaaaaaah."**

c) *Proceed immediately to the first two* **Energy Exercises (a)** *and* **(b)** *in* Chapter 17 *(under "Clearing the Aura), as well as the* **Disidentifying Technique**, *but saying "Exhaustion is present....." or a suitable word of your own choosing. Also for an immediate energy boost try the* **Instant Energy exercises** *and* **the Goddess Energy Breath** *(all from* Chapter *17). When you become more stable and confident, try the* **Tranquility Meditations** *from* Chapter 16.

3) When you want to develop your psychic, intuitive and mystical sensitivity--and not run away from it.......

a) *First meditate on the form of the letter itself--the* **"T."** *Draw it with a marker on paper or use its illustration in* Chapter 21,"The Sacred Symbols." *Then keeping the image in mind, close your eyes and aspirate the letter* **"T"** *- no sound - just with your tongue and breath forming it. You can do this fast and slow, but eventually making it very slow....* ***"Tuh,tuh,tuh,tuh,tuh,tuh,tuh,tuh - tuh - tuh - tuh -- tuh -- tuh --- tuh ---- tuh - taaaaaaaaaaaaaahhhhhhh."***

b) *Finally open your eyes, look at the* **"T"** *image again and sing forceably* ***"Tee, tee, tee, tee, tee, tee, tee, tee - tee,tee,tee,tee,tee,tee,tee,tee, teeeeeeeeeeeeeeeeeeeeeeeeeeeeeeeeeee,"*** *pushing the* **"eeee"** *sound out strongly by contracting your belly.*

U.... fearless expansion into life, generosity, limitless abundance, the humanitarian.

1) When you want to become an open channel for Universal Abundance.

2) When you need to practice generosity--of spirit as well as possessions.
When you need to learn to receive, gracefully and gratefully.

3) When you need to stop manipulating people by 'buying' them.

4) When you should stop hiding yourself away and retreating from life...........

a) *For all of the* **"U's"** *above sound (in short bursts, pushing it out as you contract the belly)* **"Uh, uh, uh, uh, uh;"** *(the same sound as in* **"up"***).*

b) *The second is quite different and begins with the powerful* **"Y"** *sound --* **"Yoo, yoo, yoo, yoo, yoo, -- yoo,yoo,yoo,yoo,yoo, yooooooooooooooooooooo."** Accompany each **"yoo"** with a long perineum/yoni contraction.[11]

V.... world issues, optimism, vigilance, social and world vision.

1) When you've become far too pessimistic and jaundiced about the state of the world;
When you need to hope and believe instead of fear and despair.......

Sound with strength and conviction - **"Vah!--vah!--vah!--vah!"** *several times then try it more quickly,* **"Vah,vah,vah,vah,vah,vah,vah,vah, vaaaaaaaaaaaaaaaaaaaah."** *Also, try to resonate the* **"V"** *as you hold your top teeth against your bottom lip:* **"vvvvvvvvvvvvvvvvvvvvvvvvvvvuh."**

2) When you need to look at **your** world vision, what **you** came here to do, to make a difference at this time in history....for the world, or for your community.......

Sound **"Vee, vee, vee, vee, vee,"** *several times (pushing the sound out from the solar plexus) then sing it much faster* **"Vee,vee,vee,vee,vee,vee,vee,vee, veeeeeeeeeeeeeee."**
Also for **1)** *and* **2)**, *do the resonating version for* **"V"** *as described in* Chapter 18, "Power Tools for the Brain."

W.... enthusiasm, sartorial splendor, pride; the motivator.

More complex than letter **"H"** (**"Aech"**when spoken formally), the prounciation for **"W"** in the alphabet presents quite a mouthful, **"dah-bull-yoo!"** The spoken letter *sounds* are all tools for the enthusiasm-raising and motivating abilities of the **"W"** energy. For additional information, read the section for **"W"** in Chapter 8, "More Letter Meanings A to Z." For interest, also look up **"D,A,H,B,U,L,Y,O,"**....in their abbreviated meanings from Chapter 6. **Note:**--since the advent of the Internet, I've noticed a curious trend with letter **"W"** - instead of saying **"da-bullyoo"** - when they give out their web-site, they say **"da-bull*yah*, da-bull*yah*, dot, com!!"** Perhaps it's easier to say quickly - who knows!

1) When you're always the life of the party, or motivate most of the neighbourhood, but you're asking, *who cheers you--or talks* **you** *up when you're down?*

2) When you don't think you're up-to-snuff and you need to develop some pride in yourself.......

a) *Use* **"Wuh, wuh, wuh, wuh,"** *slowly with strong contractions in the navel center (yes, it is vaguely like a dog barking!), try several of them.*

b) *Then change to -* **"Wwooh! wwooh!, wwooh!"** *and really purse you lips creating a strong physical feeling as the muscles of your face more intensly create the letter.* **"W"** *is very much about how you project your persona (face) and words out to others.*
Finally sing **"Woowoowoowoowoowoowoo, woooooooooooooh.'** *Also make a* **"W"** *with closed lips, hold the position and then let yourself sound like a siren:* **"Wwwwwwwwwwwwwwwwwwwwwwwww wwwwwwwwwuh."**

---

[11] For instructions on the P/Y contraction, turn to section 1 of Chapter 17, "Energy Exercises."

3) When you've come on too strong;
When you've been influencing to the point of manipulating and controlling;
When you've been stretching a point to make yourself look more grand or knowledgeable....**lying??**....*NAH!!* But **definitely** exaggerating!
When you've been proud and arrogant, lording it over others......

For all of **3)**, *close your eyes, place your hands over your ears and resonate the* **"W"** *through pursed lips. Refer to* Chapter 18, "Power Tools for the Brain" *for more precise instructions. You need to interiorize the sound--recalibrate your brain--as you think through your motivations for wanting to influence others to the point of control; for possible insights, read the* **"W"** *section in* Chapter 8, "More Letter Meanings A to Z."

X.... exceptional mental energy! Exceptionally focused (negative or positive), or scattered!

Since it's a fairly unique energy, you'll find the **"X"** *also proves itself uniquely difficult to sound. Begin by pulling the belly in with each* **"Exs"** *sound. Do it quite slowly, intentionally and as strongly as you can,* **"Exs - exs - exs - exs,"** *then sound a little faster. You'll find if you go really fast you are sounding* **"Sexs, sexs, sexs!"** *And, of course, if you do that, you may find a smile on your face - or a thought - "Oh, I wish!" You're now partaking of the sensual nature of the* **"S"** *sound and this may not be an amusing quirk of the alphabet at all--sex may well be a good solution for excessive mental compulsion! Of course, providing it was high quality, safe, supportive and regular sex--as Dr. Ruth would say, "Good Sex!"*

1) When you've taken on more than you can handle and should let half of it go.

2) When you feel totally disorganized, need to focus and stop being so scattered.
When you're feeling mentally overwhelmed and unstable.
When you've become mentally compulsive...........

For all three of the above - do the previously given sounds, but in addition try the first two Energy Exercises in Chapter 17 *(under the heading* "Clearing the Aura") *and also the* **Disidentifying Technique**, *saying "Confusion is present....." or a suitable word of your own choosing; also, do the* **Instant Energy exercises** *and the* **Goddess Energy Breath**. *When you finally become more stable, try the* **Tranquility Meditations** *from* Chapter 16, "Special Meditations" .

Y.... charismatic leader, individualist, self-sufficient, does things their own way.

The alphabet sound for **"Y"** is **"Wie,"** implying that the balanced use of **"Y"** encourages and motivates others (an attribute of letter **"W"**), to their highest creative expression (**"I"** plus **"E"**).

1) When you need to take charge and allow yourself to do things YOUR way, instead of being ordered around and controlled by others.......

Sing as loudly and strongly and triumphantly as you dare -- **"Yah,yah, yah,yah,yah,yah, yah,yah,yah, yaaaaaaaaaaaaaaah!"**

2) When you need to develop forbearance and patience with others and not insist that your way is the only way;
When you need to stop being quite so relentless and bossy;
When you need to be encouraging and use your charisma and power to inspire and guide others...........

Sound **"Wi-ee, wi-ee,wi-ee,wi-ee,wi-ee,wi-ee,"** *(the* **'wi'** *sound is the same as in* **"wild"**). *You'll feel a resonant drone issuing from the* **"i"** *sound--the* **"Y"** *energy becomes transformed by connecting to Spirit* *through the* **"i"** *energy. Finally sing an extended* **"Iiiiiiiiiiiiiiiiiiiiiiiiiiiiiie."** *The sound for the* **"iiiii"** *is the same as in* **"Sigh."**

Z.... opportunity waiting for opportunists! Watching and aligning with the play of destiny.

1) When you feel at the mercy of external circumstances and need to take responsibility for having somehow caused and attracted them;

2) When you need to challenge destiny and stop bowing down to (so-called) "Fate;" (It is **not** your lot in life--you **can** change it.)
When you want to take charge of your life and beat down the odds...........

a) *Sound* **"<u>Zzz</u>ah! <u>zzz</u>ah! <u>zzz</u>ah! <u>zzz</u>ah!"** *with strong navel/belly contractions (get that power center activated)! Resonate the* **'Zzz'** *sound forcibly behind your teeth before you release into the* **'ah!'**

b) *Also sing* **"Zeee, zeee, zeee"** *several times, pressing in the navel, then* **"Zzah,zzah,zzah,zzah, zzah, zzah,zzah,zzah, zzzzzaaaaaaaaaaaaaaaah!"** *and* **"Zzee,zzee, zzee,zzee,zzee, zzee, zzzzzzeeeeeeeee!"**

3) When you want 'closure' on something.
When you want the final authority about an issue, or BE the final authority.

For a change, try saying and singing the **"Z"** *like the rest of the English-speaking world--they say* **"Zed"** *rather than* **"Ze."** *Sound* **"Zed, zed, zed, zed, zed - zed,zed,zed,zed,zed - zed,zed,zed,zed,zed, zeeeeeeeeeeeeeeeeeed".....(the "eeee" sounds like "air").**

Beginnings and endings often interconnect. The end of the alphabet "Z," and some of its problems, also relates back to letter "A." Similarly, it would benefit to occasionally refer to "A's" different sound-solutions while also dealing with "Z's."

IMPORTANT NOTE

When working with any of the above letters and their specific needs, you may want to either draw the letter out boldly with a black (or colored) marker on a plain note pad or use the single page large letter illustrations that appear in Chapter 21, "The Sacred Symbols. In addition, I have suggested <u>extra remedies</u> for certain of the above needs in other chapters of this book and I recommend that you read Chapter 16, "Special Meditations" (it contains some very short and useful meditations, as well as more lengthy and complex ones), and Chapter 17, "Energy Exercises."

DEFINITIONS SHARED BY MORE THAN ONE LETTER

(Refer also to Appendix 3. "Some General Letter Categories.")

I'm sure you'll discover many more of these for yourself. You can either sound all of the letters indicating a similar problem, as a 'blanket' cure, or sound only the letters from your own name. But remember, just one or two attempts won't be enough--you must persevere to change an old energy pattern.

A H R Y ....for strengthening aspects of personal power.

A J K ....for increasing physical strength, resiliancy, and perseverence in the face of health issues.

A J R P Y.....for working with anger reactions and aggressive physical and mental tendencies. **"P"** develops peaceful reactions, so do the **Tranquility Meditations** in Chapter 16, "Special Meditations."

A J R Q W for developing courage, boldness and the unstoppable, daring spirit of adventure.

B E I...............for creative blocks and throat and voice problems.

C E N R......for sharpening intellectual skills, mental capacity, perception, reading and writing proficiency, analysis.

D B K S X..for helping fear of sexuality, frustration or guilt; for balancing sensual needs.

G J O Y......sound, if you lack joy and the ability to play and to wonder.

H W Y........for self-motivation and the power to motivate and catalyze the energy of others. Because *you* get going--others get going!

M L O.........to help develop interest, caring and compassion for others and other life-forms.

O B L M Nfor problems with self-nourishment--food addictions and compulsions, fear of going hungry; abandonment issues that can cause eating or weight problems; for unrequited emotional needs. (See Appendix 4, "Food Meditations."

P S T X Z...for developing tranquility, stillness, serenity, balance and surrender to Spirit.

S H...............If you feel defeated about money, social acceptance, honor, respect, success.

I R...............sound, to stop selfish and negative mental and verbal manipulation (in yourself!),to cultivate expansion of ideas and positive thought projection.

For the most part I have tried to avoid referring to the extremely abnormal and criminally destructive tendencies; these become self-evident when you begin to analyse the names of some famous criminals and insane deviates. To illustrate such problems It would take a book three times this size to list all the name letter combinations with examples of real people throughout history (including the present) - and besides, I don't wish to be that depressing! As a small example of what to look for: an excessive number of **"D's"** in a name (or **"D's"** in the Drive or Focus positions, also **"D's"** combined with several **"S's"**). When these letters are present in a name and when the person becomes **severely unbalanced** and destructive, there can be the presence of sadistic sex crimes, or a tendency thereto.
Of course, all of the letters polarize to their deviant and dangerous opposites.

OVERCOMING DISTURBING THOUGHTS AND EMOTIONS

Everyone of us at times can suffer from and 'entertain' any number of disturbing thoughts and emotions, regardless of the preponderance of certain letters in our names. Sometimes, due to tiredness or stress, we begin to doubt, fear or 'awfulize.' We can give ourselves a good "talking to" and even do the energy exercises under **Finding the Power of the Goddess** from Chapter 17 *--but we still can't turn off the compulsive thoughts!*

Letters "E," "I" and "S" are releasing sounds.

a) First use the mental command (to the thoughts), **"dissolve, dissolve,"** then slowly contract your abdomen while you sing a **very** long **"Eeeeeeeeeeeeeeeeee."** Try several long **"E's"** on different pitches, then sound an arpeggio--you need to realign your inner chord. Look also in *this* Chapter under letter **"E"** for further sounding instructions.

b) For letter **"I,"** again contract the lower belly, but now sing the short staccato version: **"I,yi, yi, yi,yi, yi, yi, yi,"** which later becomes the **E** when you sound **"Iee,iee, iee,iee,ieeeeeeeeeeeeeeee."**

c) To discharge with **"S,"** use the sound **"Saah, saah, saah."**

In addition, work with the **Disidentifying Technique,** *also from* Chapter 17, "Energy Exercises."

MENTAL SOUNDS

It's not always possible (or appropriate), to to start singing at the top of your voice whenever you feel the need.....in most public places for one thing! So you'll have to learn the fine art of Mental Sounding. *Everything you sing with your outer voice can also be sung in your head!* Ordinary thoughts (unless linked to emotions) seem rather colorless mental chatterings, but begin rehearsing a speech, poem or song in your head and you'll immediately notice the difference. It suddenly becomes heard and felt within the body. Some internal sound-switch turns on, minute muscle movements take place; and when you involve the intuitive voices as well, then the Chi body energy starts streaming into the physical nervous system--and probably engages the Light body as well!!

Sounding "internally" feels as though the energy "plucks" you like an instrument and massages you from the inside; and yes, it **is** blissful. You can just enjoy--or direct the bliss to parts of you that need physical healing, or send it mentally (along with your internal soundings) to others who might benefit from the energy. Also, if you're working to dissolve errant thoughts, try directing the bliss towards the thoughts.

Think of all the occasions when you're alone in a room yet it's definitely not the right time or place to practice sounding the vowels or other noisy exercises...and yet you wish you could! There's a way around this that lets you take advantage of the situation without disturbing as much as a fly on the wall. You go through all the full vocal motions, yet produce only the soundless sighs of your breath--instead of tones. In other words: all of the physical voice mechanisms come into play; you breathe deeply into the belly as though you are going to sing, you open your mouth and precisely form the vowels, the letters, the exercises and while you "hear" the sounds in your head--only breath comes out of your mouth!

Empaths and other sensitives frequently receive energy-impressions from locations as well as people and also pick up uncomfortable vibrations from past (or even future events). Such impressions build in them to a point above their comfort-zone. Intuitive inner-sounding always balances and disseminates this kind of energy and you can do it effectively without having to utter a sound, turn a curious head, or rattle a window!

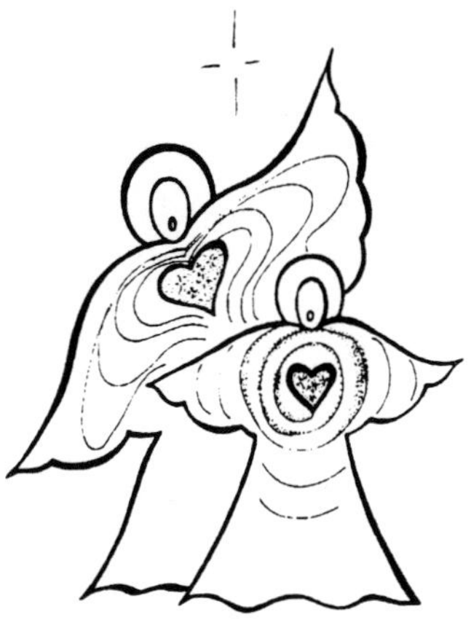

How do you wake up in the morning?

Do you bound out of bed with a leap of joy, or do you groan through sleep-stuck eyes and reset the alarm for another ten? I knew someone who, five days a week reset the alarm every five minutes for the next *twenty minutes,* then blamed his wife for not getting him up--it used to drive her crazy!

If it's a terrible chore to get yourself mobile each day and you really *want* to change, I'll help you. It may take some commitment and organizing on your part, but eventually you'll not want to begin the day without your Sounding. The sounds will set you up with energy and fill you with joy, power and motivation.

Before you go to sleep tonight, have a 'chat' with your subconscious and *tell it* that you're going to arise fifteen minutes earlier to do your Sounding work. When you're totally determined, the subliminal-self gets the message and you won't fight getting out of bed tomorrow; fix it in your mind--that first thing in the morning, you're going to follow this new pattern until it becomes automatic.

The New Getting-out-of-bed Pattern:

Immediately on turning off the alarm, and while still horizontal, stretch and wriggle thoroughly then rub-massage yourself all over. Your skin will come alive and say "Thank you, thank you!" Don't forget your face (be more gentle) and your scalp (be more vigorous!). By this time you may be over the edge of the bed and touching your toes to the floor. Next, finish off the rubbing and start slapping up and down your arms and legs with your hands, giving a final thump or two on your thymus (upper chest), to crank up your immune system. If after that wonderful stimulation you still feel "brain-dead," grasp your big toes and vigorously knead them with your fingernails and thumb knuckles. That usually does the trick! Now fully (or fairly) awake - you're ready to sound the first resonator, "**M.**"

Remember the above instructions are for the hard-of-rising. **I prefer to turn off the alarm and then lie back and instantly begin humming "M," in my wake-up tone for the day--that resonates my body fully awake! Then I stretch, wriggle, rub, slap and arise.**

Finding your wake-up Base Tone.

Begin your humming on a low note...... **"Mmmmmmmmm,mum,mum,mum,mum--mum,mum,mum, mum, maaaaaaaaaaaaah.** Hold the **"Mmmmmmm"** long enough to feel a strong vibration in the bones of your nose (nasal septum). Do this several times, any way you want to, or follow the instructions for the Resonators given towards the end of Chapter 4, "Releasing the Voice." Humming that first **"M"** gives you the base note of your initial chord for the day; this already exists within you and may be the same every day, or totally different. Sounding the note establishes an unsung chord, forming a harmonic your body wants to resonate to, in order to balance--or to *begin* the process of balancing. **The body always knows the particular note it needs to hear** and as it's the base tone for your grounding, make it as low as you comfortably can--unless your throat spontaneously sings otherwise. Following this, allow your voice to rise naturally to higher notes; enjoy yourself--improvise, but keep humming.

I always ascend from the base tone (through a major triad), in an arpeggio that ends on a forth note - an octave above the base tone. I do this as a matter of habit and because I really like to start the day by singing through my primary chord; if you don't know how to, instructions for singing the chord notes are in Chapter 12, *"Training the Outer Voice."*

Now begin humming the powerful **"N"** resonator - as you use the bathroom and empty your bladder (if it has not already been an imperative)! Having established the base note with the **"M,"** the **"N"** may want to start on a different note - we have many chords resonating within us. (Be sure to have checked the instructions and meanings for **"N"** in the Chapter, "Releasing the Voice.") *The amazing thing about the resonators is their ability to vibrate the brain and bones of the skull.*[1] *I used to wake with a dull headache (post-menopausal hormone fluctuations), and after one minute of resonating while lying in bed, the headache sounded itself away - without fail!*

---

[1] Read Chapter 18, "Power Tools for the Brain."

When you 'you've sounded the **"N"** to your satisfaction, speak and then sound the **"A"** vowels, doing both the **"Aeeeey, yay,yay,yay, yaaaaaaaaaaeeeeeeeeey"** and the **"AH"** - **"Aaah...rah,rah,rah, rah, raaaaaaaah."** This verifies the strength of your will and the power of your identity.

You might want to do all of the vowels first thing, but if you're short on time in the mornings, the above wake-up ritual is all you'll need to set you up for the day.

Obviously, these suggestions present difficulties if you share your living space. In such circumstances, you will need a more creative morning arrangement; perhaps your sounds can become the wake-up call for everybody else in the house, and who knows - you may convert some others to join you! Another idea is to sound in bed with your head under the covers--periodically coming up for air! Then there's always the basement, the shower or a large walk-in cupboard!

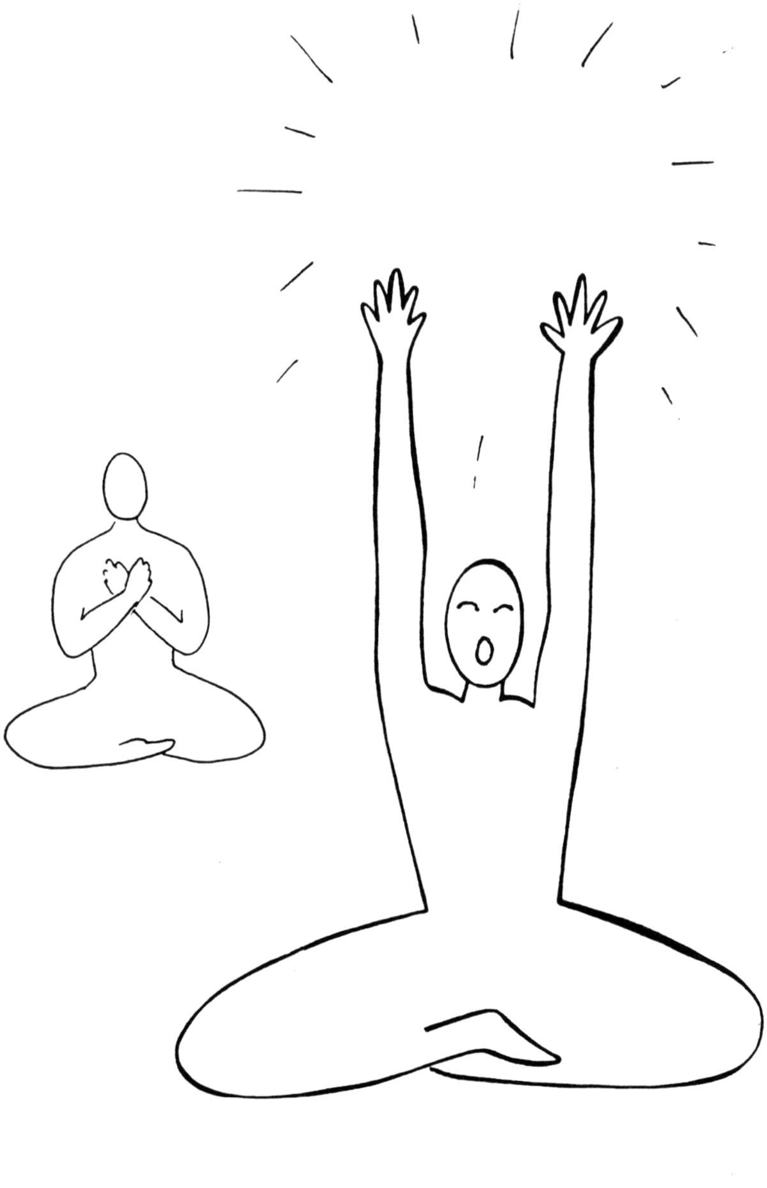

If you just opened the book at this page, it won't make any sense unless you've already read Chapter 5, "Your Name, How to Understand and Analyze it," *which explains the different parts of a name and what they mean.*

The practice of Sounding changes the vibrational rate of the cells, and often brings profound mental and emotional benefits. When you apply sound to the different letters in your name, especially the key letters, you'll begin to actualize your true potential. Also, if your name contains some of the powerful Extra Resonators[1] as the first, middle or last letters, these should be sung both ways, in resonator as well as non-resonator mode. When you're sounding, think of the letter's particular qualities that you want to activate or strengthen in yourself. At first, only concentrate on the key letters, the Drive (first letter) and the Focus (middle letter or letters), *and without doing anything else suggested in this chapter*--sounding only those two could considerably release and re-balance your life! *You can also work with the qualities of letters you* **don't** *have in your name (especially the vowels), then you benefit from those energies without actually having to change your present name.*

Name Sounding...*quick version.*

I try to sing my name every day; sometimes first thing in the morning along with the vowels. It puts me in touch with my own sound-print and I always begin with my birth certificate name--to remind me of my original life purpose.

1) For a moment, think about the *sound* of your name.....how you hear it said back to you by others. Say it to yourself several times mentally and then out loud--get used to saying it to yourself.

2) Concentrate on the very **first letter** of your first name (the Drive) and begin by speaking and then singing that letter...even if it's an odd sounding consonant. Speak and sing it the way it sounds in your name--as well as in the formal alphabet manner.
For names beginning with unique consonants combinations.[2]such as a **"C"** *adjacent to an* **"H,"** *you would say* **"Ch,ch,ch,ch,ch,ch,"** *(as well as* **"see,see,see"** *- the* **sound** *of letter* **"C"** *) - or if an* **"S"** *next to an* **"H,"** *it's* **"Sh,sh,sh,sh,sh,"** *(then* **"Ess,ess,ess"** *- the* **sound** *of* **"S"**); *and for a* **"TH,"** *sound* **"Th,th,th,"** *before making the* **"Tee,tee,tee,"** *etc.*

3) Next sing the first syllable of your first name. Some names have only one syllable like **Joan** or **Abe**; whereas **Barnaby** has three syllables, **"Bah-nah-bee."** "Bah," the first syllable, "nah," the second, "bee," the third. Sing the first syllable in your name several times before proceeding to the second, third and fourth syllables - if your name contains that many.

4) That may be enough name-work for the first day, but if you still have time and voice, follow the same idea for your middle and last names - always beginning with the **first** letter before dividing the name into its syllables.

5) To integrate the energy--just sound *all* of your names, together--as though someone had said to you, "Please say and then sing to me all of the names on your birth certificate.? *Another day, you might do the same with any legally changed or married names - but get into the energy of your given name first.*

---

[1] See Chapter 18, "Power Tools for the Brain."
[2] See pages 22 and 23.

Charting Your Name[3] .... *with in-depth sounding.*

1) This time, think about how your name *looks* - how it's spelled and written. Supply yourself with marker pens, a large blank note pad and a small scratch pad. Across the longest width of the large pad, print all your names boldly in upper-case lettering and don't forget the middle name(s). Let it be big and bold, because, like it or not, **this is the 'sound-print' for your life** containing all your potential and all your greatest challenges--and you need to see it staring you in the face! I ask that you *print* out your names, because the separate *form* of a letter reflects the meaning and power of that letter. Any feelings that come up during the hand printing, reveal your attitudes to your self, your life and what presently bothers you. Then, as you actually "sound" those letters, you'll begin to notice a change in yourself--the old attitudes move and new insights emerge. Also, meditating on the letters in your name will open up a deeper level of their meaning and power.[4]

Note: **Married ladies, and those (of either gender) who have legally changed their names--it's important to begin Name Sounding with your original name**--*the one on your birth certificate,* **that** *one holds the primary life energy information and your original sound frequency. When that name has been understood and mastered through sounding and affirmation, you then begin working on your married name, or your legally changed name.*

2) To understand your key problems, find the **middle letter** (or letters) of *each* name and either underline or circle them (preferably in some other color--so they stand out). *These mark the Focus-Challenge letters in all of your names.* Next, read the meanings of these letters so you'll know what you intended to overcome and master this lifetime - they also indicate the way you tend to challenge others. For extra sounding ideas, look them up in Chapter 9, "Sounding for Specific Needs." And to refresh your mind on the function of middle (Focus-Challenge) letters, go back and re-read that section in the earlier Chapter, "Your Name , How to Understand and Analyze it."

3) Now take up the small scratch pad and print each of the **middle** letters by themselves on separate pages (a page for each one); when you have **two letters** in the middle of a name for your Challenge, put them side-by-side on one page, because you need to sound them in unison as well as individually. Believe it or not, consonants together in the middle DO make a sound when isolated, even if it's peculiar. Example: "ST" (in the middle of We**st**on); the sibilant "S" uttered first, begins as a 'hissing' followed by the "T" which together sound like **"Ssst,sst,sst."** You can if you wish, add a sound to the "ST" by speaking or singing **"Sstah,sstah,sstah."** Finally you speak *and* sing the "S" and "T" individually, **"Ess,ess,ess,ess,"** and **"Tee,tee,tee."** In this case, you would also do your research on the separate meanings of letters "S" and "T." It amounts to double work (a double Challenge) if you have **two** middle letters!

Perhaps your Focus/Challenge energies are rather difficult, then choose to sound just one of them a day - or one for a week at a time if necessary. Use the voicing suggestions in "Sounding for Specific Needs," then read the letter's "fun" affirmation from Chapter 7, and as a contrast, look it up in the "Summary of Sacred Affirmation and Mantra" on page 191.

Follow this procedure for all of your Challenge/Focus (middle) letters until you feel there has been some movement, some empowering change in these areas of your life.

4) Now, apply the same approach to the **Drive** letters (the first letters) of all your names, which show you how you lead or push yourself out into the world around you--and finally the **Aim** letters (the last letter) of all your names, which show what you want to achieve this lifetime.

5) The following is similar to the *quick version*: look at your first name, divide it into its syllables and write them down. For instance, **Barbara** has three distinct groups of syllables - **"Bar-ba-ra,"** although some seem to insist on saying **"Bar-bra"** instead; you can sound **"Bar-bra"** if you wish, but you're avoiding the power of that extra **"A." John**, is sometimes short for **Jonathan, "Jon-a-thn"** and **Jean** is simply the one syllable, **"Jeen"** - unless **"Jeanette"** is the *real* name on the birth certificate, then it

---

3 For a sample Name Chart, see the end of this Chapter.

4 See Chapter 21, The Sacred Symbols.

would be "**Jen-ett.**" Observe the 'silent' letters in your name (if any) and sound them additionally. Notice **Jonathan** has the "**TH**" sound with a silent "**T**" and "**H**" as well as a silent "**A**" (in the last syllable), and **Jean**, also has a silent "**A.**" *The silent letters are the energies less dominant in the personality.* Also remember to include the extra letters in a name, the ones sounded instead of the written ones - such as "E" at the end of Ricky and Mary. *The extra letters add to the power of the written ones.*
Important Note: *In addition to making the letter's usual sounds, don't forget to 'resonate' those special resonating ones - particularly if they appear at the beginning, middle or ends of names. For these letters and their sounding instructions turn to Chapter 18, "Power Tools for the Brain."*

6) Finally, do the syllable divisions for all of your names. (Mine would be: "**Rin-chen-na K-har-do.**" For my last name, I need to sound the "**K**" first ("**Kuh**") followed by "**har**" then "**do.**" Unlike the stressed and rolled European "**R,**" the one in **K'hardo** is ignored and pronounced like a wide "**ah**" (as is the case with the first "**R**" in **Barbara**--it's delightful listening to a German person saying "Barbara"- they 'roll' both of the "**R's.**" It sounds like "**Barrr-barrr-rrah**"). Before sounding any 'silent' letters research the information on their meaning from chapters - 6, 7 and 8, then get some vocal ideas from Chapter 9, "Sounding for Specific Needs."

Sounding Your Name as a Meditation.

Study the instructions for the Galactic Breath in Chapter 4, "Releasing the Voice," and apply it to the letters and syllables of your name. Practice making actual sounds or silently with visualization...*see* the letter in front of you. ***If this seems like too much work....you don't have to do it all!!*** *The above covers the* ***total*** *information on charting your name with its possible sounding; you can get still good results by just staying with "Name Sounding...quick version," until you want to go deeper.*

Additional Exercises for Singers:

1) From your name, sound the letter of your choice by finding a base note and then singing the letter up and down a major **scale** for one, two or three octaves.
2) From your name sound the letter of your choice by finding a base note and then singing up and down an arpeggio for one, two or three octaves.
3) Practice the above two exercises with your name's specific syllables.
4) In situations where singing is inappropriate (you have house guests; you're traveling in a bus or plane; it's 2 o'clock in the morning), sing the exercises mentally in your head--but be prepared for the waves of bliss that begin rippling through your body!!

Sounding For Others.

Don't be content to Sound only for yourself, you can do the same for others that you know and love - in absentia. I sometimes sound the names of my children and friends as a prayer-meditation. If they're experiencing problems or distress, I concentrate on their key letters, specifically the Focus-Challenges in the middle of their names, or I may just joyfully 'celebrate' their beingness and potential by singing their names syllabically. Those of you with community concerns could decide to work on the names of your local leaders...and the trouble makers (they could be one and the same)! The possibilities are endless. Sound alone, or organize a group of Sounders.

The Challenge.

The sound of your name when honored through voice, reinstates your total "song." Old suppressed abilities and urgings (the unsung melodies of your soul), call you to recreate your life. What was it you never allowed yourself--that suddenly summons you again? What dreams did you relegate to the back-room of impossibilities?? Age doesn't come into this--there *is* no excuse - and "Too late!" is a phrase for fatalists. Even sickness can signal a protest--are you declining to be who you were born to be? Think about it! Keep sounding your name and read "Chicken Soup for the Soul"[5] to nourish your aspirations. If you think it's also too late to learn anything new - also read "The Open Mind " (exploring the 6 patterns of natural intelligence) by Dawna Markova, Ph.D. and if you're an "artist-on-hold" be inspired by the incredible books of Judith Cornell, "Mandala" and "Drawing the Light from Within."

---

[5] Refer to Bibliography.

NAME CHART EXAMPLE

Here's an example of a formal name chart I create for clients who want name analysis. You can write up something like this for yourself, family members or friends. It gives you an overview.

Barbara Joy Weston - Maiden name.

The underlined letters are the Focus-Challenges.

(Drive) B A R <u>B</u> A R A **(Aim)**
(*outer personality*)

(Drive) J <u>O</u> Y **(Aim)**
(Inner personality)

(Drive) W E <u>S T</u> O N **(Aim)**
(*environment name*)

Married Name.

(Drive) S W <u>E</u> U M **(Aim)**
(*filtered environment)*

DRIVE LETTERS ....**B J W S**

FOCUS LETTERS.......**B..O..ST..E**

AIM LETTERS..............**A Y N M**

PHYSICAL LETTERS...**A A A B B B J U W W Y**

MENTAL LETTERS......**E E N R R**

EMOTIONAL ....**B B M O O**

PSYCHIC SENSITIVE....**B B T**

WILLPOWER................**A A A R R W W Y**

For easy letter categories, turn to Appendix 3.

In some ways, training the voice reminds me of lifting weights--after all, you're just training another set of muscles. In weight lifting you begin with the lightest weights and gradually add heavier ones. Most weight lifters don't work out every day; they need recovery time for their muscles to rebuild. Applied to singing, the 'weights' you use for making strong vocal muscles are your exercises; you start with a few and add more, until bit by bit, you find yourself singing longer - as your voice gets stronger! Eventually, you increase the complexity and range of the exercises. Also, the muscles used in singing are much smaller than the massive ones used in weight lifting; tiny muscles recover more rapidly and unlike pumping iron, you can work out moderately every day--*unless you're afflicted with a throat block; for dealing with that, see* Chapter 13.

My Own Voice Training. Everything I do when I practice builds on freeing and opening the voice; that's my foundation. Each morning I pretty much follow the wake up ritual described in Chapter 10; and often while still in bed, I hum my base tone for the day and three other ascending notes, creating a major chord arpeggio. I do this with at least two of the basic Resonators (usually "**M**" and "**N**"), then I practice some of the extra power resonators[1] that happen to be in my names - including those in my birth certificate names. After that, I may follow the exact procedure of speaking and sounding some (or all) of the vowels described in Chapter 4, "Releasing the Voice." *Regarding the vowels, I find it important to read over the short affirmations that go with the different vowels so they're in your mind while you are making their sounds.* Later in the day I sometimes work more deeply on a vowel that I omitted in the morning, or do a couple of other techniques, including sounding some of the key letters or syllables in my name.[2]

With my opened Throat Chakra, I find that formal practice times frequently get interrupted by the inner voices (both male and female); they will come through and sing the exercises, then my voice takes off spontaneously in all kinds of wild and wonderful directions as though I'm being put through my paces by invisible singing teachers! To sing in this fashion brings me fresh energy and delight; I often write down the ideas to practice them again later.

How to Sound an Arpeggio.

Before starting, please refer back to Chapter 9, "Sounding for Specific Needs" under letter "**K.**" *Read the long paragraph plus the italicized one following it (between need: sections 2 and 3; I don't always repeat everything I've previously mentioned and you may want to compare both sections.*

Over many years of using the inner voices, either alone (in sound-meditations), sounding for individuals, or for large and small groups, I began to notice a distinct pattern that emerged at least once in every session. During my entrainment (to the other person or to the group receiving the Sounding), a magnificent tone of great power and clarity would arise, followed by another, then another, and finally a culminating note--all in an ascending sequence. They would issued effortlessly from my throat, with an intrinsic logic that felt significant and powerful. I noted how the tones always progressed from the lowest to the highest (not the other way around), as though reaching for some predestined completion. I never questioned the sequence and it always happened spontaneously. Then my son Ricky grew up, became a musician and attended one of my Sounding groups. He pointed out that I was singing the intervals of a major triad, with a 4th top note, creating a sequential chord--an arpeggio. As stated in a previous chapter, I sang the key signature first (the bottom note), followed by notes two and three (the triad), until on the fourth note, I was sounding an exact octave above my starting note--which of course, is the first note of the next triad in that key.

I'm trying to keep this as non-technical as possible for those who don't happen to follow music. However, I make space below for a written arpeggio, as you **do** *have to understand it. Ask some one who reads music to play or hum it for you. (If you're familiar with the Folk song "Kumbiah," the first three notes of that tune form a perfect major triad.) This sequence is all you need to know for creating*

---

[1] Refer to Chapter 18.

[2] As described in Chapter 11, "Sounding Your Name."

simple major chords from any note you may sound as your base note. The sequence and the intervals between the notes remains the same. **Chords form an intrinsic part of the body's inherent tuning mechanism; they occur naturally within us whether we hear them or not. When we intelligently sound our chords, we begin to realign the interconnecting systems of our being.**

The following is in the key of C Major and if all the notes were played simultaneously (as on a keyboard), you would hear a simple C Major chord. When you sing the notes individually and in sequence, you have sung an arpeggio. You'll notice the base note is middle C on the piano.

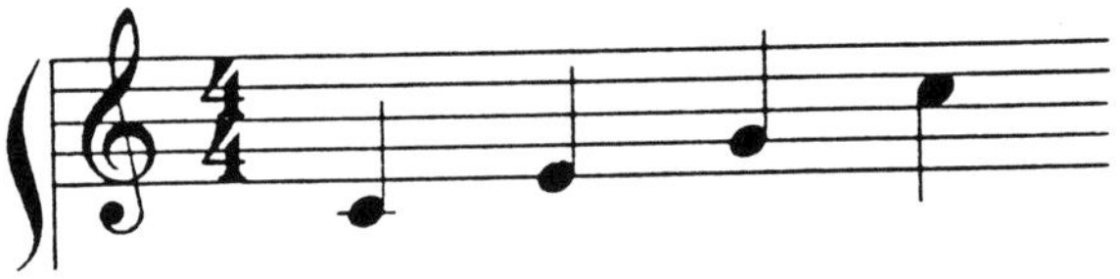

Although the inner voices usually only sing ascending arpeggios, ***when practicing the outer voice,*** *sound both up (and down if you want) through one, two, or three octaves depending on your natural range. Let your voice play with it!* The ascending notes are **receptive** and take you to an integrated resolution, whereas the descending notes are **releasing** (and grounding) draining doubts, fears and anything else that needs discharging.

Sounding Your Basic Chord for the Day.

This subject has already been addressed briefly in Chapter 10, "Wake-Up Ritual." When you hum your base note each morning (followed by the arpeggio notes of the chord), you 'wake up' and tune your brain to that frequency. If you continue in the same way for two or three minutes, humming base notes and arpeggios for **"M," "N"** and even **"NG,"** your whole being will eventually resonate to that chord. It's also important to begin working with the Extra Resonators,[3] especially if you have them in your own names. Remember, your body has many sound needs; some mornings your sound cocktail may consist of two or even three *different* base notes; you may use one base note and arpeggio for "M" and by the time you begin on "N," you may be singing a new base note in a different key. Later, when you're sounding the vowels (or even the letters in your name) and you find yourself wanting to sing a base note and chord again, it may *or may not be* the same one you resonated on waking up--and then again, sometimes it's the same for days on end, until you've sung it enough for the body's needs.
We daily create an inner symphony and the melody changes as we heal and recharge ourselves.

Originally, the chord arpeggios only emerged during my inner-voice Soundings, but once Ricky pointed out what actually was happening, I started to *consciously* sing them with my outer voice. This left me feeling more integrated with everything around me. Then I began to notice a change in the group I was teaching. Periodically we'd spontaneously sound a series of amazing chords, with our intuitive harmonizing culminating in one long note, as though we followed the same unwritten score conducted by an invisible choir master! Breathless and amazed, we'd look into each other's eyes, only to find them closing as we all sank into deep stillness. While sounding, we were united in harmony (like one mind singing), yet in the aftermath of silence, we each entered an individual space, merging profoundly with our private higher Spirits. After communion of this fathomless nature, we always found ourselves *most* unwilling to leave the deep awareness and return to class activities. I often speculated as to what would happen (how long we would remain suspended in time), if we ever allowed ourselves to stay in that sublime space!

Also, don't underestimate the power of the ***outer*** *voice when sounding the chord notes.* **For Example:** When I used to teach Sounding groups out of town, I would stay overnight at my friend Cathy's home in Portland. We had both been spiritual adventurers and researchers for many years, so I

---

[3] See Chapter 18, "PowerTools for the Brain ."

was not unfamiliar with her bathroom and frequently sang my head off in her singular shower stall. Let me describe its uniqueness for you: sliding glass doors opened to reveal an amazing array of very large to very small rocks, including magnificent boulders of petrified wood, pebbles, a shell or two, lustrous agates and pieces of amethyst mixed in with clear quartz crystals--all stacked loosely in descending order of size and completely filling the far end of the shower stall.

I loved Cathy's shower, it was the closest I could find to an outdoor pool--one almost looked for a waterfall! The rocks glistened wetly through the steam as you squirted water-jets from a hand-held nozzle, but incongruous amongst the rocks--were the plastic bottles. A great many of all sizes and colors sat around, mysterious and aromatic, tempting me to peek and sniff at their contents--many were shampoos, rinses and shower gels; you stepped over the bigger ones as you entered the shower while the rest sat on a long narrow shelf or balanced among the nooks and crannies of the boulders. *You will understand the reason for my long description in a moment.*

This fateful morning I entered Cathy's rocky enclave and began a leisurely shower, singing as I soaped. In mid-song it suddenly seemed a good idea to sound my "chord" for the day. I'd noticed in my practice, that the second note in an arpeggio and occasionally the third (not always the first and last), carried the greatest power and resonance. Sure enough, after I'd sung the initial base note, out came an utterly marvelous second note; it seemed to sing itself, so I sounded it again and again, loud and long. Suddenly my noisy ablutions were interrupted by a different noise--a little crash. I happened to look over just as one of the topmost rocks jumped forward off the stack all by itself! *"How could that be?"* I thought with suprise, *"Not my singing, surely!"* Then a rapid domino effect! More and more began jumping out, until within seconds, two thirds of the entire mound came tumbling down, showering bottles, crystals and pebbles everywhere. My astonishment gave way to alarm! Unable to turn off the water, I shouted for help as I desperately tried to hold together the boulders at the base of the stack. Cathy finally came inside to see what all the fuss was about. She found me crouching naked amidst the steam and water clutching part of the rocky disarray. "I was only sounding my chord!" I protested, "And the rocks began popping out all over the place!" She surveyed me with patient humor. "Well, I've been putting off rearranging them--and now I'll **have** to do it!" She set to it on the spot with much rumbling, rolling and scraping, while I contritely dried myself off, contemplating the unexpected power of sound!

End of story, the moral being: *be careful where you are when you sound your chord!* Needless to say, I have not dared sing in her shower since!

Sounding the Vowels.

Sounding the vowels guarantees an often immediate improvement in both the speaking and singing voice. Don Campbell, musicologist, teacher, composer and writer, advocates five minutes daily on each vowel for maximum results. *Follow his advice or find your own pace.* Sometimes I sound them all in about ten minutes; other days the time varies enormously on what I *feel* I should spend with each vowel. Suspicion grabs me if I only want to sound one or two vowels and ignore certain others. The ones I *don't* want to sing usually contain energies that I'm avoiding--and it's time for me to face and release them. The next time I practice, I <u>begin</u> with the neglected ones. And again, I can't stress enough the importance of knowing the general meaning of the individual vowels along with their affirmations and possible problems (discussed in "Sounding for specific needs" Chapter 9).

Here's a very brief Vowel resume:

Sounding the **"A's"** reinforce your identity and life purpose.
Sounding the **"E"** reinforces how you express or talk your walk.
Sounding the **"I"** reminds you to create, to receive inspiration (to *breathe* the Galactic Breath)[4].
Sounding the **"O"** reminds you to wonder and to nourish yourself with beauty and pleasure, and also lets you grieve by sounding away your pain.
Sounding the **"U"** calls you to expand your horizons, and to receive with grace, as well as give generously.

---

[4] See technique in Chapter 4, "Releasing the Voice."

When you do the Releasing Exercises, you're not only dealing with a complex set of interacting muscles but also a complicated set of emotions tied to the sounds; that's why understanding the **meaning** *of the vowels and their sounding variations proves an important part of the releasing process.*

Occasionally, when sounding one or more of the vowels, you'll feel a deep emotional reaction or unusual bodily sensation. This means that something buried has surfaced. Stay for the longest time with that particular vowel *and the note* that triggered the reaction, until every sensation and feeling has been discharged through the sound. When discharging in this manner, try rocking from side to side, or forward and back, while you're singing. Continue to feel the sound in your body long after you have stopped vocalizing. Next day, when you sound it again see if the emotional charge has gone from the vowel--it often has.

Discovering Your Range.

Do you believe you have a certain range? You must have some idea what your top and bottom notes are--in other words, your singing limits? Once you begin daily vowel releasing, your range may take off like a rocket! Mine used to vary from day to day, establishing itself afresh every time I practiced. *For now, get a fixed range out of your head--get gender limits out of your head!* Think more in terms of an expanding, fluctuating range and don't be put out by the fluctuations. I have a deep voice (a female baritone, I like to call it!). Once in a while I suprise myself by rumbling softly on the *second* **E** flat bass note below middle **C**; other days I'm only able to sing low **B** flat, seven semitones *above* the previous low **E**.....but still quite low for a female voice. Naturally I'm not given to high soprano performance, so I'm often delighted to find myself singing a strong high **A** flat instead of my usual **F** or **F#** (and the occasional high **G**.)

This all pales in the light of a remarkable and long dead voice teacher, Alfred Wolfsohn. In respect to human voice potential, he became an unparalleled master. His life still inspires me and I greatly lament the unavailability of his musical knowledge today. Wolfsohn created a psycho-physical method of vocal healing and voice development in London, England during the 40's and 50's. He demonstrated a range of eight octaves in male and female voices regardless of age. His pupils were in the Guinness Book of Records because of their phenomenal vocal abilities. Unfortunately, his singing work came to an end with his death in 1960. Successors carried on, but not in the field of singing, only the speaking aspect of voice as it applies to theater--unless someone trained in his method has begun to teach singers again?

Finding Your Lowest Note. Strengthening and Extending Your Low Notes.

Perform some head rolls followed by shoulder crunches; open your mouth very wide a couple of times, then relax; now take your attention inward. Feel your Center in the middle of your chest.

a) The best vowel for low singing is "**O, oh, ow,wow,wow**." Try it. Slacken your lower jaw and feel the note inside you, then take it as low as it wants to go. If you have a piano, it's interesting to find the note you've landed on and to see if you can possibly make it any lower. *Feel very relaxed as though the tone is rolling out from the very bottom of your throat and vibrating your chest.* The sound doesn't have to be loud and booming, you just need to be ON the tone softly and steadily. Then take it one note higher and feel if you have more strength of tone; if you do, try and bring that same resonance to the lower note. If you can't - you may be able to after the following exercise.

b) Now from your lowest tone, sound upwards very gradually, a semitone at a time. Begin with a long "**Ooh,**" - extend the sound by stretching your mouth to "**Aow**" - the same sound as in "**now,**" or "**cow,**" pulling the tone in and out by widening and narrowing your lips and the space inside your mouth, ending with one very long note. Perform two or three of these extended tones on each ascending semitone.

c) Continue upward in this manner through five or six semitones from your lowest note. Take deep breaths between each tone and keep relaxed.

d) Now again sound your previous lowest note and notice the difference--there's usually a distinct improvement. In my case, I can frequently go another two or three semitones lower than where I began. It also helps to drop the jaw and incline your head slightly towards your chest while you sound the tone...*but eventually you have to be able to produce the same tone with your chin in the normal position.*

e) A further exercise begins from your lowest note and *ascends* eight notes through a perfect major scale; sing this with very long repeated **"Oh's"** (one **"Oh"** for each note). Then take the same scale *down,* returning to your original note.

Variations:

e1) Take it more **rapidly** up and down **one** octave, maintaining purity of tone.

e2) Take it more **rapidly** up and down **two** octaves.

We have been working the very lowest end of the vocal range; the interesting part is that your lowest note could be quite different tomorrow! The above exercises strengthen this area of the voice and encourage the development of 'male' voices within the female range and richness and power of tone within the male range.

Finding (and extending) Your Highest Note.

Immediately following the low range exercise, relax and as you switch directions mentally breathe to the spaces in your skull around your eyes and think of high sounds and lightness. Pause, and practice the Galactic Breath for several moments *(see page 9).*

a) Now return to your low range and from your base note, commence to sing just *a little higher,* where your voice feels more strong and vibrant, then start sounding very short bursts of **"Kah, kah, kah,"** -- the tone ascends with each **"kah."** *Don't worry about the individual notes - just glide quickly upwards.* The higher you get, the lighter the tone, until you can't sing any higher; the **"kah,kah,kah,kah"** ascending scale can only go so far, at that point you end with one long **"Kaaaaaa-aaaaaaaaah."**

That feels like your top note, correct?--wrong!

b) Following your extended high note, pause, take a breath into your belly and sing another long **"Kaaaaaaah"** <u>one note higher than the last.</u> And as you do so, send the **"Kaaa"** through the top of your head and out into space to the center of our Milky Way galaxy (as in the Galactic breath). After that, you'll feel yet *another* note higher again--that you *know* you can sing; pause, take another belly-breath and **"Kaaaaaaaah"** the next highest one (out to space).....and so on until you've attained a new apogee.

c) Try several upward swoops of **"Ka,ka,ka,ka,ka,"** to your high notes, repeating the sequence from **a)** to **b).** *You'll be amazed at how much higher you can reach with this technique. It also stretches your belief system and enables your throat to open, so after a while your preliminary ascending* **"Ka,ka,ka's"** *will reach higher each time.*

Note: The "Kah" sound loosens up the higher voice because it has the energy of the bliss arising from the sexual centers behind it. The bliss releases creativity and joy.

The Feline Approach! Sorry, for cat owners only.

Another more playful technique for opening the throat to higher tones depends on your cat--and if your cat has a high enough meow! *I am serious.* I enjoy the company of a pure bred, tortoise shell Persian with a squashed-in face. Whether the inbred flat face has anything to do with my cat's high-pitched meow, I have no idea. (This story *does* lead somewhere!) At one point in my struggles to release a stubborn throat block, I began trying to imitate the exact sound of my cat's meow. When I could duplicate the sound and voiced the top **"Ow"** (which I discovered was seven semitones above the initial **"Me"** in **"Me-ow"**), something inside me reasoned, *"If you can* **speak** *the meow perfectly, you should be* *able to* **sing** *the top note of the "Ow."* I tried and instantly could do it. The spoken "meow" loosened up my throat and that's when I hit my first **A** flat in 35 years! My cat doesn't always meow that high, but it gave me confidence and removed my boundaries to singing higher than I ever thought I could. However, I think cat's voices depend on the personality and the breed, you'll have to find out for yourself.

Regardless of your feline's genealogy, If you start following your cat's voicings with the object of imitating them, you'll frequently hear a reversed tonality in the "Meow" - sometimes the cat puts the highest pitch at the beginning instead of the end. Practice sounding and 'saying' the meow both ways. It's a marvelous exercise for stretching the upper soft palate and the very back of the throat that tends to tighten up with doubt when you want to sing very high. In lieu of a cat, the ascending **"Kah"** will also open the throat.

With regards to overloading the vocal cords, always be your own judge to monitor how your throat feels. Don't force, rest frequently and intersperse exercises with the Galactic Breath from Chapter 4.

Finally for new singers--you might consider obtaining a delightful and useful video about voice called "Learn to Sing Overnight." It will give you all the basic rudiments of singing technique...which you could then apply to the ideas and exercises given in this Chapter.[5]

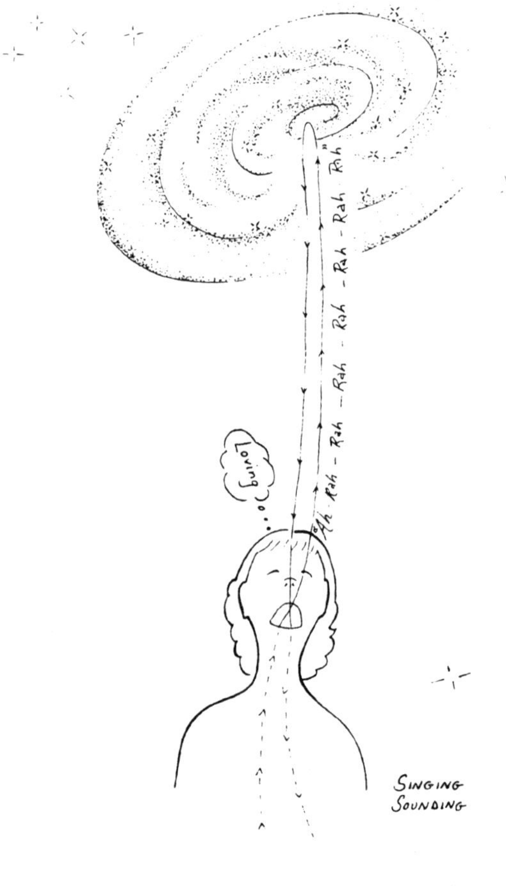

[5] Send to: Overnight Music Series, 78-080 Calle Estado #2A, LA QUINTA, CA. 92253-9963.

13..... RELEASING THROAT BLOCKS

A throat block restricts the amount of energy available to the throat, causing vocal weakness. **Classic throat block signs:** a preponderancy towards colds, throat infections, laryngitis; self restraints to creativity, plus a nagging feeling of being limited, unworthy and of not 'having a voice' - often due to childhood conditioning, abuse or trauma.

Some people carry blocks only in respect to singing; ordinarily, their voices seem normal and strong; to hear them speak you'd never dream they couldn't carry a tune or their throats close up whenever they attempt to sing. I've also heard the opposite story--of glorious professional singers whose speaking voices sounded weak and reedy. A third variety includes persons who can neither speak *or* sing well--the extremely restricted! This category has two possibilities, the first includes the genuinely traumatized or neurotic; the second represents a class of beings set apart by either mental or creative genius; they endure the required social-banter but psychologically there's no point in them speaking - "Hardly anyone can understand where I'm coming from--or can communicate with me on my level--so why bother to speak?"

When we speak, we each have a personalized range of tonal expression--it's the normal way we deal with the outside world; it's how we verbalize when we interact with strangers, chat with friends, call the dog or hail a taxi. The singing voice however, is another matter entirely. Countless people go through life without ever using--or ever *desiring* to use it! Song arises from a completely different place, a deep creative core that releases us into expressive joy--or poignant sorrow. It also provides the easiest and most powerful link into higher Spirit through the inner-voices. Actually another voice block does exist (one that has been *my* personal challenge), with it you have the freedom to sing from the inner realms, but struggle to sing with the ordinary voice.

This Chapter contains a large number of different techniques, all useful in understanding and releasing throat blocks. Choose the ones that appeal to you, but above all - rediscover your lost voices. These include the weird exploratory sounds, the squeals, yells and cries of your infancy, childhood and even your youth and maturity--all the sounds that were "shushed," shouted down or otherwise suppressed. They form the words you never spoke, the songs you never sang and remain bottled in your being, impacted in your cells. Deeper still lurk the voices of your sub-selves (past lives?) that speak out and sing forth when you open the channels to their expression....giving women deep and resonant male voices, and men astonishing alto and soprano tones! In the following exercises you'll have the opportunity to release your inner sounds and investigate the total range of all your remarkable voices.

All varieties of throat block share the same core origin--a damaged Emotional Body.

For some, the damage can be traced to infant (pre-verbal) rejection, abandonment and abuse; others track theirs to remembered put-downs (usually from childhood/youth), and even severe childhood and adult molestation. A deeper and more inaccessible source can lie in past life experiences. *(A great body of work has now been written on past life therapy by the therapists themselves. As a sampler, try to find the classic from the 60's, "Many Lifetimes" by psychiatrist Denys Kelsey and his wife Joan Grant, or "Past Lives Therapy" by Morris Netherton, Ph.D. and Nancy Shiffrin (an interesting book from the late 70's), and one from the 80's--also by a psychiatrist, "Many Lives, Many Masters" by Brian L. Weiss, M.D.)*

Physical Clearing.

Although you think you're releasing your throat by exercising the voice, the damage doesn't just lodge in the throat, it extends throughout the entire physical and emotional body in the form of a general holding-pattern (or a series of holding-patterns). Combining sound with movement helps break up and loosen those patterns. But first, turn to Chapter 17, "Energy Exercises" and try the series of movements under section **1...a)** called "Clearing the Inner Field." Then proceed to the excellent instructions for releasing the upper body in Chapter 4, do these first before adding sounds.

Grounding the Crud with Sound.

As you sound, visualize all of your miseries and complaints draining out into the ground.

1) **Moaning DOWN** ....Stand, feet shoulder width apart for balance, then hang your arms, head and torso forward from the waist, swaying from side to side. Now make sounds; begin with a series of freely expressed groans, moans, sighs, squeals, screams and roars (whatever bursts out of you), let it *all* come out!

A note for the more Ample Bodied. *If you're blessed with a paunch that won't let you comfortably hang over it (or you have back problems) - rather than dangling your arms down to the floor - bend your knees a bit and hunker down supporting your hands on your knees with elbows out. Begin the following exercises in this position and see how much movement you can add to it.*

1a) Sounding UP ....Take a deep breath or two as you return to an upright position. Now instead of groaning and moaning begin to make all kinds of freeing and wonderful tones and noises, and keep your head high and torso moving, arms swinging, stretching, wriggling and shuddering.

1b) Sounding DOWN ....Bend from the waist again, hang your head down and sing your sounds upside down. Finish upright with at least three deep, sighing breaths.

Upward Release.

This reminds me of those delightful Buddha statuettes with their arms flung high in the air.

2) **"The Joyful Buddha:"** Begin by hanging down again from the waist; start singing on a low note - then glide the sound up, simultaneously straightening and flinging your arms high in the air as you hit your top note!

Repeat the Upward Release two or three times.

All this physical posturing helps you free yourself from holding-patterns that affect your voice; you don't have to do it every day--although in the beginning stages, it might be a good idea! You're trying to activate your total sound instrument not just the vocal cords.

Dissolving Holding Patterns by Sounding Vowels.

One of the most powerful ways of generally opening and empowering the voice appears in Chapter 4, "Releasing the Voice" (inspired by musicologist Don Campbell's vowel voicings - I have added the *meanings* of the letters along with additional voicings). In this Chapter we'll concentrate on the vowels especially tailored for releasing throat blocks - **"A" "E"** and **"O."**

Vowel A - the power of identity - the sense of ego strength or ego loss.

Equivalent body parts - **face/eyes/brain** and the function: **perception** - reveals how you perceive your world and how you register all your ego reactions. The main reactor being the face...."his face fell" or, "his face lit up." **Think of:** loss of face, an about-face, facing-up, putting on a 'new' face, and face forward. Personal insults and put-downs are literally taken 'face first' and cruel remarks are often called "a slap in the face," so our faces come in for a tremendous amount of emotional punishment, most of which gets stored in the cheek muscles. The following **"A"** exercises release blocked facial energy and open you to a new sense of your own self worth.

Crinkle your nose and stretch your mouth into an exaggerated smile revealing your upper teeth and gums--then sound the most forward version of the letter **"A"** *(as in* **"at"** *and* **"apple"***), but make this normally short sound very long and sustained for the duration of the breath.....***"Aaaaaaaaaaaaaaaaa-aaaaaaaaaaaaaa."** *Hold this mouth position (with the crinkled nose) for all of the following exercises.*

a) Begin by making this 'flattened,' extended **"A"** in the form of a long, breathy, (voiceless) sigh. For me, this sounds like the tide-surf, pushing its frothy fingers up, up, up the beach, then pulling them back again to the tumbling sea, only to rush madly shore-ward again at the tips of the next thrusting wave. I call these sounds "wave-sighs." When you breathe forth the **"A"**....it's the wave-tips rushing up the sand; when you breathe in again....it's their returning to the sea. You can even lean forward and back as you breath in and out. Try this visualization-motion-breath several times, until you feel soothed and relaxed. *Tap your cheeks all over with your finger tips to release any tension.*

b) Next, picture an old, neglected wooden door. Use the same flattened "**A**" (as in "**at**") but make the low (audible), rumbling, tentative, sometimes squeaky sound of a creaking door, a door that's just being opened after a very long time of shut-tightness. Gradually hear and feel the door opening wider and wider (while still maintaining the same mouth position). This sounds more like a deep 'rumble' in the throat, rather than a pure tone and when you grumble to a stop, there's usually breath left, so let it out in a strong expiration--the sound of the air rushing through the newly opened door!! *Finish by tapping all over the face.*

c) Other flattened "A" sounds to play with:

1c) The thin, intermittent (yet maddeningly persistent) whine of a mosquito.

2c) A race car gathering speed as it comes towards you (steadily raise the pitch).

3c) The race car rushes past you (increase and lower the volume **and** the pitch.).

4c) Combine the last two ideas continuously (you're watching the Indi-500!).

5c) A factory siren. A World War Two air raid warning. *Have fun - be a noisy five-year-old! At some point during these and your own explorations, a tone will arise as* **'the'** *most powerful and resonate--that's usually your recharging tone--the one that releases; it doesn't necessarily have to be a pretty sound, in fact, it could be gratifyingly strident!! For all of the above, keep the* "**A**" *flattened and forward.* When sung in this manner (with lifted upper lip and cheeks), you will eventually experience a slightly painful, yet marvelous stretching-release that proceeds from the point where the cheek muscles insert themselves each side of the nose, and extends across to the outer cheek bones. It also opens the passages behind the nose, and (when using higher notes), exercises the soft palate. After sounding, you'll feel blood rushing into the area - as though some long-held identity pattern (established by holding-in the face) has been released. The sinuses may even tingle for some time after. A new energy will be present in your face. It will feel more alive.
Now sound the "A" in the other ways suggested in Chapter 4, "Releasing the Voice."
Work with "**A**" *when the sense of self has been wounded, suppressed or denied.*

Vowel E - the power of speech, the ability--or the inability to communicate freely.

Equivalent body parts - **throat/larynx** and the function: **voice/speech** - reveals your degree of self confidence through the way you speak and otherwise express yourself. **Think of:** he gave voice to; the voice failed, spluttered, screeched, sobbed, pleaded, raged, giggled, grated; the words gagged, stifled, strangled in his throat; her throat stopped; she had no voice in the matter.
When the throat is blocked, a lot of other things are blocked as well. Ask yourself...are you expressing yourself, your abilities, your life, in the way that **you** want? Frequently this kind of block spawns an intense fear to think, speak and act from your core-self, to **be** who you really are, to create freely and to share your ideas with others. These factors connect also to the holding-pattern in the face.

The face-releasing exercises already given for letter "**A**" also apply to letter "**E;**" just sound "**E**" instead of "**A**" - and again, you use the flattened **'e'**-sound (as in "**extra,**" **elephant**" and "**eloquent**"). In this case, an extended "**Eeeeeeeeeeeeeeeeeeeee**" would have a similar sound to "**air**" **(but without the 'r' at the end)**, or how you say **'e'** in the word "**egg.**" Remember to do the exaggerated smile with the lifted lips and crinkled nose. All the exercises are the same, begin with the whispered "wave-sigh" on the beach, then progress from the creaking door through to the other noises and don't forget the 'face-tapping' after each series of sounds.
Now sound the "E" in the other ways suggested in Chapter 4, "Releasing the Voice."
Work with "**E**" *when there is an inability (or fear) to speak easily, clearly and strongly and/or to create and express in other ways--be it in music, art, literature or anything else that you need to communicate.*

Vowel O - emotions, the power of nurturing, the ability to receive and give pleasure; to wonder, and when reversed**--neediness and sorrow.** Equivalent body parts - **stomach/ breasts** and the function: **nurturing/digestion** - reveals your nurturing skills towards yourself and others. **Think of:** she/he gives me a gut's ache, makes me sick to my stomach; it was like a blow to the stomach; it left me with an empty feeling in my guts; my stomach ached at the thought of it; I have no stomach for this task; the situation is hard to digest; I cast him from my breast - received him **to** my breast; she felt a yearning in her breast - she beat her breast in anguish.

The most potent letter for getting in touch with suffocated emotions, vowel **"O"** also releases the core-pain from being denied a mother's emotional support--and any other disappointing mother-surrogates you may have attracted. This inner core-pain will show up at the darndest times! Sometimes you're going about your business feeling fine with the world, then out of the blue, you're hit by a strong commiserate reaction to someone or something. Anything will do it, from an "in your face" experience," a book, newspaper or magazine, a film or TV program. In these odd instances (through empathy), you're actually touching the tip of your own emotional iceberg and can use these reactions to your advantage to release some of your own unresolved pain. Next time you get one of these very strong feelings, try and sustain it while you gracefully retreat, grab a soft pillow (or a stuffed Teddy bear) and begin to **"Oooooooooooooooooooooohwww"** with a vengeance! Public places aren't the best for surrendering to paroxysms of grief! I can remember after a particularly potent film ("Shadow lands," the life of C.S.Lewis with actor Anthony Hopkins), trying to sustain my intense anguish all the way home in a friend's car!!

Refer also to the sounding instructions for "O" in Chapter 4, "Releasing the Voice."

Work with **"O"** *when you look back on your life and see more sorrows and emotional needs than joys; sound it daily as a grief-relief until you feel all of your moans and tears have been uttered, then begin to sing its other more joyful and "wondering" sounds.*

The Diaphragm.

We spoke briefly about the diaphragm in Chapter 3, "The Body as a Musical Instrument," here we'll consider it as the muscle that can suppress emotion. Author Ken Dychtwald's interesting book "Bodymind,"[1] contains a section on the diaphragm in which he describes the way it blocks uncomfortable feelings (containing them in the lower body) from flowing upward and being fully felt. He also points out that pleasurable responses will also be dulled along with painful ones, eventually leading to a muscle armoring that freezes the diaphragm into a permanent 'holding-pattern.' A supple and strong diaphragm plays an essential role in the production of a free voice; I include my own exercises below for releasing this muscle. Curiously, whenever I'm singing and notice a weakness or lack of steadiness in certain tones and then do the diaphragm release, there's always an immediate improvement--which leads me to suspect those particular notes of hiding unresolved traumas.

The Diaphragm "Bellows-Breath" Release.

In this, you expel the breath upwards from the midsection with a sudden and forcible contraction of the diaphragm - much like the strong puff of air you get from working an old fashioned pair of bellows; but not only that, it's also important to move the muscle down as well as up.

The downward movement.

1) Take something heavy (such as a weighty book), lie flat on your back with your knees up. Place the book across your midsection just below the rib-cage.

2) Now breathe **in** deeply - **down** into your belly; then breathe **out** and **upwards** with a soundless **"Ha,"** as though shooting the breath right though the top of your head to the stars - to the center of the gallaxy itself!! (Also breath **in**, as though breathing *from* the center of the gallaxy.[2])

Give yourself about ten breaths, try to make the object on your belly move and wobble, rise and fall. If necessary PUSH your stomach out as you take the breath down into it!

---

[1] Refer to Chapter 5, "Abdominal Region and Lower Back."

[2] For more information on the Galactic Breath, see Chapter 4, "Releasing the Voice."

Discontinue the downward movement floor-and-book routine when you've got the idea of "breathing into the belly" and concentrate on the **upward movement** *exercise.*

The upward movement.

1) Get up from the floor and stand tall.

2) Now bend over and hang from the waist, knees slightly bent, your arms dangling.

3) In this ungainly posture breathe **deeply into** the belly.

4) Then, with a strong contraction of the belly (this is the "bellows" action) shoot the air **up** through the chest as you say **"HUH!"** Occasionally, do it rapidly as though you're panting like a large dog that's just chased a car! Stand up straight periodically so you don't drain too much blood to your head! *Alternately, this can also be done while bending forward and grasping the knees for support.*

5) Continue to do this (deep-belly-to-upward-movement) **"HUH"** breath, initially, with or without adding sound - although the effort of sounding may release more--so aim to eventually make some kind of noise with every **"HUH."** You'll know when you've done enough. And yes, you *will* have a sore diaphragm at first, until you've released and strengthened it.

The most noticeable benefits occur on your thinnest sounding, weakest notes. Try an experiment. You'll need a piano/keyboard or other instrument. Play the note that you want to improve on, sing it in your usual less-than-perfect way, do the "Bellows Breath," then immediately sing the problem note again. You'll notice a marked improvement; the emotions weighing on that particular tone will continue to dissolve as the diaphragm changes from a barrier into a doorway. Relax and repeat several times, then apply the **Galactic Breath** technique from Chapter 4. Once the note has become clear and steady, you can further develop its strength with other exercises.

Sounding Your Name to Release your Throat.

Next to the vowels **"A," "E,"** and **"O,"** the sounds of your own name (its letters and syllabic sounds) are enormously important. Many times, the cues to releasing throat blocks lie dormant and waiting in the energy of your given name (the one on your birth certificate). Turn back to Chapter 11, "Sounding Your Name," and to the section at the very beginning called "Quick Version." Singing through your name in this fashion reconnects you to your life's purpose and you'll begin to access and unlock its energy; also, be sure to look up the meanings of all the letters in your name. (Refer to Chapters 6, 8 and 9.)

Dealing with Anger.

A damaged emotional body brings sorrow, regret, even anger and blame; these feelings block the throat (and your life) from receiving pleasure, joy and delight. Practicing the previous exercises helps throw out emotional gunk, but for some of us, a deep intense anger lurks beneath our tears. If this describes you, your throat block contains more rage, frustration and despair, than sorrow! And certainly some of us combine the two--sorrow *and* rage. *Here follows some rage-diffusing techniques - if you're game enough to try them!.*

Growing Your Canine Teeth.

Let your upper and then lower lip muscles flex and stretch, then imagine your gums swelling as your canine teeth grow into enormous fangs. These are your animal weapons and your feelings of rage and fury have now come **into** *your teeth and lips. Your eyes will feel a new energy in them and will either widen or narrow into slits.*

Sounding Your "Animal" Power.

Still feeling this marvelous power in your face, curl your lip and begin with the almost soundless, threatening, spitting, snarl of a large wild cat - **"Aaaaahrr."** *Try several of these and deep in your throat growl some final warning* **"Aaaaaaaahhrrrr's"**! *Now you're ready to sound forth your anger and frustrations with sung or shouted* **"Aaahh, rah,rah,rah,rah,rah,rah, raaaaaaaaaaaaaah's."** *Vary the tone* *and the pitch according to your emotions. Remember old frustrations, incidents--even faces! Feel and release the rage, then open wide and roar like a triumphant lion. Keep "roaring" until a sense of satisfaction and even glory fills you.* These sounds resonate the nasal septum and at times you'll seem to be singing from the corners of your eyes! The procedure may stir up and loosen thick mucous in your throat, if so, gently clear it; cough if necessary, swallow several times and take a few sips of cold water. Next, scrunch and release your shoulders, move your head from side to side and stretch the back of your neck to discharge any tension you may have built up, then take several deep breaths. Finally, allow yourself to relax completely for a few moments and practice several healing Galactic Breaths (page 9).

Dealing With Fear.

It's a familiar story.....you feel propelled to move in certain directions, but failure and self-sabotage always interfere. Why such a struggle to sustain free-expression and success? Have you accepted 'failure-programming' but don't realize it? Some of us fear success and the responsibility that it brings more than anything. "How could I handle being successful, I'm not worthy!"....or, "Then I'd have to give up all my blaming and excuses!"

This fear intrudes into speaking and singing because the voice reflects our freedom to express ourselves and fear constricts the voice. Even the most earnest desire to speak and sing will hit a wall of resistance when fear lurks in the background. The harder we try, the more strongly the throat closes and any calculated use of the voice (such as preparing to give a speech, or trying to learn a song) shuts it down. Result - frustration and despair! If you suffer from a long history of throat blockage, the old resistance most certainly will rear its ugly head when you attempt regular singing lessons and vocal exercises--and it's hard not to give up when.....*"Darn it, there goes my throat, closing down again as usual!*

The next time your voice fails ask yourself if it's happening out of fear, or interference from pre-conditioned sub-selves. Many of our wounded inner-selves (including past life personalities), periodically commandeer our voices with their hidden fears and doubts.....particularly when we're attempting to overcome their practice of restricting our throats. The traumatized inner-child and our 'selves' from the past (with their hidden vows or curses!) need healing as much as our surface personalities and are often responsible for certain inexplicable and uncontrollable emotional responses, compulsions and cravings.

Disassociation for the Voice.

Be very aware and feel the fear or block to your singing/speaking then say:

(Part One)

"Fear of singing (speaking) **is present, (**or **resistance** is present,)
I am not the fear-resistance ,
I am the Infinite Spirit of effortless song (and powerful speech)**."**

Breathe deeply and evenly and repeat several times until you feel the resistance diminish.

Now you can also add if you wish:

"I am the glorious Voice of Spirit.
I am the Infinite Word of peace and power."

*BUT, when there is very little response to these efforts, you can assume the presence of pre-programming in the form of sub-selves, so **to** your resistant sub-personalities say:*

(Part Two)

"Fear of singing (speaking) **is present, (**or **resistance** is present,)
You (or we) **are not the fear-resistance,**
You (we) **are the Infinite Spirit of song and speech."**
You (we) **are the glorious voice of Spirit.**
You (we) **are the Infinite Word of peace and power."**

Emotional Healing for the Voice.

While holding your throat with both hands, begin first with Part Two of "Disassociation for the Voice" and proceed to the following:

> **"I acknowledge that in my essence,**
> **I am the Infinite Voice of higher Spirit.**
> **And I acknowledge that in *your* essence** (my sub-selves),
> **You are *also* -**
> **The Infinite Voice of higher Spirit.**
>
> **Whatsoever in the past has separated us**
> **From freely sounding our voice,**
> **I now accept - for us,**
> **I now forgive - for us,**
> **And I now release us -**
> **To live in the Light as the Sound of Love.... So it is."**

The above exercises are <u>*the most effective and unfettering*</u> *when you find yourself in the* **actual** *grip of a serious throat close-down. Example:* you have just been singing gloriously or speaking magnificently, *"Wow!" you think..."I'm really doing well this time!!"* But suddenly you begin to cough for no reason. The coughing increases and you notice with some alarm that the spasms seem to be steadily closing down the air passages to your lungs. The raw fear of not getting enough air takes over and you even dry-retch in an attempt to clear the psycho-physical obstruction....but the histamine reaction only increases! **You are now directly in touch with deep throat-block fear.** Immediately, command yourself to relax and in order to tamp down the rising panic begin to breathe VERY gently and try not to cough. *At that moment* - hold your suffering throat with both hands and repeat first Part One and then Part Two of the "Dissociation" several times...followed by the "Emotional Release." Soon the feelings in your throat will change completely; the fear abates, the muscles and tissues return to their normal state while warmth and energy extends into the face itself - as though it's being massaged and rearranged! (A somewhat terrifying experience, particularly when it happens in public--but with a very powerful release if you do the above....*and one which I can personally attest to!!)*

Releasing with the "N" Resonator.

The following are expansions on instructions (for **"N"**) *already given in* Chapter 4. *They help you defy conditioned suppression and allow you to say "No" to the internal voices that persistently sabotage your efforts. Actually, you'll be sounding* **"Na"** *- which means the same thing.*

1) Commence by clenching your teeth together and sounding a long sustained **"Nnnnnnnnn."** *Remember to bare your teeth in a continuous snarl of defiance.* Try several long **"Nnnnnnnnn's"** on different notes; then sound it as though you're 'revving' up an engine: **"<u>N</u>nn--<u>N</u>nn--<u>N</u>nn--<u>N</u>nn"** finishing with another long **"Nnnnnnn."** When doing the "engine revving," contract your belly strongly with each 'rev' to push the sound out. Do this sequence until you feel a strong vibration in your skull.

2) With your bared teeth <u>still clenched</u>, begin with the **"Nnnnnnnn"** and then turn it into **"Na,na,na,na,na,na, naaaaaah."** (Try the engine-revving on the **"aaaah"** sound.) *Still keep your teeth clenched and be sure to establish a strong inner resonance.*

3) Again start with **"Nnnnnn,"** and continue into **"Na,na,na,"** but this time <u>*open your mouth*</u> to sound a fully *open* **"Na,na,na,"** finishing with a long, loud, wide **"Naaaaaaah!"** If a disapproving face (or faces) come up from your past--snarl **"Na,na"** to those face(s)! *Repeat this to your heart's content.*

Extra "N" Exercises.

Now that you've done the defiant and discharging work of this letter, you can sound it from its mode as a "bringer of balance." On the days when your voice seems fresh and there's no inner resistance, try these stretching, balancing - and fun exercises.

1) Using the **"Nnnnn"** (and being as smooth as you can), begin low and **"Nnnn"** rapidly up and down a long scale of two or three octaves. Take a breath and repeat. Keep relaxed and repeat several times. Enjoy the inner sensations as you make the sounds.

2) Still using **"N,"** begin on any note and repeatedly take it up and down a very *small* scale.

3) Still sounding **"N,"** begin with a note in the middle of your range, then sound **"N"** *down* as far as you can go. Repeat several times.

4) Do the same as **3)** but in the opposite direction - *up* as far as you can go.

All of the above **"N"** *work makes the soft palate flexible and opens the nasal sinuses. You can try them with the assistance of a piano, an electronic keyboard - or just approximate the scales in your mind and let your own voice play!*

5) If you happen to be learning an actual song, instead of singing the words, sound **"Na, na, na"** (one **"Na"** for each word). This extends, exercises and strengthens a great many very small muscles in your voice mechanism that you never dreamed existed. You'll find it quite a workout and on returning to the words, they'll be easier to sing!

In the past, my own throat-block sometimes reared its ugly head when I did the "N" exercises. My upper palate and inside my throat would tighten and swell (as well as my nasal passages) with a histamine 'fear' reaction. Something inside me seemed to whisper *"You can't defy the powerful person!"*-- and then my voice would begin to close down. At that point, rather than push it and end up strained and frustrated, I would immediately stop - do a "Fear of singing is present, I am not the fear..etc." and when everything had relaxed, I'd make another **"N"** attack; persisting with several attempts at doing the exercises throughout the day if necessary! *All this was extremely frustrating in the light of my effortless and joyous sounding with the inner-voices!!*

The 'Semi-Silent Treatment.'

When you first decide to overcome a stubborn and ingrained throat block, just one practice session can give a serious shock to the vocal mechanism. Best take the next day off to let the throat recover and sing only on alternate days until your voice becomes stronger. On the days you don't sing, set aside a similar amount of time in which to expand your breath capacity by blowing into large empty bottles, playing your pan-flute (if you have one) and stretching and moving your face and jaw muscles -- *and by practicing the Sounding exercises mentally.* When you sing soundlessly inside your head, the vocal muscles still carry out minute movements similar to actual singing. Many athletes use 'mental practice' techniques for improving performance - and not only athletes! Years ago in Europe, a female opera singer was in preparation for an important role but had to undergo unexpected throat surgery and as a result, could not use her voice for a number weeks. During those weeks, she practiced mentally every day and at the end of the imposed silence sang her role to perfection.

You could also use a piano or some other instrument and play the notes to give you an external reference while you sing them in your head. After a couple of weeks of alternating sound and silence days, begin to sing with full voice on the first day and 'softened' voice on the second. Eventually you'll graduate to singing effortlessly every day as you relax more and stop being afraid. **For fear, also do the Disassociation Exercises commencing on page 105.**

After you've finally cleared away the emotional blocks, you're dealing with the purely physical level--and all throats are not equal! They vary in capability from day to day, so please remember when practicing to let your muscles fully recover before another burst of singing. If your speaking voice sounds thick and scratchy, don't try to sing again; it's too close to your last practice and the muscles haven't recovered enough. Wait until your speaking voice returns to normal. *Also, at first keep your practice times short. The secret to strengthening muscles is to let them rest and rebuild after the pressure of exercise.*

Brahmarie Humming to Strengthening the Voice.
Claimed (by Indian Yogis), to "strengthen and sweeten the voice," you'll find this Hatha Yoga technique described at the end of Chapter 4. For me, it opens the upper head passages and vibrates the skull, leaving me with a very clear and expanded feeling. It also extends the breath capacity and re-calibrates the brain if I'm feeling dull or head-ache-y.
But remember, if it hurts your throat to do it, you're not performing it correctly!

WORKING WITH GEMSTONES.

Using the gemstone malachite to Clear the Throat.
This dark green, striped, semi-precious stone is often used by crystal healers to draw blockages and impurities from the body. Small inexpensive specimens can be obtain from rock-shops or Gem Shows. For use on the throat, I fold my malachite up in a piece of silk, soft cotton, or just a narrow silk scarf and wrap it around my throat with the malachite positioned on the lower part of the throat (at the "V" notch above the two collar bones).

The Meditation.....*you can sit or lie down for this.*

1) Place the fingers and thumb of one hand on the clavicle (collar) bones that sit just above (and to each side of) the throat notch. Rapidly tap the bones with your fingers several times, then slide your fingers and thumb into the notch and stroke the throat firmly with an upwards motion over the thyroid area ending at the voice box (larynx). Repeat gently but firmly several times. Finally, tap the entire lower throat area lightly with your fingers.

2) Tie the malachite onto your throat.

3) Imagine a glowing malachite-green light surrounding your throat. It's as though this remains constantly around your neck and shoulders waiting to nourish you. Now, with each breath, breathe the deep green light **into** the area just massaged and where the piece of malachite is now resting. Ultimately you'll receive so much light that it flows in and out without depleting the glowing color you've imagined around your neck and shoulders.
As the malachite clearing breath is a preliminary to opening the Throat Chakra don't be suprised if the entire area begins to feel tingly and warm.

Wearing Amber to Unlock Emotions Held in the Throat.
This information came to me via a warlock, well, not personally--but you'll understand when you hear the story. Several years ago in Oregon, I had a friend whose husband created jewelry. I used to visit their shop and gaze longingly at the display of unset gems and semi-precious stones. One day I paused to stare at something quite new and amazing....it looked like a large pear-shaped, golden drop, with tiny, delicate leaves imbedded inside. I was about to ask its name, when to everyone's suprise and my own astonishment, I suddenly burst into tears. My sobs gasped for no reason and tears spilled down my cheeks! "My goodness--what IS that stone?" I managed through the waterworks. "It's not a stone," came the reply, "It's amber from the Baltic sea." I stepped back and just as suddenly--all tears ceased. The husband looked at me quizzically, "And you seem to have made quite an emotional connection, that means you're bonded to it now!"

I discovered that amber is really petrified prehistoric pine tree resin. Millions of years ago, it oozed out of trees as sap and in the process, sometimes entombed the insects and vegetation of those ancient times in its sticky gold. This particular piece of amber completely fascinated me, especially after my unbidden outburst of tears, but the 'gem' was not for sale, unless I also commissioned the craftsman to create a piece of jewelry around it. I went back several times to the tantalizing specimen and if I got too close, the tears would inexplicably appear! Totally puzzled and also frustrated that I couldn't just buy the amber and take it home, I finally related the incident to an acquaintance who said she had studied mysticism for several years in L.A. under a warlock (a male witch).

She told me that amber was a 'specific' for the Throat Chakra and had the power to release emotions trapped in the throat!

Needless to say, I now possess quite a lot of amber, and yes, a necklace *was* created for me out of that memorable piece....it became a Christmas present! I do recommend amber for the throat, but it needs to be worn quite close to where you feel the block. Earrings and necklaces are all very pretty, but they're usually too far away from the problem area. To aid your process, I suggest you purchase a couple of medium to large amber beads, string them on a cord and wear them around your neck for an indefinite period, or wrap a piece of amber in a turquoise silk scarf and tie it around your throat when you go to sleep.

The Amber Breath of Light Meditation.

1) Pinch-grip the lower throat (above the "V"-notch), slide the fingers and thumb up the entire length of the neck. *Repeat 3 or 4 times.* This stimulates the Throat Chakra.

2) Tie amber onto the throat.

3) Lift your arms and hands high above your head and breathe from an upper *Golden Light source* down to the amber at the throat. After establishing the breath, lower the hands to hold them in front of (but not touching) the throat.

Affirmation:

"I speak and sing (breathe in and down)....

....as the Voice of Light." (Breathe out and up to the golden light.)

Finally place your hands in your lap, keep the affirmation going - breathe from the throat UP to the light above the head and DOWN into the throat several times. Fill your body with golden light, then project it out into the world.

4) When going to sleep and wearing amber at the throat, do the above meditation but without the 'arms above the head' motion (or holding the hands in front of the throat). With the breath, simply establish the flow of golden light from above the head and down through the amber into the throat.

During the practice of this meditation, the Crown center on the top of your head may become sensitive or activated in some way and you could encounter a sudden expansion of awareness that is NOT clear, bright and pleasant - but foggy, discombobulated and uncomfortable. The throat is the 'gate' between the physical energy system (with its switching mechanisms in the brain) and the out of body Chakras above the head (with their connection to various expanded mind states and interdimensional realms); meditative work on the throat sometimes stimulates and opens these higher Chakras and we are not accustomed to the resulting sensations. The energy needs to be grounded to help us integrate the over-stimulation.

Grounding techniques.

Should discomfort continue at the Crown, behind your eyes or elsewhere in your head, stop instantly and try discharging with sound. Do the Brahmarie exercise (mentioned previously), then hum an arpeggio to the **"M"** *or* **"N"** *Resonator (beginning on a low note) to re-calibrate the brain;* ***then turn to something completely physical:*** *thoroughly massage each of your big toes and thumbs (energy meridians from the brain terminate in the thumbs and big toes); go into the garden, walk on the grass in bare feet; if the weather's inclement, walk with the rain on your face; eat something to ground the energy (bread and grains are best); jog, trampoline, play your drums--if you have some, or put on a tape and dance!* ***The process of integrating our other dimensional capacities unfolds gradually. The test is invariably the same: always remain sharply aware and in charge of your body!***

General Voice-Release Affirmations

I am a free and joyful singer.
I am a clear and powerful speaker.
I am the glorious voice of higher Spirit.
I am the Infinite Word of peace and power.
I am the limitless voice of higher Spirit,
I am the Infinite Presence of glorious Sound.

To end this Chapter we'll look briefly at the two other vowels **"I"** and **"U"** and their relationship to voice production. **"I"** not only energizes the third-eye/brain, it also governs the lungs, the breath and our ability to incorporate Prana (Life Force, Chi) *with* the breath.[3] The Prana brings bliss and unites us directly with Spirit. When we sing *as Spirit,* our voice is transformed. **"U"** governs the lower belly and Root Chakra, grounding us through our feet to the Earth Mother. It marks our firm foundation--our base for living in the body. When you breathe the Life Force in, you swell the lower belly and connect the energy through your feet to the core of the earth--here the voice finds its base support and solidness.

By now, you probably realize that a throat-block isn't necessarily just one thing; it's usually a combination of several factors and the above techniques address some of those factors. But here's a thought--your lack of voice strength might be hiding behind something entirely different. For me, I was refusing to paint or do any kind of regular art work....in spite of the fact that painting and sketching had been one of my great joys in the past. Within a few days of allocating myself the time....I was painting *and* singing joyously! So you *want* to be a singer--what else are you denying yourself? What other 'fear-of-doing' blocks have you placed *in front of* your voice. Allow them to happen--and the voice could automatically release. All self-expression links to the throat and to the Root Chakra; *this means:* the inspiration to create (or just to **be yourself** and **do your thing**) must be grounded, brought down (from speculation) and acted upon--if only for your own satisfaction and delight at having done something!!
Then, will your heart sing.

Finally, a more fundamental point of view based on the connection between the bones of the body and the Chakras (from **"The Body is the Barometer of the Soul, so Be Your Own Doctor II,"** *by Annette Noontil...see Bibliography) places all throat conditions in the category of "judgment" - in relationship to yourself and others. Stop judging (yourself and others) and the energy will flow freely through the thyroid area.*

To Release from Self-judgment:

"I accept - that all I have done in my life has been necessary.
All of the 'failures' were not really failures!
I have wasted nothing,
I have learned from everything."

To Release from Judging Others:

"I accept - that everyone
I have related to in my life,
Has been a necessary part
Of my learning process."

And this is the tough one....

"I attract everyone I need to learn from,
Regardless of who they are
And what they do (to me)."

"<u>I am responsible</u> for creating my life!"

---

[3] See "Accessing Instant Energy" beginning on page 159.

For a moment, let's translate the body into a metaphor - think of a vase, perhaps an elegant amphora from ancient Greece; the narrow neck of the vase (or jar) represents the throat, a gateway between the body and the higher Chakras. Physically, we are nothing more than *containers* stuffed with conditioning in the form of desires and karma from the separated-self known as "soul." The throat hides a secret--when ***its*** Chakra opens--so also does the door between the tangible physical body of the soul and the invisible, ineffable Light body of the higher Spirit.

Most traditions refer to a *descent* of Spirit into man. It's vibration appears to arrive from above, penetrate the top of the head then gradually (or suddenly) fill the body with power. Spirit (like God) is always thought of as UP....above our heads, somewhere in the heavens! *A correct perception as far as direction goes,* but instead of the old personification of deity coasting in the clouds, it refers to the extra-dimensional powers of our *own* being coming from out-of-body centers **above** the head. *(The ancient Chinese and Persians listed up to 8 extra power Chakras above the head and a present day visionary and international healer, Colin Bloy from Barcelona, Spain, works with 9.)* The descent of energy into the throat (and heart) opens channels between these upper centers and the rest of the body, with the "throat-gate" being the valve. This "fire" or power aspect of Spirit has a natural affinity for the Heart Chakra, where, united with the Inner Beloved,[1] it fuses an important link between the higher centers and our physical world.

The previous Chapter "Releasing Throat Blocks," does not address opening the Throat Chakra, although the meditations from that section can serve as preliminaries. *Occupying somewhat the same area, the throat and its Chakra normally function from very unrelated energy systems.*

A throat block manifests in the physical speech organs, circumventing the power of will and restricting the external speaking or singing voice (or both).

An unopened Throat Chakra restricts the interdimensional voices and although these voices *use* the physical speech organs, their ability to make sound originates from little used frequencies in the Life Field, including "the Higher Sound Current" and also the Third Ear within the Chi-body.

As already mentioned, many levels of inner voices exist. Mediums and psychic Channels generally use only minuscule levels from the frequency range available; they may channel one or maybe two voices from other dimensions, or as in the case of many Mediums, speak primarily for the earth-bound dead, or from teaching-entities in their own Life Field. In these cases, their Throat Chakras *do* function, but only marginally--and sometimes at the cost of total consciousness (when deep trance occurs). With a fully opened Throat Chakra, one does not enter a trance, instead, the usual awareness greatly expands--sharing center stage with a superior cognition not available in ordinary consciousness. From that very clear and energized state, the enhanced intelligence discerns and monitors the various forces wanting to sound through us - whether a disembodied entity needing assistance to exit the earth-plane, an inner-self guide giving encouragement or help, a Devic life-form communicating from a nature realm, Angelic Presences, or the transcendent tones of our higher Spirit.

When functioning from this rich and multi-level dimension of the inner sound--always, always be fully present! Within transcendent Mind, your ordinary mind remains clearly aware and even in total Self-union (although changed), you should still remain aware!

Only the "Fire from above" (or Spirit **as** fire), can initiate the total opening of the Throat Chakra. As intimated, this electrical-like energy descends from the upper Chakras and flows into the brain-nervous system, connecting the more refined Light Body energy into the physical and Chi energy grids. It brings shock waves of recharging bliss to the entire system and unlocks the "throat-gate" as the higher power centers in the heart.

That's an abbreviated description, I hope it doesn't sound too alarming - more precise details follow!

The sign that marks the opening of the throat in this manner has been known for centuries and called "the gift of tongues" (or glossalalia). Bewildered onlookers of old called it "The ecstatic stammerings of men and angels." Providing you keep the Chakra open in the days and months following this

---

[1]See Chapter 16, "Special Meditations," section 4.

profound event, you will start receiving other physical phenomena. These frequently begin in the lower back where you'll feel a periodic expansion of heat bringing wave-like vibrations flowing all over the body; the same thing can happen in the chest (or the chest and back simultaneously). You're now plugged into a new power socket! This higher octave energy seems to have a mind of its own and investigates the corporeal almost on whim; its task is to integrate the upper Light Body frequency with your two other major energy systems--the outer physical (combustion/electromagnetic) and the inner non-physical Chi (or Ki). At other times, your throat may become the focus of Spirit's attention and will tingle and burn with a strong (not entirely pleasant) heat. When this happens, stabilize the area by breathing turquoise or golden light into the persistent heat and tingling, also wear a piece of Amber[2] at the throat notch for a few days.

To further develop and maintain this union between your three different energy systems, I strongly recommend a daily "Sounding in the Spirit" - but first the 'opening.'

THE OPENING

Background: In several religious and esoteric traditions, Spirit has been regarded as a **single** *external* entity rather than a natural (though hidden), component of every human energy system. A confusion, perhaps, with the Ground of Being that comprises all things--including us--and could be more aptly called "Infinite Source" or "Presence." (You might say, "By that--don't you mean "God?" In a sense "Yes," but not the anthropomorphized version!)

Traditional 'Tarrying.'

These earlier historical gatherings devoted themselves to spiritual union in the fullest sense *in that they looked for an eventual physical transformation* and practiced the spontaneous uttering of glossalalia, (the sign of Spirit's presence and an opened Throat Chakra), as an aid to that transformation.

People wanting the opening would 'tarry' with several others who had already been initiated. They met for the express purpose of speaking in tongues and entering different states of ecstatic bliss caused by the powerful collective sounds recharging their three energy systems (the physical, Chi and Light bodies). This communal practice sometimes catalyzed even those with *unopened* Throat Chakras! Naturally, the larger the group, the greater the power! Modern ecstatic gatherings of this nature also generate enormous amounts of healing energy, especially if that's the meeting's intention; but the credit for any recoveries always goes to a pre-designated *external* deity or other archetypal power.
(A tendency occurring in 'civilized' as well as primitive societies.)

To assist the descent of Spirit into the heart and throat, traditional techniques use a familiar (New Age) idea - they set up a magnetic field. For this to happen, you must act and speak *as though the higher Spirit has already been received.* In the charismatic Christian method, they begin with the ordinary outer voice--singing phrases such as, "Alleluia, alleluia," "Thank you, thank you," or "Praise God," etc., until the higher energy (Spirit) descends from the upper Chakras and the inner voices begin to speak and sing.

Because your Light body and personal Spirit form a natural (through neglected) part of your *own* nature and your *own* super-physical energy, you can feel confident to welcome and receive this powerful part of your being - with or without archetypal invocation!

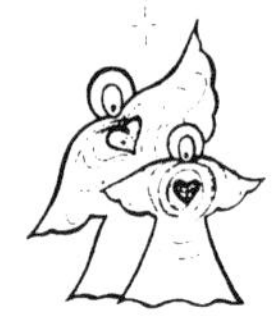

A PRELIMINARY

Sometimes the heart needs special preparation to receive the fire aspect of Spirit.
Refer to Chapter 16, "Special Meditations," <u>section</u> **4,** and decide whether you may want to actually open the Heart Chakra *before* attempting to bring in the higher Spirit.

---

[2]Refer to section on Amber in Chapter 13, "Releasing Throat Blocks."

Opening the Throat Chakra

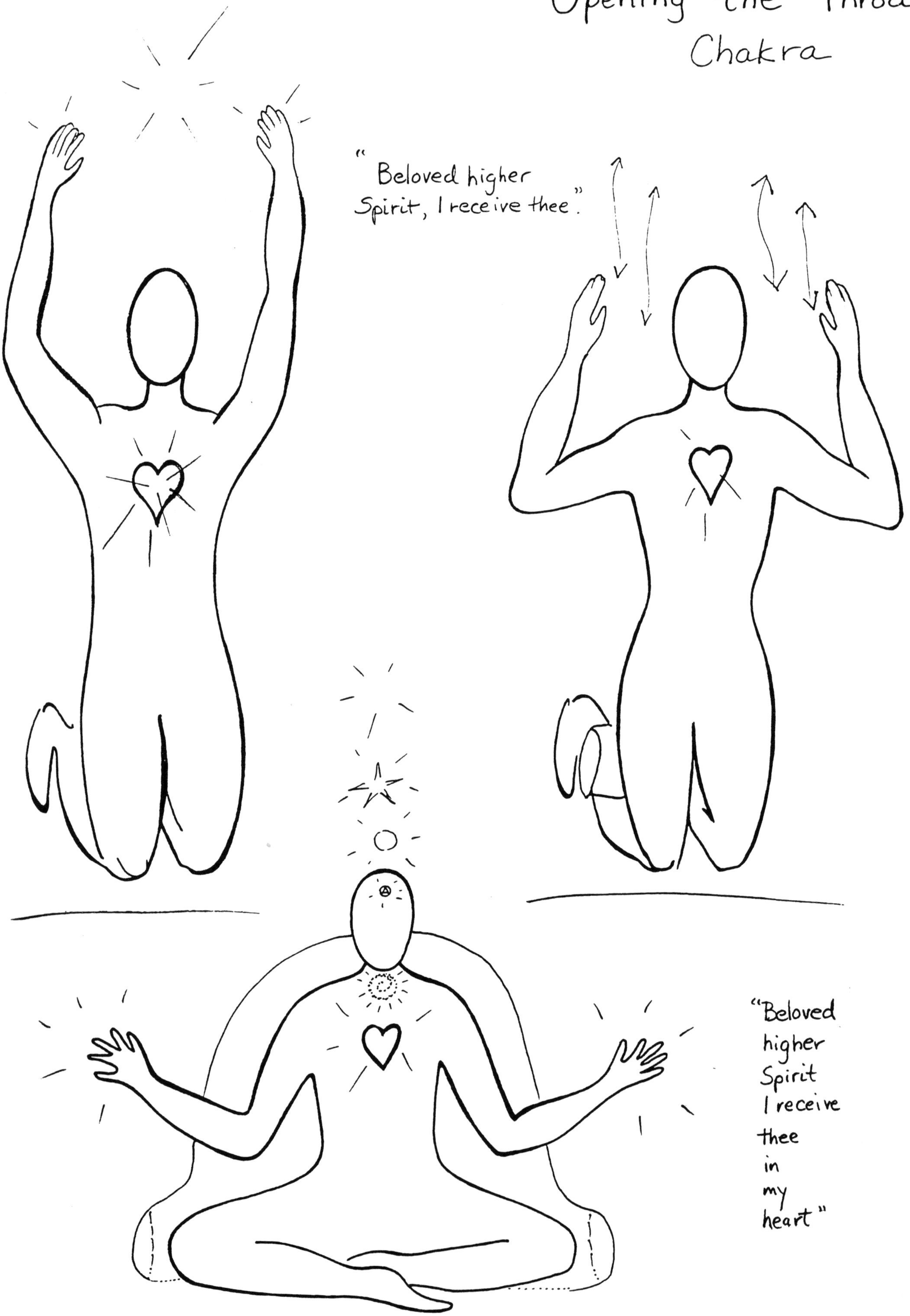

"Waiting on the Power."

That's what you say if you haven't yet opened to the power of your higher Spirit--you're "waiting on the Power." It took me six weeks of "waiting" 45 years ago to receive mine! Today, everything has speed-ed up enormously and I've had the joy of facilitating the process for others in seminars and workshops. Group energy provides the secret ingredient--when two or more agree to invoke their higher Spirits together, the power becomes greater than the individual sum of the parts. You might try and convene your own group of spiritual adventurers willing to give themselves this experience, but failing that, try at least to find *one* additional person to work with on a regular basis.

1) Whether you all decide to sit on the floor, up on chairs, or even kneel on the floor (and rest your elbows on the seats of your chairs), **it is important to keep your spines straight.** Your posture then assumes the perfect conducting rod for the upper energies to descend into the physical system! Now **lift up your hands to about level with your head**; *these are the antennae for your spinal conducting rod.* Hands contain magnetic centers (mini-Chakras), one in each palm and when you lift them up, the posture activates the extra Chakras above the head and provides an entering pathway for Spirit. The following invocation engages and aligns your emotional energy. Repeat it several times mentally until it warms your heart and fills you with a feeling of sweetness and joy. Your lifted hands and the crown of your head may begin to tingle and stream with energy.

INVOCATION TO THE HIGHER SPIRIT

Eternal lover of my soul,
Thou, who yearns to make me whole;

Immortal Spirit of my heart,
Return and claim thy broken part.

O Love, who shines eternally,
Restore my heart as part of Thee.

Lift your hands up even higher and feel that you are breathing the upper Light of Spirit **in and out** *of your hands as you mentally repeat several times:*

"Beloved higher Spirit, I receive thee."

(Lower your hands and rest your arms for a moment.)
Now lifting them up again - breathe **in** *through the hands as you say:*

"Beloved higher Spirit,"

Then direct the **out-breath** *down your arms and into the heart as you say:*

"I receive thee in my heart."

Repeat several times breathing the energy from the hands into the heart.

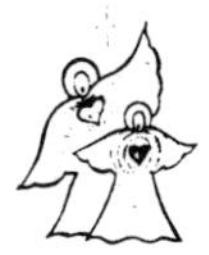

<u>While you're mentally reciting the above:</u>

1a) If you're kneeling up against a chair or other support and need a temporary change of position - place a small cushion across your lower legs and sink back on your heels, or use one of those tiny padded meditation seats that you slip your feet under. You can lift your hands up just as well while sitting back on your heels (or on the seat), but as soon as you feel rested, assume an upright kneeling position again. *The Spine should be in a straight line from the knees.*

1b) Periodically bring your hands high over your head--hold them there for a moment or two, then gradually move them down almost to your ears; repeat the movement several times; eventually, just keep your hands at shoulder height, or if you're leaning up against a bed or something similar, anchor your elbows on it with your hands up.

1c) For those of you preferring to sit, choose a lounge or large padded chair to seat yourself well back into; your raised arms (bent at the elbows) can rest comfortably against the lounge or padded back of the chair.

<u>What you are doing</u> with your antennae-hands is slowly pulling the upper Field down. You'll feel the energy first as a tingling in the palms, followed by a 'rippling' sensation on the scalp; even the air surrounding your head and shoulders becomes charged. Eventually, little energy currents run in waves down your head, shoulders, arms and back. *A whole group of people doing this can become positively electric!*

2) Once you feel the build-up of power, you *must* engage the throat and make audible sounds! Otherwise, the powerful upper energies will just charge through all your physical circuitry without opening the throat to the inner voices. A traditional term for this part of the process is called "Taming the unruly member" (the tongue)! Your ego/intellect must stand aside and surrender the audible voice to the power of your Spirit. The difference between the *conscious* sounds you'll be making and the highly energized inner sounds will prove quite unmistakable. Truly spontaneous sounds don't happen freely until after the throat has been fully opened; you begin by 'priming' the outer voice with something familiar, which is discontinued as soon as the power descends and releases the inner voices.

2a) You might like to start by repeating (or singing) the Jewish/Christian sound of praise, **"Hallelujah!"** - powerful in its own right as a 'bringer down' of Spirit, but if you don't like anything connected to organized religion (and some people don't), here's something simple and repetitive without religious connotations:

2b) Repeat (or sing) continuously **"<u>Kee</u>-ah, <u>kee</u>-ah"** (stress the underlined syllables) together with perineal/yoni contractions[3] and a pulled in lower belly (this engages the Chi energy); the ensuing bliss will often bring down the higher Spirit.

2c) Also try **"Ee<u>kee</u>-al-*ahh*, ee<u>kee</u>-al-*ahh*."**

2d) Another one to use with lower belly contractions: **"Y<u>ih</u>"** ("Yih" sounds the same as "sigh"), **"Y<u>ih</u>ee, y<u>ih</u>-e, y<u>ih</u>-e." Sing it rapidly and continuously, spontaneously changing pitch.**

Sound these both slowly and quickly, and don't give up your efforts, as it may take some days to some weeks of persistent practice to trigger the opening. Only by sounding the inner voices can the throat fully open and the upper energies release and integrate with the lower!

---

[3]Refer to Chapter 17 "Energy Exercises."

Not everyone reacts in the same way to the energy of Spirit. Some hear the inner sounds and voices in their heads (before they sound them); others experience gentle warmth in the chest, back and throat with blissful 'overtones' in several of the Chakras; and for a few, the incoming power is disconcertingly intense, beginning in the chest, where strong heat and vibration build up before rising to the throat and jaw causing trembling, shaking, stammering and even explosive coughing.

The Christian mystics say "Quench not the Spirit." If you have received any or all of these unusual body signals--**Spirit has already visited your throat's door.** You need to open the door by allowing yourself to speak and sing through your inner power and if the power has been "quenched" through ignorance or fear, **you need to call it down again!**

Restoring the Power (if you had it once and lost it):

From the preceding pages follow the instructions **1)** *through* **2d),** then relax and stretch the back of your neck to loosen any stiffness or tension; gently turn your head from side to side and move your jaw up and down several times (quickly and slowly). When the inner power rises and causes you to stammer, do so! Stammer until it becomes waves of incoherent jabberings. **This is the initial loosening of the speech organs** and a very positive sign of progress. *Don't be alarmed by how strange you feel and sound--you're almost there!* Take courage, make a leap into the unknown and allow yourself to utter whatever wants to come out (no matter how peculiar), this opens the pathway for the inner voices. You'll be immediately filled with indescribable rushes of surging energy--and with an ecstasy that can *only* resolve itself through sound! Regardless of whether you speak or sing, your throat will feel stronger and more powerful with each outpouring. Soon the words will flow in complete phrases. It doesn't matter whether you understand the languages or not; allow yourself to be swept along by sound...your separateness dissolving, your voices soaring! Finally the bliss waves and sounds subside, leaving you transformed, recharged and refreshed. Everything you consist of has been affected, your mind/emotions and your physical/super-physical systems--from the molecules within your cells to the outer reaches of your life Field! *The sounding process becomes easier each time you invite your higher Power of voice to fill you.* As you progress, you'll find yourself singing with amazing facility, sometimes in long and powerful passages, the tone and range far surpassing anything your outer voice has ever done before - unless you're already a professional singer, but even then your abilities will be greatly augmented!

During Sound workshops, I have seen people red in the face and almost apoplectic with their unsung higher energy. Unaccustomed to our own paranormal power, we don't know what to do with the energy when it comes into us! Of course, the solution and the *resolution* lies in the actual release of the energy **as sound**. When individuals reach this stage in my classes, the group energy makes it much easier for them to let go. All I usually have to say (to anyone quivering on the brink) - is, "Stand up and sound!".......and much to their amazement, they do!

Each time you surrender and allow the Chakra to open, the languages and melodies become stronger and clearer; they are the integrative voices of your past, present and future, from your sub-selves, your inner guide-teachers and your own highest Spirit sounding the songs of transformation.

The above descriptions give you some idea of the initial opening; of course, once this has happened, you must keep the Chakra operational by allowing the inner voices to sound on a regular basis; it's called "Sounding in the Spirit" and you can do it alone or with friends of like-mind.

Sounding in the Spirit.

Before you succeeded in opening the Throat Chakra, you probably programmed your day to include a practice time...you waited with upright spine and upheld hands, drawing down the energy and invoking the inner voices. Regular sounding in the Spirit is no different, except now the response is immediate - you've already uncovered the pathways - *Spirit responds in an instant!*

After my initial opening and for my own sounding practice, I chose the same spot to meditate in every day. I would wait, saying words of invitation "Hallelujah" (etc.), until I felt the energy begin to tingle around my hair and start its delicate dance on the frontal lobes of my brain. Then my breath came ever so gently until a growing warmth entered my heart and rushed into my throat--and I became once more transported into soaring sound! Neville, my first husband said he could hear me four blocks away as he walked home from work - back then, I 'sounded in the Spirit' regardless of neighbors - now, I'm more circumspect! I've issued neighborly warnings that I teach voice empowerment and periodically administer a noisy kind of sound therapy (which is easier than saying "I'm a Voice Shaman"). One person living behind me however, remains convinced that I'm an opera singer, practicing my exercises!

Spirit has many modes in the body. Sometimes the power remains strong and hard to contain, yet you feel quite blissful, that's when you spontaneously speak and sing and the energy integrates very rapidly. The sounding is always natural and glorious! At other times, the experience begins subtly with a gentle suffusing warmth and rippling sensations flow to different parts of the body, leaving you refreshed, energized and filled with ineffable joy and peace. The voices aren't necessarily always present, but there's always the presence of Spirit.

During a sound practice, you may just want to rock gently back and forth - or from side to side; for some strange reason, the motion seems to aid the flow of energy through the top of the head--and it certainly feels wonderful! Then occasionally, in the middle of all the surges of sound, the faces and names of loved ones (and even unrelated people in trouble), will flash across your mind. The focus and intensity of the inner voices immediately changes and you feel as though a limitless power is reaching out to those in need...as you speak and sing.

Also, you might be absorbed in a mundane activity, like making a bed, washing the dishes or working on an assignment, when you notice the unmistakable signs of Spirit (waves of energy and undulating bliss). You're not even meditating--so what's going on? It's like being unexpectedly called by your lover to an immediate assignation.....what a pleasant suprise! I usually drop everything and sit or kneel down, accompanied by note pad and pen. When 'summoned' like that, I may go into powerful tongues and song, but invariably, I will also receive valuable information and insights that need to be written down. Higher Spirit frequently plays the trickster and catches you unawares, calling on you at inappropriate (?) times, startling the outer mind into the realization that you now enjoy a two-way communication. It's not just *you* invoking the Presence, or demanding information; be prepared to receive when you least expect it; learn to flow and respond to the energy or you will miss opportunities of unparalleled magnificence and usefulness. *"Quench not the Spirit!"*

As mentioned elsewhere, the inner voice strength sometimes spills over into the regular speaking voice, then the normal resonance changes dramatically, as though something inside has switched over to a vastly superior sound system. This happens mostly when I lecture or give workshops and it's not anything I can turn on or off at will--it's part of my higher Spirit's agenda, but I always mark the spot when this takes place in a private conversation. It may happen mid-sentence, without warning, causing my voice timbre to alter noticeably--drawing the immediate attention of the other person. Certain words (in this mode) actually seem to *generate* energy - as well as bring special emphasis in that particular conversation and to that specific person. You're vocally plugging into higher Mind and in the same mode as when the inner voices speak and sing through you, but on these 'ordinary' occasions, it's your *outer* speaking voice that becomes enormously empowered. *You should consider all this as a natural and legitimate part of your own super conscious physical, mental nature--although a socially banished and greatly neglected part!*

The inner voice languages are mostly unknown, but sometimes when sounding the energy for larger groups or doing individual work, you'll sing or speak in a language that **is** known to someone there. *You* won't understand the words, but the other person does....and the words are especially for their ears! Your conscious mind stands aside while your throat becomes a vehicle for the higher Mind *of the other person.*

Case in Point: Thirty years ago, I lived in London, Ontario (Canada) at my Yoga and Art studio; one of my students and friends was a local artist, a beautiful dark haired woman, born in central Europe. On this particular evening I heard a knock on my door and on opening it, there stood my artist friend and a companion I had never seen before. After greeting me warmly she said "This is a dear friend and compatriot from my own country and I think you have a song for her." That suprised me, I'd been absorbed in a painting and didn't feel *remotely* like sounding for anyone!"

You always have a choice--to allow, or to say "No." I chose to allow. The three of us seated ourselves in a cross-legged circle on the large empty floor where I gave Yoga instruction in the day time. I sat directly in front of the visitor to tune into her energy and I closed my eyes so I wouldn't be distracted by her smiling, receptive face. Within seconds the power of Spirit filled me and I began to speak confidently in an unfamiliar tongue; "it" talked away animatedly for several minutes, then burst into a beautiful song in the same language. The song continued for verse after verse - after verse, never hesitating, altering the beat or missing a note of the lovely melody. Finally my outer mind, which also enjoyed the song, decided that I had better call a stop, or it might go on all night! When the energy subsided, I opened my eyes and was quite suprised to find the visitor crying quietly into her handkerchief, while my friend had a comforting arm around her shoulder. What had I done--the song had been so happy? They told me the words spoken first had been in the Latvian language and were filled with comfort, hope and encouragement, and the long melody following was an old Folk song, cherished greatly by the stranger--her Grandmother used to sing it to her when she nestled in her lap as a little child! The language and song only came through me on that one occasion--from the life Field energy and Spirit of the other person. *When we sound for others, we don't just utter our own inner voices, we also sound* **their** *inner voices.* Quite frequently the person you are sounding for, will remark with wonder, "That strange language made me feel so marvelous, I don't know why, but I'm vibrating all over--and parts of it sounded *very* familiar to me!"

Translating.

A further expansion of the "tongues" comes when you suddenly find yourself translating. You may have just spoken several phrases in an unknown tongue, there is a pause - and with the same feeling of detached awareness, you find yourself speaking again (for approximately the same amount of time), but now in English! At first it would only *appear* to be the translation, but eventually, you'll encounter the phenomenon in a situation where someone present will understand the language and confirm the interpretation! Direct and *separate* interpretation only occurs periodically (for me); mostly I may be speaking in a strange tongue while another part of my mind simultaneously 'hears' the translation and later, I'm able only to communicate the 'sense' of it--only what I was able to *remember* hearing--during the time the language was being spoken! In other words, the translation is concurrent with the tongue--you'll be speaking or singing in an unknown language, and you'll be hearing English words in your head at the same time! I have been in groups containing individuals with the *separate* "gift of interpretation," they rise in the power of Spirit and give the 'translation' after someone *else* has just spoken in tongues--they don't hear the words until they stand to speak. *It makes you wonder who and what we really are, and what our potential is, as fully developed and aware spiritual beings!*

At the moment, we're still infants and barely out of training-pants! For the most part, the glossalalia circumvents the intellect and we need to disengage the ordinary mind to receive the energy coming from the higher sound-centers.

Sounding in Your Own Language.

The hardest thing of all is sounding directly *in your own language!* - it's easier to speak in a language you don't understand--than in one you do---the outer mind wants to interfere and argue with the message because you understand the words. The power of Spirit flows more readily when the outer intellect has been set to one side. This energy is quite different from the experience of "translating" (explained above), which occurs effortlessly and powerfully immediately after (or while) an unknown language is uttered. When English comes through as part of general sounding, it can be spoken as well as sung and to prevent your intellect editing the message, you generally receive only single words or phrases at a time - as you speak or sing each small phrase, the inner energy then releases *the next* word or small phrase! It's quite scary to the outer mind because you literally don't know what you will say next! The process does get easier and as you learn to relax and trust you'll find yourself giving more normally delivered phrases. You allow English to sound through you in the same way that you allow the unknown tongues - in a detached yet fully aware manner.

With an opened Throat Chakra, we're supposed to surrender **all** of our words to higher Spirit and no longer speak from conditioning; our destiny is to become "The Word," the sound-vehicle of superconscious Mind. The periodic practice of inner sounding (Sounding in the Spirit), must spill over into our everyday lives; our voices should reflect the new and integrated center of our being. Part of this requires the *constant* practice of Inner Listening. We learn to listen inwardly for what another soul *needs* to hear from us--not what we think we have to say to them. Outer mind can't read the thoughts of others--but higher Mind can, if necessary! When we align with that Mind, we don't actually spy on another's thoughts, but we speak and respond from a level far beyond our ordinary understanding. Many times, we must act as intermediaries between the disowned higher Spirits of others and their everyday minds. *It's all a matter of knowing that the inner level exists, paying attention and learning to access it at will.*

Another Example: Many years ago, late at night, a certain relative came through the front door 'plastered' out of his mind, very sorry for himself and complaining bitterly! Having a comfortable conversation with this person when he was sober was difficult at best--let alone when drunk! I felt a split second of fear and panic, knowing I could *never* cope with him in his present condition, but in the next second I sent a firm mental call to higher Mind: "Help me, what on *earth* do I say?" Staggering into the room, he saw me standing there and began whining in my direction. I spoke to him kindly and firmly from my "other" Self. He stopped dead, as though a shock had passed through him--then an incredulous smile broke across his face. His mind seemed to clear and instantly his whole body relaxed and softened. "Oh, you *must* understand how I feel," he uttered passionately, "Or you could *never* have said that!"

No, "I" could never have said that! My outer mind received the empowered words from within and allowed them to be spoken. To this day, I have no memory of what those words were; they came out of my mouth for the *other* person's ears, not mine, but their effect was immediate, calming and healing. *We desperately need to be able to speak with such discernment and only the higher Mind can bring such wisdom into ordinary consciousness.*

The power of the Light body and the Inner sound resides within us all as the hidden multilevel nature of mankind.

This Chapter provides tools for a personal opening to the higher Power of Spirit and the inner sound frequencies, and also for the maintenance of the experience after the event; Chapter 15, "Healing with Sound and Sound Power Groups," gives you a wider application of the Sound and Light Energy.

And through it all, remember to breathe the Galactic Breath.

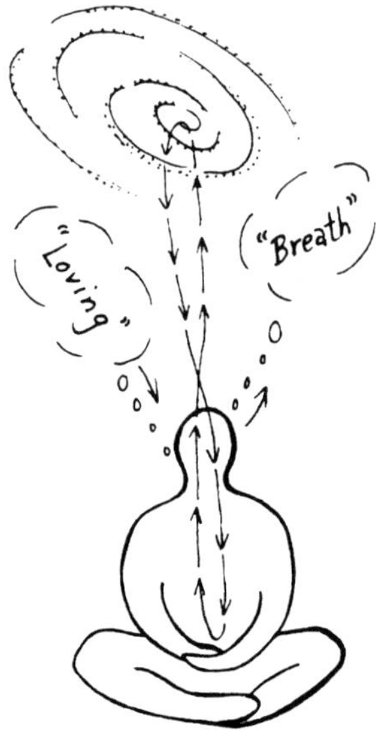

15.....HEALING WITH SOUND & SOUND POWER GROUPS

The power of sound to heal has always suprised me. I recall over twenty years ago in Everett, Washington giving an inner sound demonstration to a group of about fifteen people. Most were my students, but on this occasion, some had brought along friends as their guests. They occupied every chair in my front room; the overflow sprawled on the floor and stared curiously up at me. I explained the need to be extra quiet and receptive so I could tune-in and translate my impressions into sound. I also asked them to note any unusual physical changes (like flowing energy, tingling, heat) that could result from the sounding. Directly after closing my eyes to concentrate, tones and spontaneous songs welled up in me; I probably sang for about five minutes. When the sounds ended (and I came back to earth), I was suprised to find a guest on the floor right in front of me, collapsed and weeping across the lap of one of my students! The rest of the group looked uncomfortable, curious or puzzled! "For heaven's sake what happened?" I demanded. The collapsed person gradually sat up, rearranged herself and wiped her eyes. She spoke. "For the past six weeks I have been terribly depressed and my friend (*indicating her sympathetic neighbor*) persuaded me to come here tonight. As you sang, my depression lifted...and...I'm crying because I'm so relieved!" There were other interesting reactions to the sounds that evening, but hers--I remember the most.

This happened in the early years of my moving to the US. from Canada. I had just cautiously begun to work with my voice in America using demonstrations and sound experiments. On another Everett occasion, my husband arrived home from work one afternoon with a buddy. "I've been telling Al about your sounding," he announced. "See if you can help him, he's got a funny pain in his foot." With that remark he went out the back door and down the stairs leaving me alone with his friend! Disheveled and grimy in work overalls, Al sat on a chair and began to remove his boot. While he struggled with his laces, he explained that his pain felt as though a fine needle was embedded in his foot. Yet, no amount of X-rays or doctor-probing had discovered anything concrete and every time he inadvertently stepped or stood on it in the 'wrong' way, an excruciating pain shot through his foot.

His explanations over, Al proceeded to locate the exact area by firmly prodding his stockinged heel. "***Ow*** - found it!" he exclaimed. "Here, give me your finger and I'll put it right on the spot....that's it, right there!" I knelt on the floor and grasped his suffering foot with both of my hands (a finger firmly on the troublesome spot) and mentally asked for the right sound to release the pain. In due time, a single bell-like tone came out of me; its resonance rang strong and pure and I knew this was the note I had to keep on singing. Every time I'd run out of breath, I'd inhale deeply and start over again. Finally, in mid-breath, Al interrupted me. "Wait, wait," he said. "I think you've moved off the spot, I can't feel it any more." He once more took my finger and pressed it repeatedly into his heel. Then looking puzzled, he brushed my hand aside, peeled his sock off and began probing vigorously for himself. "Darn!" he muttered with frustration, "I seem to have lost the spot." After a few more moments of fruitless hunting he finally realized the pain had disappeared. "I can't believe it!" he burst out incredulously; "It's gone!" *Indeed it had--and it never returned!*

These two straightforward examples illustrate first, the effect of general sounding on a *group* of people and second, the effect of combining specific touch and sound for an *individual.* Sounding in response to simple problems can have surprising results, but the results are even more surprising when sounding the complex energies of (so called) past lives!

Case in Point: Prior to my interest in Name Analysis, I spent several years researching and teaching the improbable subject of palmistry. (A chance encounter with a British book on medical and traditional palmistry had originally piqued my curiosity.) All students who took my lessons made ink prints of their hands to constantly refer to in class and it was during one of these group palm-printings that a student announced she didn't seem to have a destiny-line. It was true, I confirmed its absence and everyone rushed to look at her hands and examine her ink-prints. With few exceptions, the destiny-line on most hands shows itself as a fairly straight North/South groove running through the middle of the palm and supposedly indicates one's path in life. After a number of weeks attending regular classes, this particular student phoned me up one night with a request--would I please do a sounding for her? She'd heard from the others that I did some kind of sound therapy and wanted my assistance.

Since the end of her marriage eighteen months ago she had been suffering from a strange and inexplicable reaction. The marriage of two years had not worked out and both she and her husband had agreed on divorce - an amicable divorce; but once it became final, she went into daily spells of prolonged crying, in spite of the fact that she felt no remorse or loss whatsoever from the severed relationship! Cry she did--and she couldn't stop it!! A psychiatrist and group therapy had also been tried, but to no avail. Much to her disgust, the therapist had finally said (after weeks of therapy), that there was nothing the matter with her and all she needed to do was pull herself together, start reading detective novels and get her mind off her divorce!

We set up an appointment and she arrived at my door three days later. I sat her down on a straight-backed chair in the middle of the room, lowered the lights and told her to close her eyes while I checked out her Life Field with my hands explaining that in the process, I would locate any blockages in her energy and re-balance her Field - and that during the process I was likely to burst into long tones, song, or strange languages (when I hit pockets of energy that needed clearing). We began.

On aligning with her Field, I became assailed with vivid mental pictures of tribal Africa--an Africa long before the invasion of the white man. *Visual impressions are not my strong point--this was getting interesting!* As I circled her chair and moved my hands methodically through her Field, I was frequently halted (by the strength of her energy-Field) to speak in strange guttural languages or sing in rhythmical chants. Meanwhile, my eyes 'saw' an enactment of the (possible?) past life reason for her reaction to the recent divorce. Then I began to directly re-experience her agony with emotions of great sorrow and poignancy; almost overwhelmed--I found myself sobbing, moaning and railing!! In the midst of all of this, my witness-mind questioned "*Whatever must she be thinking--listening to all this strange mumbo jumbo??.* I continued to sound until the energy and the remarkable pictures ceased.

This was the story I mentally saw and emotionally felt: In those days, it was apparently the custom for the local villages to offer chosen females as gifts to the King, a powerful Chief, who by lineage ruled over many villages and tribes, including tribes he had vanquished in battle. My student (then a burgeoning young beauty) was thrilled to be chosen by her village as a 'gift' for the great Chief. She traveled in a special party to the Royal Compound with other new wives being sent as gifts. It was a tremendous honor to be thus sent, but the greatest honor occurred, if you subsequently gave birth to a royal *male* child--then you were entitled to live in the enclosure of huts reserved for the male-bearing wives of the harem. Two years passed, during which the King mated with her on several occasions, then for no reason (other than he no longer found her pleasing), he sent her home to her original village -- rejected, divorced and pregnant! The tribe also ostracized her - for it had been deeply humiliated by the royal rejection. She was banished to a tiny hut on the edge of the village, where she lived out her life in bitterness and sorrow with her son. Yes, the final irony - she had given birth to a male. With a royal son, she should have been living in the King's Compound as one of the most honored wives!

The man whom my student/client had recently divorced had supposedly been the King-Chief in that previous lifetime. They'd married again (repeating the karma) *and* for the same two year period, but even though the severance this time had been amiable (a plus), it nonetheless triggered subliminal memories of unresolved emotions and deep disappointment--in her. I found my input from her sound-session remarkable--I rarely experience such detailed and chronological information about a person's past life. Usually I get just enough to understand and endeavor to change the energy; this time, as her surrogate, I saw, felt, spoke and sang her story! It had been an intensely vivid, powerful and energy filled experience for me - and, I expected an equally strong reaction from her also - but there was *none*! I stared at her in disbelief--I had felt everything, she had felt nothing! People who'd previously received my soundings always felt *something* - physical tingling and chills, emotions or reactions to certain tones, languages or songs.

A relatively new palmistry student, this lady had never heard me talk about past lives; so in the light of her singular lack of reaction, I held my peace! "Are we finished?" she asked pleasantly, half rising from her seat. "Yes, quite," I responded. In leaving, she said how much she had enjoyed the experience, thanked me warmly and, waving over her shoulder walked down the stairs to her car. I remained considerably puzzled, especially as she stopped coming to class. About a month passed before she phoned me. "You'll *never* guess what has happened!" Her voice bubbled with excitement. "Remember that sound balancing you gave me?" *I most certainly did!* "Well, immediately after it, the next day in fact, I stopped crying - just stopped - and haven't cried once since; then several days later, I happened to glance down at my hand, and I couldn't believe my eyes" (*pregnant pause*), "I had grown a four inch long destiny line in the middle of my hand!" -- *I gasped!* -- She continued. "I've waited to make sure it didn't vanish again overnight, but it seems to be here to stay. Please can I come back to class next week and show it to everyone?"

She returned in great triumph, the center of every one's interest, physically demonstrating something that up until then, I had only read about: the hand can grow (and also erase) lines in response to significant changes in consciousness. In her case, the primary changes had taken place in the subconscious and had been instigated through the power of sound. In class, we made fresh palm prints to compare with her old ones; there the evidence was unmistakable and in black ink prints for everyone to see! The other great testimony to the transformation was her new and sparkling personality, some definite blockage had dissolved away. From then on she became an avid student and (to her further amazement), when she gained enough knowledge and confidence to read the palms of others, she showed remarkable psychic abilities that went above and beyond her basic palmistry skills. She now truly had a new 'destiny.'

This experience taught me that when you sound for others, there didn't have to be a reaction or even **a** *response--in order for them to benefit!* Since then I have witnessed many other mental, emotional and some physical releases as a result of sounding for groups as well as for individuals.

Before passing on to actual techniques, here's one more example I want to present. It involves a present day *physical* affliction that had an apparent past-life cause.

Sibyl (not her real name), came to me for Name Analysis and midway through the consultation, I found it necessary to give her a sounding. It happened quite by chance. In the course of our conversation she showed me a very large ganglion on the palm of her hand immediately under the index finger, saying it was quite uncomfortable and due to be surgically removed in a few days. I wanted to see what effect the sound would have on it, if any, and offered her the experience of a sounding. She readily agreed.

I gave my usual warning remarks (of the likelihood of hearing strange sounds and languages coming out of me), then stood behind her chair with my hands on her shoulders. Immediately a feeling of dark foreboding and evil filled me. I let out a sudden, horrified "Oh, my gosh!" as my hands pulled back in alarm. In the seconds before their hasty retreat, a stark and desperate scene had flashed across my inner vision. I saw a small band of pirates quarreling violently on a beach piled high with crates of plunder; rain squalls lowered in the sky above and a gray surf thundered behind them. Suddenly, the flash of knives and Sibyl (then a male and one of the pirates), fell bleeding to the sand with a mortal wound! I looked carefully at my client; she was petite, very feminine and quite charming - no vestige of a pirate there! "I can't do another thing" I said carefully, "Until I create a barrier around you." Hastily I did my Cross of Light[1] ritual in her Field and finally the strange and menacing vibrations abated. Sibyl looked at me enquiringly; unlike my student from the other sounding, she felt that she had lived before in other lifetimes.

"I'm sorry to have startled you," I began, "But it appears your ganglion connects you to a rather unsavory life and demise as a pirate; perhaps you were murdered then at the approximate age you are now, and the growth on your hand might be a reminder of the unresolved incident." The white, pointed lump looked engorged beneath the delicate pink of her hand. "May I gently touch it with my fingers?" She nodded her consent. "I'll try and find the right tones to disperse the karma." The notes came easily, along with some interesting songs, during which Sibyl felt a large amount of energy flowing through her body - the ganglion, however, remained the same...as large and pointed as ever. We returned to the Name Consultation and spent the rest of a pleasant session together.

She left and the event went to the back of my mind. Then one day, at least two years later, I received an interesting phone call - it was Sibyl phoning me long distance from central Oregon. At first I couldn't really place her, so she had to remind me with some details. "I was the pirate who got murdered on a beach because of a treasure dispute, and you sounded for a painful ganglion on my hand." Then I remembered! She continued. "Yesterday, while going through some old tapes, I found

---

[1] See page 126.

the Name Analysis you did for me some time ago, and listening again to those marvelous sounds you sang, I thought you deserved some feedback--I get the feeling you don't often get much." *She now had my attention!* "What do you mean by feedback?" I asked. "Well....I never did go to the doctor and have that operation--the ganglion vanished a couple of days after your sounding--thought you'd like to know!" *The frustrating thing about sounding for specific problems is there are no guarantees, results are always in the Lap of the Gods! Your Spirit, higher Mind and the inner-voices give you the sounds and you can only trust that* ***some*** *good will result.*

A reminder: when you sound for others, you not only use *your* inner-voices, but *their* inner-voices as well. The best general description of this process appears at the end of Chapter 2 - and because of its relevance to healing with sound, I've repeated it here:

"To do a 'balance' for someone else, you begin by aligning with the person's Life Field, then instantly your sounds become dual in nature - not only do your inner-voices sing and speak (whenever inclined), but the sub-selves of the person you're sounding for will also speak and sing through *your* throat! In effect, you have assumed the role of a sound-surrogate and in the shamanic tradition, you "journey" empathetically into the other person's past, directly experiencing their emotional, mental and physical states (as well as their voice frequencies). Part of this process involves actually *seeing* events and *feeling* emotions from past-life traumas that relate to present-life problems; another part involves releasing entities and other interdimensional life forms that may have become attached or trapped in the person's Life Field."

A similar result takes place in past-life hypnotherapy, when by recalling a relevant life under hypnosis (and subsequently reviewing the information), it acts to relieve a present day illness (or emotional stress).[2]

SOUND HEALING TECHNIQUES.

HEALING 'ONE-ON-ONE'

a) Combining Touch and Sound.

1) Have the person lie face up on a couch or bed, or something you can kneel next to (if you don't have a massage table). Cover them with a light blanket if they are cold, then tell them to close their eyes and relax and (so they won't be startled), say you will probably begin by laying your hands on their solar plexus to see if they will 'take' any energy through your hands. Explain that you're only a conductor for the particular frequencies they might need and that you, yourself, will **not** be depleted in any way. Also warn them you may at times make sudden noises, long tones, or speak strange languages, chant and sing--while on the other hand--you may not utter a single sound!

The same applies to the energies coming through from the Ki body - everything always depends on what the other person needs and subsequently draws through you.

2) Sans a massage table, kneel beside them on a cushion or folded blanket (be kind to your knees!) and unless otherwise directed by intuition, lay your hands gently on their solar plexus. Wait a few minutes in this position to allow for entrainment[3] with their energy.

3) Begin to breathe **in** through the crown of your head and then breathe **out** of your hands and **into** the other person. Give yourself several breaths to see if your Crown Chakra opens and the energy starts flowing down. When it does, you'll feel an energy current passing through your body and into your hands, which then become hot and tingling. Sometimes many different pulses channel through you; as stated above, it always depends on what the other person *needs* to receive. At some point in the treatment, you begin to automatically 'ground' the energy through your lower extremities, and even when you're kneeling with the soles of your feet facing out, they will still tingle when the grounding flow begins.

---

[2] Refer to "Past Lives Future Lives" by Dr. Bruce Goldberg, published by Ballantine Books.
[3] For understanding "entrainment" read Itzhak Bentov's "Stalking The Wild Pendulum."

Healing One-on-One

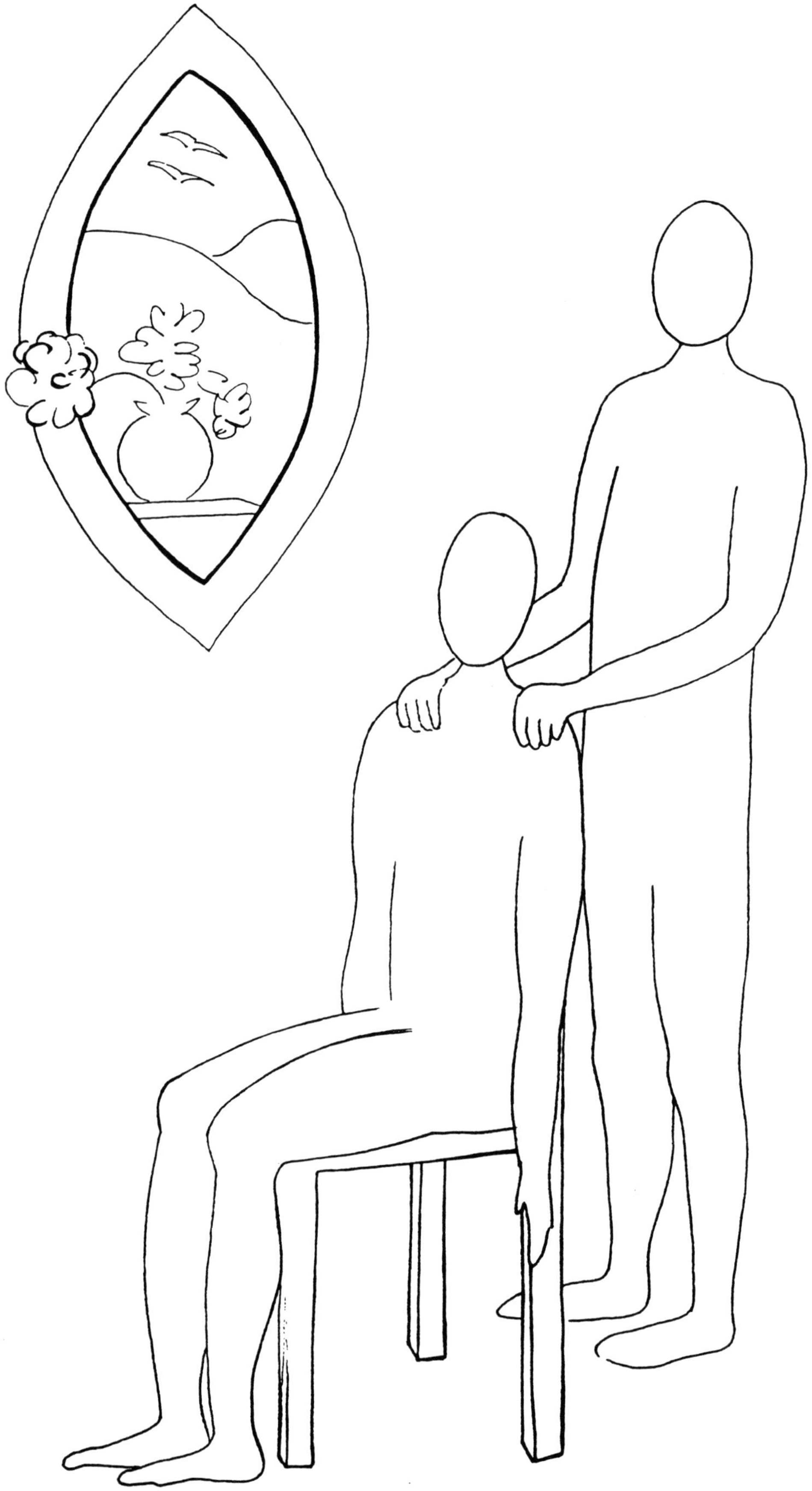

Tuning in

You both receive each other's energy.

One person working on field

4) At times your hands will separate and rest on different parts of the body simultaneously. If you happen to be an empath, you'll also receive (from the other person), aches and pains in your *own* body as you work--*no, you are NOT taking on their afflictions,* you're registering physically **where next to lay your hands on them.** The 'trigger' pain stops when you have sent enough energy into the indicated area.

5) As the energy begins to increase, you'll more powerfully release the charge through your hands by sounding long resonating tones and speaking in tongues (should they arise). The receiving person usually feels an increased flow of vibration and/or heat during and after a sounding. Tune in to where your hands need to be placed at any given time (and note the nature of the energy passing *through* them), also be aware of the power filling *you* from the inner-voices and align with the energies that need to translate into sound.

6) Sometimes the other person will have a specific pain or problem area they want you to work on. Lay your hands where they request and see if the energy will flow there. **Leave your hands in place on an area for as long as the energy continues to pass through them.** Both you and the person you're working on will know when the treatment has run its course; the energy simply stops flowing from your hands (the other person no longer feels any heat or vibration and neither can you) and there are no more sounds wanting to be spoken or sung.

Each person you work on is unique and draws through you--the precise frequency they need to recharge or heal themselves. Did I mention there are no guarantees? One person will pull in volumes of energy, enough to refresh you both! Another will also draw in large amounts (in that you feel hot and vibrate all over), but most of it wants to remain in *you* and very little seems to flow over into the other person - or they just don't appear to feel it or accept it openly, even though their higher Self has summoned it. With other cases (as already illustrated), **you** may experience a great deal--the person being worked on feels nothing--yet a transformation still takes place in them, or, results are delayed for hours or days. I always tell the person that it takes three days to a week for the full effect of a sounding to come through to them.

We are not the machines that science once thought we were; we are individual souls, inhabiting and modifying our 'containers' according to personal karma and social conditioning--and also awakening our capacity for becoming functioning spiritual beings in transformed bodies.

Beginning Healers. Even if you have never facilitated healing before, just your compassionate *intent* will open your latent channels.[4] An excellent textbook on touch healing to read: "The Therapeutic Touch" by Delores Krieger (Ph.D,R.N.). Use it as a basic text but allow your intuitive connection with higher Mind and Spirit to always guide you - and of course, combine your touch with sound.

HEALING 'ONE-ON-ONE'

b) Clearing and Balancing the Life Field (Aura) with Sound.

1) For this, the receiving person sits upright in an armless, straight-backed chair. Make sure their unshod feet touch the floor (but not each other); if necessary supply a flat cushion to go under the feet - some people are short. Their backs should be held straight, not slouched, but resting firmly against the chair, and their arms must hang down to discharge any blocked energy *(no hands clasped in the lap please!).*

2) Ask them to close their eyes and pay attention to the effects of the sound in their body, rather than trying to analyze it. "*Feel,*" tell them, *"Not think!"* Stand behind the chair and explain that before clearing their aura/Life Field with the magnetic centers in your hands (and with sound), you are first going to place both your hands on their shoulders and 'tune in' to them.

During this short time of relaxed receptivity (on both your parts), one of several things may happen:

2a) As you receive their energy, your hands begin to tingle and you start to receive insights and input from their higher Mind. This information could be several sentences, just one or two words, or

[4] Read the inspiring story beginning on page 40 of "Chicken Soup for the Soul" compiled and written by Jack Canfield and Mark Victor Hansen.

merely emotional and visual impressions that need to be discussed and interpreted. All of it may be meaningless to you--but quite significant to the other person, or it may *gain* meaning as the sounding proceeds.

2b) Your hands become instantly uncomfortable the moment you touch their shoulders - even to the point of an increasing pain that moves through your hands, wrists and up into your arms. When this happens, ground any excess energy by firmly stamping both your feet on the floor (warn the person first, or you may startle them!); then, visualize the pain energy changing into a "healing power" and 'breathe' it back down your arms again. You might need several breaths to return it all, depending on the pain's intensity; it also helps to picture the transformed energy as a green light traveling through your hands and into the body of the other person. (The shade of the light varies with the needs of the person receiving it...but green is an excellent balancing color.)

2c) As you tune in with hands-on-shoulders, your Crown Chakra may open suddenly and draw down a powerful energy charge resulting from the two sets of merged higher Chakras--yours and theirs; this immediately flows through your arms and hands and into their shoulders. If the energy dramatically increases and you **both** become ecstatic and blissful, transfer your hands to the top of their head (*their* Crown Chakra). Their Spirit may be choosing you as a conducting rod to allow the other person to experience, for first time, their own higher frequencies!

2d) You have placed your hands on their shoulders but discern little or no energy. This could mean a very compacted, closed Life Field (due to various blocks and traumas), or a very unreceptive, closed down or unaware person. In these cases, you just note the situation and proceed to balance and open the Field with the rest of the procedures.

2e) If, on tuning in, you instantly feel a pain (slight to intense) in any part of *your own* body, you have registered an important key area (needing to be worked on) in the other person. Immediately transfer your hands to **that** part of their body to receive further impressions--or to impart energy. If you receive more than one of these personal physical-triggers, place your hands on them in the order of their appearance (in you). When you no longer feel any of these sensations in yourself, return your hands to their shoulders for further impressions.

2f) A final possibility - you could encounter a very rapid and very powerful entrainment with their energy - *both of your Life Fields instantly align giving you immediate access to several (if not all) levels of their being.* Completely without warning, Incredible cascades of sound will burst out of you, (usually much to your--and their astonishment)! Allow the sound (songs, voices, tones) to subside before proceeding, giving you both time to integrate and if necessary discuss the event!

3) **<u>You are now ready to balance their Life Field.</u>** Place both hands, palms facing downwards, about four inches **over** the top of their hair (or scalp, if they don't have hair!), *but don't let your hands touch their head.* Pause, while you wait for the energy to build; at the same time (with very small movements), begin moving both hands up and down in the air above their head, but not more than four or five inches higher (than the head). Soon your hands will begin to tingle as an energy field builds between your hands and their head. They may say, "Wow, I can feel something happening up there - what are you doing!?" You have activated their Crown Chakra and initiated the rest of the entrainment process within their aura.

4) Maintaining your hand position, step back slightly, giving yourself more room to sweep their Field with your hands. **Now wait for the next instructions.** *(You are about to continuously sweep their Life Field from above their head, then down to the floor and up again, in a circle all around them -- finishing where you began -- which was directly behind their chair.)*

5) Begin as before, your hands held with **palms facing downward** about four to six inches above the person's head and (*while you continue to feel the active charge in your hands*), pull the energy from their Crown Chakra down to the floor at the base of the chair behind them, being careful to follow the contours of their body with your hands while maintaining a four to six inch distance. By the time you have completed your first downward sweeping movement, you will be bent from the waist and your fingers will now point almost to the ground, with the **backs** of your hands facing the

Balancing the Life Field

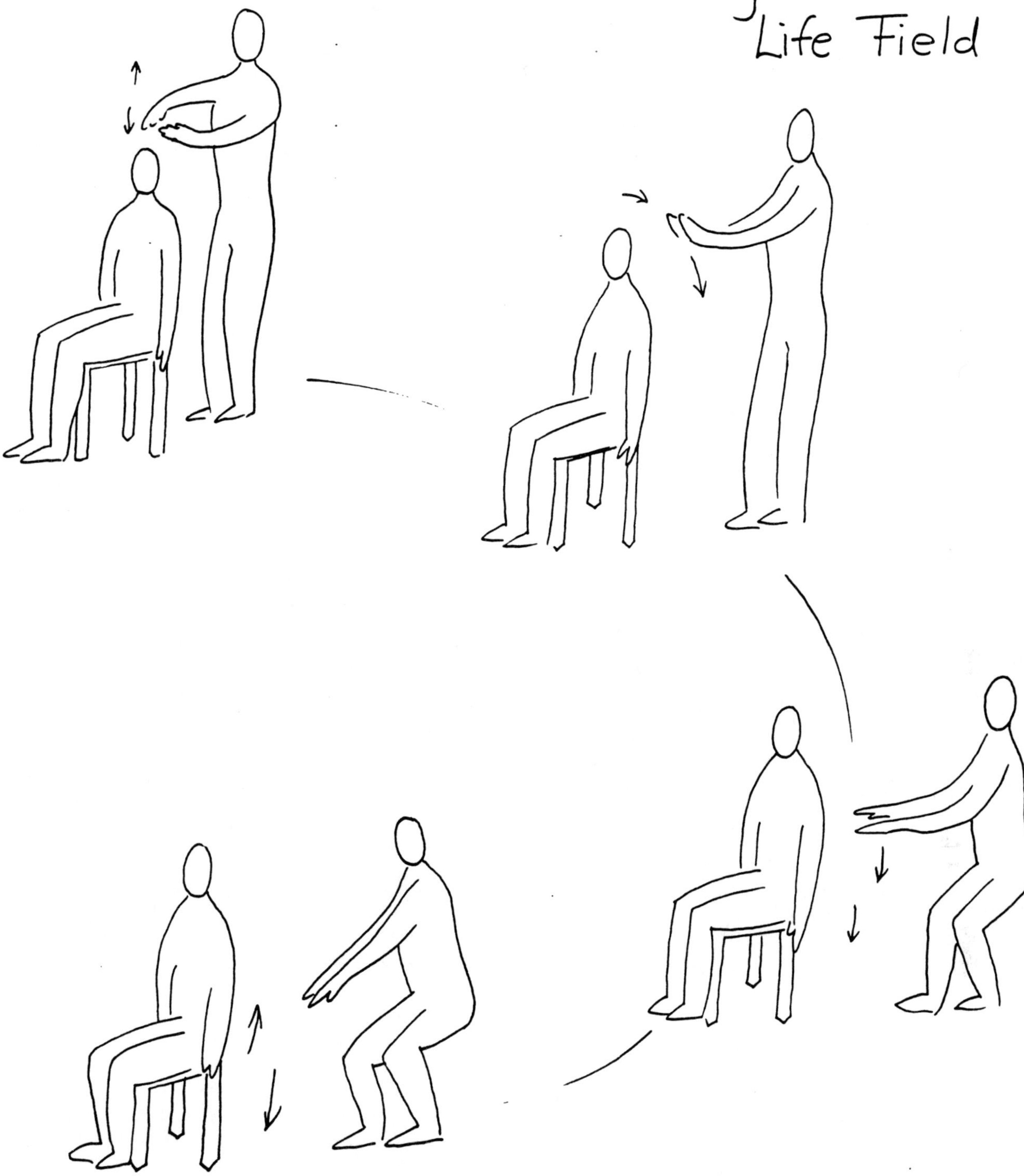

chair. At this point, gracefully begin your upward return (with the *backs* of your hands beginning the sweep and following the contours of the body), until the palms once more face down towards the head at the starting position above the Crown Chakra. *To reiterate a little differently: the palms begin by facing the body above the head, and on the downward sweep (about half way down), you'll find only the finger tips are facing the body and three-quarters of the way down only the backs of the hands are facing with the fingers pointing to the floor; coming up, the order is reversed.*

6) Repeat the above up/down movement **once** (two times in all), then step slightly to the right, no more than a foot, and repeat the entire sweeping procedure. Continue doing this (stepping eight to twelve inches to the right and then sweeping up and down twice) around the person until you have made one complete circle and you are back where you started - standing behind them. The up/down sweep can be fast or slow, depending on the 'feel' of the energy. At times you work very rapidly, at others, so slow, it's like pulling your hands through a heavy fog--or thick syrup!

7) Now do a second pass of sweeps completely around the person, but this time *pull the energy out to about a foot away from the body before you begin the sweep.* In a final pass, you can pull the Field out to almost three feet - but only if you have the space and time to do so.

The above sections, numbered 5, 6 and 7, describe the basic physical movements for clearing and recharging the Life Field. They can be done again (one circumnavigation), at the end of the session to seal the aura, but this time, move to the *left* around the person instead of to the right.

In all this, where does the sounding part come in? Again, it always depends on the needs of the person you're working on. There are no predetermined tones or sounds; sometimes you'll perform an entire circle of "sweeps" before the energy builds to a point where you know you have to stop and allow the sounds to come out. Again, at other times, the power of the inner-voices can strike without warning, with languages and songs gushing forth like a multi-layered fountain of sound; in this event, you barely have a chance to place your hands on their shoulders before the sound-dam bursts, sometimes with shattering force (as mentioned in **2f** above)! In the past when this has happened, people subsequently tell me they were not expecting to hear such volume and intensity, but after overcoming their initial shock-resistance and relaxing themselves, the tones became glorious and transforming. Now, I try and remember to warn beforehand - that sound may erupt suddenly and vary greatly in tone, intensity and volume--but sometimes I forget! Generally, as you move around and perform the aura sweeps, the energy builds gradually until it veritably 'stops you in your tracks' at certain juncture points in the Field where you have activated specific blockages and information pockets (even "doorways" into other dimensions appear in aura). When this happens, simply stand still, pay attention and allow the inner-voices to sound through you. After all the energy for *that particular* area in the Field has been translated into sound, you can then share with the person (you're working on) whatever visual, emotional impressions and insights you may have collected while you were singing or speaking in tongues (especially if they were exceptional and powerful). Then you ask them if *they* received any unusual input--emotions, sensations, vibrations, visual impressions or instructions?

After your mini-discussion, you go back to sweeping the Field at the approximate point where you left off before the sounds interrupted you, and you continue until you're stopped again! It may take fifteen minutes to sweep around the circle just once, if the energy keeps commanding you to stop and sound. On the other hand, in certain instances, the primary balancing comes from the aura re-balancing and you may just sound two or three times during the sweeps, or only once while standing behind the person at the completion. **The procedure always adapts itself to the needs of the person receiving the treatment.**

Some Life Fields are so debilitated that instead of extending outwards, they remain closely compacted near the body and when you work on them, you might sweep both the inner and outer layers and feel nothing - or hardly anything - not even in your hands. In these instances, the person's aura contains one or a series of barriers, or remains weak for undefined reasons and before any further work can be done, you need to perform the following drainage ritual to clear the obstruction(s).

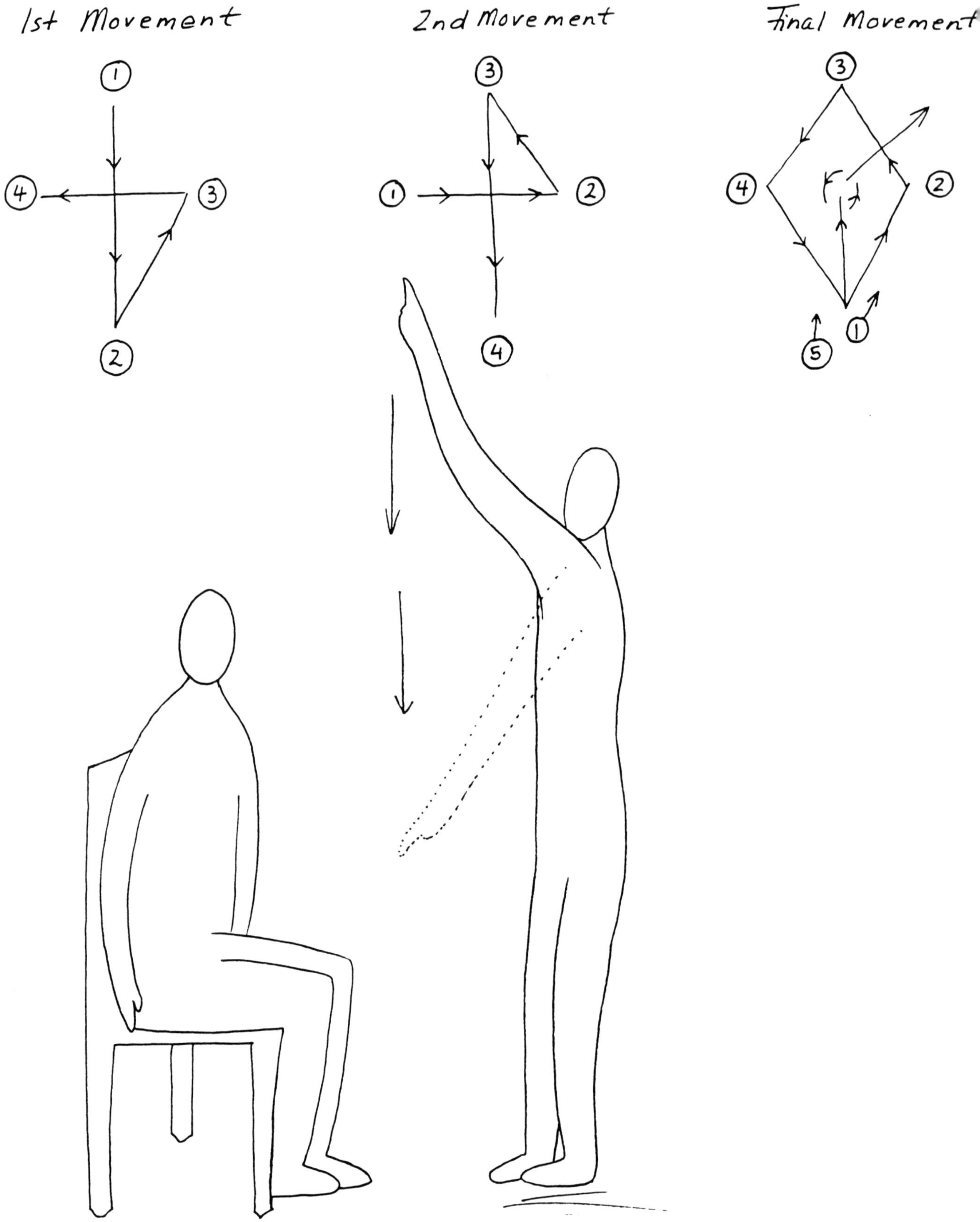

Beginning the Cross
-1st movement-

Drainage Cross of Light

DRAINAGE CROSSES (Double Crosses of Light).

They say "Necessity is the Mother of invention," and most of my techniques appear out of thin air in response to some situation I find myself facing for the first time. The drainage crosses concept came spontaneously in the middle of a difficult sounding for a student, who appeared to have a rather negative entity attached to her Life Field. On detecting its presence, I thought "Uh-oh! What do I do now?" I needed to open some interdimensional pathway for it to leave the earth plane--instead of being attached to my student's aura. Their connection to each other (entity attachments are rarely random) supposedly came from a Christian mediaeval time-frame, so my mind flashed to the most powerful icon for overcoming evil in those early days - the Cross!

I made the traditional Sign of the Cross.....not in front of my *own* chest, but in the air facing my student sitting in the chair. My hand went up, then down (from heaven to earth) - then from left to right - (being left handed, that's *my* way, but you may go from right to left if you prefer) and I imagined, as I drew it in the air, that I was creating the symbol with "lines of light;" then instead of finishing the Cross after making the traditional 'sign,' I found myself repeating what I had just done--partly in reverse - *which I thought very unusual!* (Now, after years of experience, I know it's a useful power-symbol for returning earth-bound spirit-entities to their own dimensions.)

Let me explain the reversal: *Use your own hand and try making it for yourself as you read; this will help you follow my instructions.* To get the idea, make a sign-of-the-cross in the usual way, but make it facing out into the room. You have now completed the final hand motion--from right to left or left to right--it doesn't matter! *Then instead of stopping there,* immediately re-point your finger in that same spot (on the right--or left) and move it across to the opposite side - then once more point your hand up above and down below. It's like a superimposed cross of light in reverse.....but my hand didn't stop there, either. From my last hand gesture (with finger pointing to the ground), I moved it up and out to the right and continued around the cross, making a big diamond shape joining all the four outer points, as though I was drawing an old fashioned paper kite in the sky - **this formed the image of the final Power Icon**! *(Refer to illustration.)*

All this came to me quickly, as my student sat waiting on the chair, so I immediately drew four double crosses of light around her....one at the back of her chair, followed by another one directly opposite--in front of and *facing her;* then I did two more...one facing her left shoulder and then one facing her right shoulder. Also, as I completed each cross with its diamond shape--I then swept my hand up through the center of the cross to an imaginary point of light, way above her head. (I did this for each cross). When they were all in 'position' around her, I stood again behind the chair, and once more raising my hand on high, mentally linked all the crosses into one white 'path' terminating at a point of light--the symbolic doorway between dimensions. Then I commanded the entity (attached to her Field), to pass between the crosses and go up the pathway to the point of light - where 'he' could go through and progress in another dimension (this can be invoked in silence or spoken out loud). As I breathed, I pictured him walking up the path until he vanished. He did - and so was born a technique I have used for many years as a clearing device for specific or general obstructions in the Life Field, such as earthbound entities and misplaced nature spirits....and several of the other odd things that sometimes get stuck in human Life Fields!

NOTE: *The hand movements for the Cross of Light are* ***very*** *large, as expansive as you feel like making them -- not the minute movements usually indicated across the chest when making the Christian sign of the cross (from the forehead to the heart and then touching the left and right shoulders); you are setting up Power Icons to surround the person sitting on the chair--icons that function like shields as well as doorways.*

These symbols can be created mentally when you find yourself in difficult situations that cry out for clearing or defusing; such as in the outdoors where the land has been traumatized; in a crowd where the mood is tense or ugly; in the waiting areas of airports--especially when a flight has been canceled; in houses that need re-balancing or exorcising (put crosses in the middle of a 'problem' room and in each of its four corners, as well as on stairways and in halls and passages. These

situations also respond to "internal sounding"[5] when it's in a public place and inappropriate to use your outer voice).

While driving their cars, two of my students make very small, very rapid crosses to release the spirits of road-kill animals; the same two ladies recently set up an enormous cross at the beginning of an access road to a popular nature reserve--with the injunction that all those who passed through it would appreciate the beauty of the land and honor the trees. Another student, while watching the news on TV responds to scenes of death and violence by making Crosses of Light .

The following invocation should be used in conjunction with the Double Crosses of Light.

THE CROSS OF LIGHT INVOCATION

"I now command,
All negative and misplaced influences, entities and vibrations,
To pass through this Cross of Light,
And return to where you came from."

or,

"And return to your original Spirit," or, "Return to where you will go forward."

or,

"And return to where you will be at peace."

Repeat the invocation either aloud or mentally, after the four crosses have been set up around a person, or when several have been set up to change bad vibrations in a house, room or other location. (Say the invocation for each room in which a cross or crosses have been placed.)

If you find making the drainage cross too complicated (*it's much simpler to demonstrate directly),* **adapt the idea to an icon of your own creation. I'm just sharing my story of what works for me and others who use the doubled Cross of Light icon.**

CREATING SOUND POWER GROUPS

First, you're going to need a group of interested people, and hopefully, at least *one* of you has opened your Throat Chakra - it only needs one person to catalyze the rest! Try to meet regularly (once a week?), it keeps the momentum going. Have a group intention of sounding for each other, as well as working on special projects, such as distant healings, earth stabilizations, difficult urban areas and even nations and their leaders in these troubled times.

General rules for group soundings.

Try not to sing from the intellect (from your knowledge of music or voice production). Formally trained musicians generally know too much! Instead, "Trust your instinct" - to quote from Star Wars! But seriously, allow your sounds to arise entirely through intuition. The group beginnings may be croaky, squeaky and cautious, but at some point you will all find yourselves making very resonant and ringing tones. When this happens to each of you, sing the (resonate) tone until it moves (of itself) to another resonate tone; if you lose it, return to the one that previously rang out strongly and let your voice flow into a spontaneous *interaction* with the sound of the group. You must find your individual place within the chorus and intuit continuously just when you are to blend your sounds in harmony with the rest or when (on feeling a compelling power), you are to sing out strongly above them all in obbligato! As you all become accustomed to this interactive process, every one's sounds will begin to 'take off' bringing a recharging and transforming benefit for those present....even the non-singing observers on the side lines! At a certain point in the joint harmony or cacophony (in the beginning it doesn't matter which), you'll feel when the sounds want to finally fade--let them fade (although sometimes they swell and fade several times before the actual culmination). When the group really gets in tune with itself, invariably, everyone stops singing at the same time; followed by an unmistakable group-sigh of completion. Sometimes the effect of the sounding has been so profound and so moving - that without prompting or hesitation, everyone goes into instant and deep meditation!

---

[5] See "Using Mental Sounds," page 87.

1) To begin each meeting (and clear away the effects of the day), everyone should run through the Aura Recharging from Chapter 17's "Energy Exercises," also spend a few minutes of stretching, including the neck and shoulders, the mouth and jaw. Then go into a free and noisy sound work out, described in **Chapter 4,** "Releasing the Voice;" this will limber up the group 'voice' and charge up any flagging spirits.

2) Next, form a circle (you can all be sitting or standing) and after doing a general invocation[6] (only if everyone wants to!), tune in to receive and sound - your inner sounds.

3) Follow your communal-sounding with a few minutes of sharing and discussion. Discover what each of you experienced; there are often breakthroughs, insights, emotional releases.
Now that the general mood has been greatly elevated, you are ready to work on each other...or an invited guest .
Note: *It's easier to sound intuitively for someone else seated on a chair, than to sit in a circle of people and sound as a 'floating' interactive choir--that comes with practice; you are then aligning yourselves with a group Life Field energy containing merged higher Spirits that direct the sounds and insights of the group as a whole. Encourage yourselves to surrender and flow with that energy.*

Group Sounding for Another Person.

You'll be using a technique previously presented in this Chapter. Refer to section **b) "Healing One on One,"** Clearing and Balancing the Life Field (Aura) with Sound beginning on page 123. Under that section, look at paragraph number **3** - but instead of only *one* person sweeping the Field for someone sitting on a chair, you'll now have an *entire group* sweeping the field of one person sitting on a chair! Which of course, makes it considerably more powerful! Actually, it can become too crowded with more than six to eight people doing the clearing sweeps. If your regular membership is in excess of that, divide it up and take turns; some stand and sweep the Field, while the rest sit or stand behind in a non-moving circle that can project energy through their hands to the working group. Every time a different person sits on the chair for a turn at being worked on, the backup and aura-sweeping groups can change places.

1) So now there are six or eight of you ready to sweep the seated person's Life Field and one of you should be standing directly behind the chair. This is how you'll always begin and end your moving circle--with the same person behind the chair. If you all want to practice tuning-in, the (behind-the-chair) person begins by placing his/her hands on the seated person's shoulders and after a few moments of receptivity, moves over and lets the next one in line have a turn. You can continue with this and allow everyone in the circle to directly experience, via the shoulders, the seated person's energy--it's a practice that develops and improves psychic sensitivity. Directly after that, it's a good idea to discuss and share the group's impressions (including the person's on the chair) before proceeding. However, the 'hands-on-shoulders' doesn't really have to be done when you're working in a group; it simply takes up too much time, but it's good to practice occasionally because you need to do it when working one-on-one.

2) Activating the Crown Chakra. After tuning-in (if you all decided to), take up your positions in the circle again to commence sweeping the Field. Start together with all of your hands above the person's head, then begin moving them up and down (remember, in small movements) above the head, to pick up the feeling of the Crown Chakra energy.

3) Balancing the Aura. When most of you notice the tingling in your hands, commence all together to do the first down/up sweep; *repeat once more,* then **all** move a step to the right and do the second down/up movement; repeat again and move on until you have (as a group), circled entirely around the person in the chair.

---

[6] like the one at the beginning of Chapter 16, "Special Meditations."

While you are circling and sweeping, remember to watch for any build-up in your personal energy. It can take the form of extra heat in the chest and an altered breathing pattern, or you may start to feel very heavy and have difficulty moving your arms up and down--that means **stop**, *tune in, the energy is compelling you to* **sound**! *Some members of the group will register the sounding signals more readily than others and those persons generally end up being the key energy-sensitives, the ones to say:* **"I think we have to stop now and sound."** *At which, all stop, pay attention to their inner energy and allow the sounds to arise. When each spontaneous sounding concludes, pick up where you left off working the Field and continue sweeping it until someone, or all of you together, feels you need to stop again and sound some more.* **The outer non-moving group (the one that's standing and projecting energy), should *also* sound along with the inner circle.**

3a) Having made the first orbit with every one's hands six to eight inches from the receiver's body, all now step back and draw the energy 'out' to about eighteen inches distance and repeat the entire procedure--sounding when and where necessary. Each time any interesting impressions come up mid-stream, let everyone pause for a mini-discussion and then continue on with the sounding--or the impressions tend to be forgotten in the heat of the activity.

3b) Finally, If there's room and time, do a circle three feet from the seated person's body, otherwise seal the newly balanced Field by doing one sweep in the *opposite* direction (left instead of right). *The distances from the person's body are only approximate, with some people you may want to come in closer - three to four inches on the first circle, a foot on the second and two feet for a third.* **Remember, if the person you're treating seems stressed or otherwise emotionally upset, elect one or two from the group to set up surrounding Crosses of Light and speak the invocation before going on with the sounding.**

4) During the various sweeps of the Field, if anyone (in either the sweeping or outer circle) begins to pick-up strong physical sensations, aches, pains, or marked, intense emotional reactions - the sweeping circle should immediately stop balancing and the person who got the impressions, then comes and lays hands, or *one* hand on the corresponding body part of the person whose receiving the treatment in the chair. *Interestingly, sometimes two or three people pick up the same area of affliction, while others discern a pain/problem in a different body part.* Try not to smother or overwhelm the seated person; several hands (from different people) can be placed (gently) one on top of the other, and others are held two to three inches away from the in-place hands. Now, with one accord, all direct energy into the selected body-part (or parts) - with, or without sounding. Those who are "see-ers" often pick up colors while working in healing situations; these colors can be shared with the group so everyone can mentally project the color along with their sounds. More than one color might come up for use. *All energy, whether color or vibration is projected through intention and the breath.* When painful emotions arise, the receiver (or receivers) may find themselves directly experiencing and releasing the emotions on behalf of the person. being treated. When such interludes have been resolved by the group, they should return to balancing the Life Field--unless everyone feels that the session has been successful - although only thus far completed.

5) When you've finished a group sounding, let the receiver remain seated for several minutes allowing them to 'come back to earth' in their own time. Also, the entire group may need to take a break - a rest time to further discuss and integrate the energy. At this point, glasses of cold water would refresh everyone. Water taken after interdimensional healing work integrates and clears the energy. Those who channeled a great deal in the session may also need to run cold water over their hands, wrists and forearms--this has an instant re-balancing effect. If anyone in the group happens to feel disoriented or in an *uncomfortable* altered state, bring them a small pinch of salt (sea salt is best) and a half glass of cold water; this combination will restore them immediately.

Other Power Group Projects.

Experiment with distant and surrogate healings. Distant healings can focus on out of town relatives, absent loved ones, public figures, international leaders, areas of local and world tension, misunderstandings and war. Bring photographs or newspaper articles to serve as focusing points; place on a small table or low stool, over which you make *a single* Cross of Light (plus invocation); then the group gathers around in a circle to project energy, color and sound to the surrogate object. If not sounding to a specific (absent) person, arrange the sound-projects into categories and make one or several piles (of papers and photographs), then sound to each pile in turn. Area and world maps can be 'dowsed' with the hands to send stabilizing energy into oceans, geographic fault and volcano areas. *The curious color most frequently occurring for earth stabilization resembles a deep gold-yellow, like the color I imagine in the center of the galaxy..or the gold of the setting sun.* Use this technique for all kinds of locations, local or overseas--a map or photograph is all you need. With an involved person assisting, I once sounded (from my home in Oregon, to a very large haunted house located in France. All we had was a photograph of the house and my friend's direct connection with the location--on her frequent visits to France, she mostly lived and worked in that particular house...you could say, she knew it and the 'ghost' rather well! Some months later she returned to France and confirmed that we had been successful in putting the spirit to rest. *Which brings us to surrogate healings:* these happen when a friend or relative of a person absent (but needing help), sits in the center of the Sound Healing circle and receives the energy in lieu of the missing person. (While in the process of 'receiving' for someone else by proxy, the surrogate mentally projects the energy *to* that person.)

Inner City Sound Stations.

I close this Chapter with a healing vision for the crumbling inner cities and for the young people within them who live in an atmosphere of despair and violence. Their empty hearts have no vision; they don't know themselves as physical and spiritual beings of great potential! Mostly they remain lost in their animal instincts. Yet, essential for our survival, this animal part drives our bodies and grounds us to the earth demanding space, fresh air and light for the health and balance of our total being. Otherwise, we revert to a vicious jungle law of roaming in packs, marking out territory and preying on others. Many inner city kids live like this, just to stay alive in a failed social system - in a state of bitterness, hopelessness and rage.

There are now gangs in the once gentle city where I live, a small, beautiful College town, known for its open, natural and healthy lifestyle. The youth of this former pristine city have clean air to breathe and space to spread themselves, but many are homeless, having left or been abandoned by their birth families. There are no longer positive patterns or heroes that inspire them in the outer world, so they create their own--that is all the hope they have--to resist what they know and have been taught because they feel it has failed them.

The Sound Warriors.

My call goes out to those who have opened their Throat Chakras (have become Light Singers and understand their triple bodied nature), to go in the power of their song and teach our youth to become Sound Warriors. There must be old warehouses or school auditoriums that could be set up as Sounding Stations--havens of sound, where the young and angry could discharge their fury and deep underlying sorrow. There, they could reconnect to their creative potential and Spiritual Power by sounding **out** their rage and sorrow and sounding **in** the hope and wonder of who they really are--through the vowels and the key letters in their names, they could be taught to heal each other and their communities with the inner sounds of Light.

Considerably more can be taught and directly experienced in a hands-on class or workshop, but the above Chapter covers enough basic information to get you started. In my own work, I use additional "tools" like different crystals under the person's chair or between their feet to aid in grounding and to bring in other energies; then I also have different drums, rattles, feather-fans, Australian 'clicking-sticks' and an American Indian flute, but all of those are just extras--and not even necessary--your voice is the primary tool and that's all you really need. *Remember, your higher Spirit and your connection to the inner-voices will guide you the rest of the way. But please begin. The world is waiting for the Light Singer healers!*

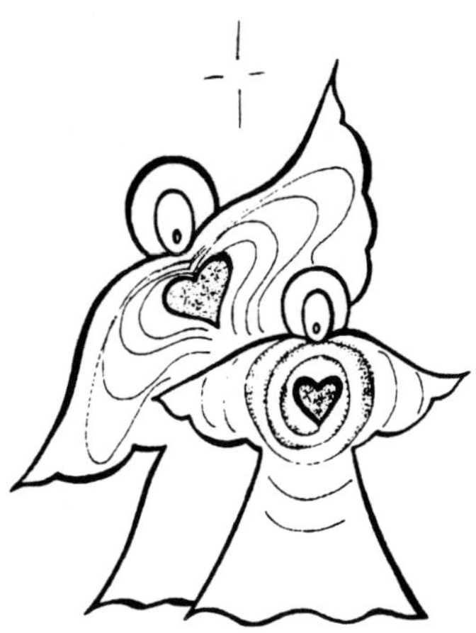

16..... SPECIAL MEDITATIONS

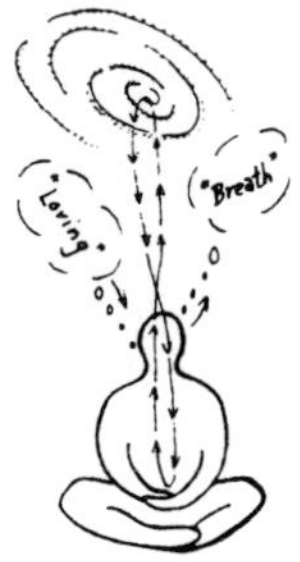

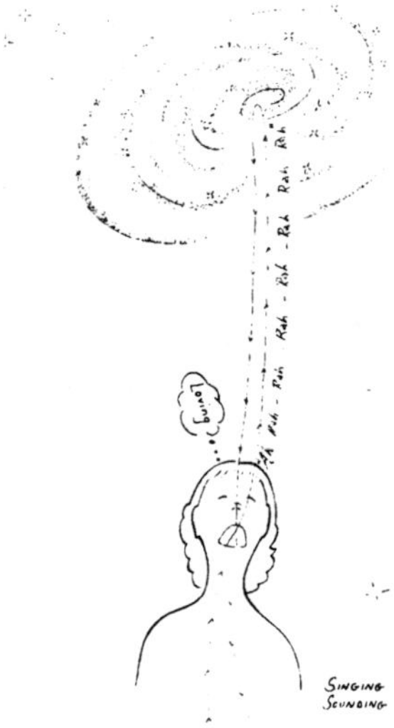

POWER AND PROTECTION INVOCATION - ONE

(Repeat each sentence once if doing this in a group and twice if alone.)

For this day I,...(your name) now call forth my power and may I use it wisely.

I align with my Holy Spirit and the Source of All that Is.

I align with the Universal Consciousness.

I honor my parents for giving me birth; I honor the Earth Mother and all of Nature.

I ask for direction and assistance from my Guides and helpers from this and other dimensions.

I call upon my Angels of Light.

Protect and guide me this day and unfold my life into its greatest potential and fulfillment - for my benefit and for all those whose lives I touch.

Supply all our needs and surround us with every opportunity for growth and joy.

May we join each other in the Universal Consciousness,
And may we include all beings and creatures.

Keep us always in the greater Presence,
And keep us aware of that Presence surrounding and filling us
until we realize that we also are that Presence.

So it is.

The above is an example of an invocation that one usually hears or presents at the beginning of meditation gatherings - or that one recites for oneself. In the following more intimate version, the essential meaning is retained, but the words and rhythms engage you more deeply in accessing your own hidden powers and those of the interdimensional beings surrounds you.

POWER AND PROTECTION INVOCATION - TWO

"I,.....(say your name)..stir up my powers and gifts - to bless, heal and transform."

"Beloved Holy Spirit, I open and receive your power."

"Infinite Source of All, I feel your sacred Presence."

"I enter the web of universal consciousness
Where I connect to............." (here, I see the faces and 'name' the names of loved ones or others I wish to pray for, or send healing energy to.)

"Thank you dearest parents, for the life you gave me.
(Thank you Mom and Dad, for all your loving care.")

" Thank you blessed Mother Earth for sustaining me."

"Untiring Guides and unseen Helpers, nudge me with your gentle counsel."

"Angels streaming from the Light, protect and keep me on my path."

"May I use each special moment,
As a chance to shower blessings."

"For everyone I see today, remind me to return them all
To their rightful place within the Conscious Web of Higher Mind."

"Help me to accept all life-forms with respect."

"Let me live as the Presence of Light, let me love as the Presence of Love,
Show me each day, the sacred way, to remain in Oneness with all Life. **So it is.**

Now follows an in-depth discussion of each section given above - what it means - and what you can expect to experience as you progress into the powerful energy of the individual meditations.

"I,..(say your name)..stir up my powers and gifts - to bless, heal and transform."

These refer to your gifts and talents--the strengths and abilities that you were born with...and may be neglecting or avoiding. Remember, as you unfold yourself, the world becomes a better place.

"Beloved Holy Spirit, I open and receive your power."

The Holy Spirit is your higher power and descends from the upper Chakras through the Crown, and/or directly via the frontal lobes of the brain to the Ajna (situated in the middle of forehead) from where it recharges all of the body's Chakras. You will feel it sweep through you as continuous waves of bliss! Or it may concentrate on and fully activate only one or two of the Chakras, such as the heart and throat in turn. It will trigger the inner-voices and songs through the Throat Chakra when that center opens.

"Infinite Source of All, I feel your sacred Presence."

The Source energy manifests through all of the head centers and is strongly sensed first as a **separate** *"Sacred Presence" - a pervading cloud of numinosity that surrounds and extends out from the head and over the shoulders.... a protective overshadowing....reminiscent of giant wings! The Source Presence (the All-pervading Intelligence) augments and expands consciousness, so that eventually one penetrates the inner duality and attains the Luminous Mind - or the All-encompassing expansion. If you don't at first experience the 'sacred Presence' you can use your hands to open the pathways. Sit peacefully and 'frame' your face with your hands...the wrists join under your chin, your thumbs rest in the groove behind the angle of the jaw below the ears and the fingers rest on the cheek bones at the sides of the*

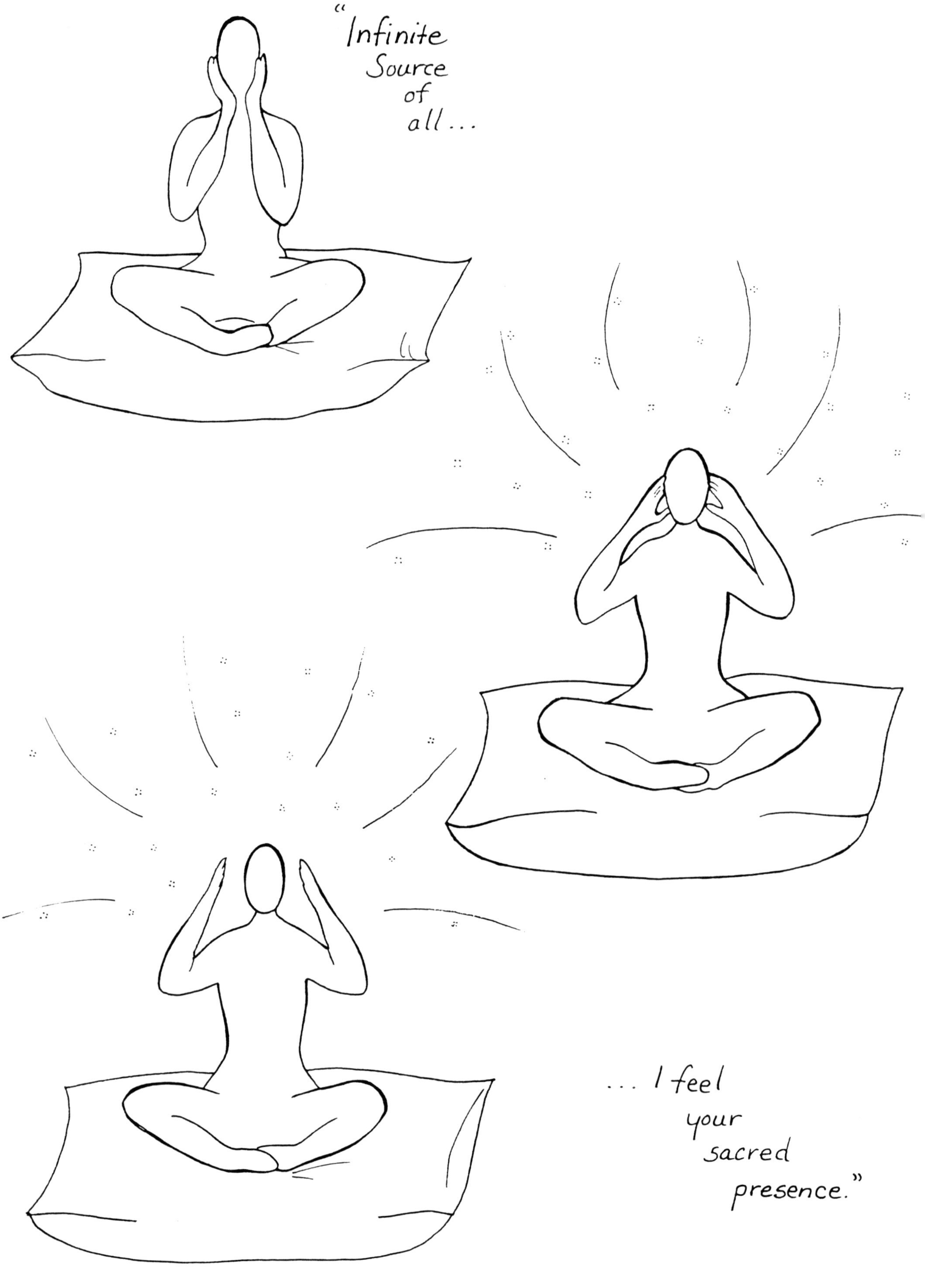
"Infinite Source of all...
... I feel your sacred presence."

face (just in front of the ears)....now open your wrists and lift your hands out sideways until just the finger and thumb-tips only are resting on the sides of the face. Just hold them there and repeat several times the powerful mantra that begins Psalm 91 from the Old Testament (King James version)..."He that dwelleth in the secret place of the Most High - shall abide under the shadow of the Almighty." Next, lift the fingers two or three inches entirely off the cheek bones and just hold the hands (like antennae) each side of the face. Within seconds, the Crown and other head centers will open and you will find yourself breathing in and out of the upper Crown. When the 'Presence' descends, lower your hands and resume the original affirmation......"Infinite Source of All, I feel your sacred Presence."

"I enter the web of Universal Consciousness
Where I connect to....." (here, I see the faces and 'name' the names of loved ones, or others I wish to pray for or send healing energy to.)

It takes an actual 'shift' in awareness--an intention, to enter the vast and subtle mind-matrix where every human on the planet is linked as one intelligence. It is the easiest place to go to when praying for others. Try visualizing the Universal Consciousness as a giant interconnecting web of golden pathways containing the higher Minds of all souls on the planet, as well as their past life sub-selves. Call up the names and faces of those you love (or are praying for) and they will appear on the golden web before you. (I find the background color to be a deep green, but you may perceive it entirely differently.)

"Thank you dearest parents for the life you gave me.

If you **can't** *say "dearest parents" you may need to practice the technique called "Emotional Healing - Relationships" under Section 5 of this Chapter (page 145).*

Thank you blessed Mother Earth for sustaining me.

Acknowledge and honor the Earth Mother/Goddess - her sacred land and waters, and the creatures we share her with - and you will not want for sustenance or be without shelter.

"Untiring Guides and unseen Helpers, nudge me with your gentle counsel.
Angels streaming from the Light, protect and keep me on my path."

If we do not ask, we cannot receive. Those who assist from the inner planes need us to consciously invoke and engage their energy. This is simply a matter of frequency-linking. In order to match their frequency we must petition them, thus opening the pathway to their influence (or if we won't, or can't - others can ask assistance on our behalf--just as we can also petition help for the needs of others).

"In this new day, guide, protect me; let me know each special moment
As a chance to shower blessings."

Our enlightened place in this world is as 'conducting rods' between dimensions - and as transformers of gross to refined, dark into light, and the restoration of spirit into form.

"For everyone I see today, remind me to return them all,
To their rightful place within, the Conscious Web of Higher Mind."

In the earlier 'web' prayer, you penetrated the Universal Consciousness for the purpose of sending goodwill and energy to those you know or are concerned about; with this prayer, the relationship changes. You enter the web to become a conscious part of the matrix and to draw others in with you. When next you're alone in public, try taking a deep breath and relax your surface thoughts, then soften your eyes and say to yourself...."I now enter the universal mind-matrix"....you will instantly find yourself in the 'higher-group-mind' of the human species. Notice how your perception shifts. Something in you has expanded into a larger energy field. You look at your body and it appears the same, but another part of you has become vast and boundless. In this new awareness your response to the people around you has shifted also. And it doesn't matter where you are--you could be with strangers in the street, in a restaurant, bus, or waiting room; this much greater part of you embraces them all equally and for each one you mentally repeat....."I place you in the Universal Consciousness." Then those that walk by no longer seem like strangers. You will look in people's faces and they will pass you smiling - linked through your eyes to the vast mind-web of mankind; a separated part of them (and yourself) has been reconnected.

"Help me to accept all life-forms with respect."

You will discover to your suprise that the nature forms and animals also have their own group matrix and will welcome you there when you 'visit'....they of course are already one with their higher group consciousness. Only humans walk in isolation. (For healing with the inter dimensional Spirits of herbs and plants refer to the unique book written by Eliot Cowan called "Plant Spirit Medicine.")

"Let me live as the Presence of Light,
let me love as the Presence of Love,
Show me each day, the sacred way,
To remain in the Oneness with all Life. **So it is.**

2....TRANQUILLITY MEDITATIONS

The experience of transcendent stillness emanates directly from the Root Chakra at the base of the spine and is your physical and mystical sign that the Chakra has opened. It means that your highest Spirit has descended to the coccygeal center and united with your physical essence in the Root. (Your Root center anchors you to the physical plane.) It may happen spontaneously for no apparent reason, or arise through meditation and mantra; someone else's energy may also activate it. Whichever way, you must recognize and surrender to the initial sensations and allow the manifestations to attain their fullness. You always have a choice--to experience Spirit (in this case) as stillness and connectedness to the earth, or turn it off and remain in your usual thinking/feeling mode.

My first spontaneous experience of this happened while chatting with Joan, a visiting associate and friend. In mid-sentence and for no reason, I suddenly stopped speaking. The Crown Center had opened on the top of my head and as energy moved through me, I found myself swept into a profound and deep stillness beyond anything I had ever experienced before. I remained observing my friend's familiar face, but I watched from a mute and fathomless place within myself - my body a living statue, my arms and hands fixed in a frozen gesture before me. Though Immobilized, I felt totally comfortable and at rest! Finally Joan spoke. "What's happening?" she asked me quietly. Words arose unbidden (by *me*) from the depths of my arrested body; I could hear them and knew they needed to be spoken and with some considerable effort managed to summon up my faintest voice: "I....have...to say...this," (pause). "Be still...and know....that...I am God." It was a phrase from the Old Testament![1]

After repeating the phrase once more, I reverted thankfully back into the silence. Joan just sat watching me; she had seen me 'process' before, but nothing quite like this. Several more silent minutes elapsed. With still no desire to move (or to ever move again for that matter!), I felt exactly like a rock - as though I'd entered my core-center. The silence continued and I remained serenely frozen in time; then very gradually my motility and voice returned and I haltingly tried to describe a feeling so vastly *beyond* what I had ever thought of as peace--that in the end, words absolutely failed me! "The peace that passeth understanding?" Finally with extreme reluctance, I returned to my usual awareness.

Before the mystery of names began to fascinate me, I had previously read about the English poet Wordsworth who attained an expanded state of consciousness by using his name like a mantra--that is, he repeated it as a power-word over and over for an extended period of time. After I gained my present knowledge on the meaning and value of names, I began experimenting with Wordsworth's idea (for myself) and was quite suprised to re-encounter the "stillness" experience as a result. In addition to repeating my name, I also added the mantra: **"Be still and know that I am God-Goddess."**

Invoking the Stillness.

Sit in a comfortable chair with your feet placed flat on the floor and your back held straight. To make the recitations flow more easily get yourself an Eastern rosary of 108 beads (called a mala). *You could even be creative and make your own.* **For every recitation (no matter how long), move one bead.** *Do at least two rounds of the mala every day (216 recitations), or do 108 on your name and 108 on "Be still and know." Increase the number of rounds if desired. Bead shops (for supplies) are almost ubiquitous; but failing that, there's always the alarm clock to time your meditation.*

Initially, I separate the mantras, repeating my own name for five minutes, followed by "Be still and know" for another five minutes. Eventually, I combine the two in a final meditation.

---

[1] Psalm 46. verse 10.

<u>**Here's the combination:**</u> *Begin with your name.*

"...(say your name), " *then* **"Be still and know that I am God (....or God-Goddess)."**

If your sub-selves resist, you say: "Be still and know that *you* are God-Goddess."

Close your eyes and relax into the mantra as it goes around in your head and the beads pass through your fingers and fall around your hands. The stillness may at first elude you, or only surface once - *once may be all you need*--but the other benefits will prove enormous. With the meditation on the **sound** of your name, you will ground your identity into your body and into the earth--and begin to walk with a new found confidence. Further, as you become more and more deeply the expression of your higher Spirit, *you will know and feel who you are in a new and powerful way.*

The Nostril Breath.

This meditation rests the outer intellect and takes you to the 'inner cave' of higher Mind. Before you begin, disengage your eyes; do this by relaxing them and repeating mentally to yourself:

> **"Soft eyes,"** - *breathe into eyes.*
> **"Gentle eyes "** - *breathe out of eyes.*

1) Repeat the above a few times, *then focus attention away from your eyes and onto the tip of your nostrils. At the nostril tip, be aware of your breath gently coming in and out.*

2) When you are at rest in this procedure, repeat mentally, two words:

> **"Calm......."** *as you breathe* **in** *to the nostril tip,*
> **"Peaceful.."** *as you breathe* **out.** **That is all.**

Repeat for as long as needed. *Use wherever and whenever you want to become calm and detached, or set aside a daily time to practice this as a formal meditation.*

When I first practiced this several years ago I initially enjoyed a new found tranquillity, until a dramatic change occurred in the meditation. One morning, after beginning the breath and entering the inner space, I was startled to receive waves and waves of information pouring into my head, information pertaining to my research and writing--fresh and important ideas that had never occurred to me before! I had to interrupt the meditation to write them down! This phenomenon ensued without fail on every subsequent session. *What had happened?* I finally realized the mediation had given me a stilled and focused outer mind that allowed the Inner Knower to 'download' information; I had established a direct pathway to my higher Mind to help me fulfill my life's work. This may not necessarily happen to you, but at least you will gain inner tranquillity with the practice!

3....OPENING THE HEART MEDITATIONS

The natural qualities of the Heart Chakra are compassionate love, kindness and caring. Unfortunately, our hearts tend to collect unhappy feelings--disappointments, yearnings, tormenting passions and jealousy! As adults, we connect through our hearts to old pain stored in the belly center from our unrequited inner child. Spirit has many natural 'seats' in the body, the primary one however is the Heart Chakra. This non-physical center has been described as the 'second heart,' because of the strange activity in the chest when the higher Spirit descends and attempts to open the Chakra. The heart then appears to move erratically--to beat differently. A secondary pulse may even announce itself, as though you have two hearts in your chest, one beating out of phase with the other (at least initially). During these visitations (of Spirit to the heart), heat, vibration and a sensation of expansion can permeate the entire chest area. Should this come upon you unexpectedly, you're in for an alarming time--to say the least! Also, when you happen to harbor unsatisfied love or emotional disappointment, it's possible to experience intense or stabbing pains in the chest when the center begins to open. I know personally of several people who, under the impression they were in the throes of a heart attack, admitted themselves to the nearest hospital Emergency Room where everyone became terribly puzzled when their test results were normal! ***I'm NOT saying here*** *that you shouldn't give yourself the benefit of the doubt when your heart's health seems seriously threatened.* **Please rush to the hospital--either way--you need to know**, but if nothing is the matter, your Heart Chakra could be trying to open!

Closely linked in location, there appears to be both a physical heart of flesh and blood and an etheric 'heart'- the actual Chakra! These mysterious centers (the Chakras), exist both inside and outside of us acting like superconductors between the visible heat-combustion physical body, the invisible energy-double (Chi body), and the equally indiscernible Light Body (consisting of out-of-body Chakras above the head). **The inter-connectedness of this entire system takes place through the primal energy force commonly referred to as "Spirit."** As most humans only live in one third of their potential form (and see life exclusively from the physical combustion-body point of view), they remain oblivious to the other two thirds--their Chi and Light bodies; consequently, the direct experience of higher Spirit as the integrating force between these three bodies is largely unknown. Many people equate the term "soul" with Spirit; however, soul and Spirit are **not** one and the same! The idea of 'soul' more accurately relates to that part of (limited) consciousness known as ego/will...in which resides the veiled *potential* for expansion into Source Awareness - and again, very, very, very few have realized the Source Awareness--let alone live effectively within the non-ego state![2]

One of the manifestations of Spirit, called the "Fire from Above," actually signals the first descent of this higher energy system into the physical and Chi body complex; It's an almost masculine power that comes down from above the head and then sweeps through the entire system in the form of rushing waves of power, heat, expansion, vibration and ecstasy. When this first happens, accompanied by the throat opening and "tongues," it's called (in Christian mysticism), "The Baptism of the Spirit."

Further effects of the higher Spirit on the human organism are as follows:

1) In the Heart Center specifically, the energy awakens us more gently (but no less warmly) to non-judgmental, unconditional acceptance and love, and releases our supernormal faculties of compassion and healing power.
2) In the Throat Chakra, it opens us to the inner power-voices (the glossalalia), with their songs and sounds of healing and transformation.
3) In the ordinary mind, Spirit connects us to higher Mind, to supernormal knowledge, insight, inspiration, wisdom, and finally to the luminous Source Consciousness.
4) In the nervous system, muscles and organs (when dire need dictates), it activates the raw power of the Chi body and floods us with superhuman strength and vigor--above and beyond the capability of a sudden adrenaline rush.

We concentrate now on the heart, because once Spirit returns in force to the heart (its natural home), it heals our deepest emotional pain and begins to enliven the rest of the energy centers.

All this seems totally foreign to our culturally programmed thinking. Even my many years of direct experience didn't help me explain to others how they could receive their own higher Spirit. I finally found a way, through a 'magical game,' a game that lets us open and become once more the innocent, trusting child. Remember the ancient saying: "Unless ye become as a little child, ye cannot enter the Kingdom of Heaven." Heaven may be as close as your unused Chakras, especially the ones above the head! Periodically throughout history, we draw to us great teacher-messengers who express such compassion, insight and love, that our hearts and minds revive; but over time and distance, their memory and messages (in the hands of powerful rulers), turn into manipulative ploys to engender fear and elitism rather than openness and love. The powers that control us today still desire to keep the human race in ignorance and division. Even our present physical form may have been a calculated design of biological interference from ancient alien techno-gods[3] (a genetic deviation created from a super-intelligent, intergalactic being and a primitive, programmable, evolving life form).

---

2 Read "Collision with the Infinite - a Life Beyond the Personal Self" by Suzanne Segal.

3 Scholar and translator, Zecharia Sitchin in "Genesis Revisited" and "The 12th Planet."

But enough of speculation! Let us return to the heart, the place of healing and restoration.
Before beginning any procedures for the heart, one should first establish a foundational relationship with the polarities of the crown and root Chakras - the God-Goddess archetypal energies. Please refer to all three parts of **Section 3** *(Finding the Power of Mother-Father, God-Goddess) from* Chapter 17.

The Magical Game.

The child in us who needs love relates to a trustworthy, loving adult, whereas our grownup self relates to a loving equal, usually of the opposite sex. The 'game' we will play rolls all of these needs into one archetypal image--the Inner Beloved, epitomizing a love so perfect and all-encompassing that we will find ourselves opening, receiving and totally dissolving into it. (Our hearts ignite, when the Spirit returns as Love.) Children call such games "pretending," grownups call them "intending." As physical electromagnets, we establish unerring magnetic signals--just by being persistent in imaging and intending the results we want.

The thought of the Inner Lover sounds a bit farfetched for most of us. But we *can* relate to the perfect lover/mate.....if we haven't given up entirely! Most unattached or unhappily attached people don't mind believing and affirming that Mr.Right or Ms.Right could one day come into their lives. I've heard quite spiritually aware people say, "Forget about the Spiritual Beloved, I want the **real** flesh and blood one--let's work on that!" And certainly you must, if your heart inexorably yearns for the ideal relationship in which two people dream, work, play and progress together spiritually. It's usually called..... "A companion along the Way."

So for those of us who hanker for a companion along the way, and one has not yet appeared, here follows ***The Perfect Love Affirmation*** *to bring such a love into your life. (You always affirm that your intention has actually been fulfilled.)*

Intending the Perfect Love Companion.

Sit with your hands resting on your thighs (or gently in your lap), palms facing upward. (The gesture of openness and receiving.) Your hands magnetize to the Heart Chakra.

Begin by saying: **"I...**(say your name)..... *breathe* **in** *and* **out** *on your name....*

Now draw to me (breath in)
My (in every way) perfect Love, (breath out)
In the form of another (breath in)
Spiritually aware (breath out)
Totally caring (breath in)
Passionate person. (breath out)
And I see this beloved (breath in)
Already at my side." (breath out).

Then devise your own breathing pattern and mentally recite the following
Perfect Love Affirmation:

"I have an amazing and marvelous love,
A love beyond compare,
A mental, emotional, physical love,
A spiritual union fair.
Together we're one in the world,
To create, to play and to dare.
Together we're one in the world,
To explore, to heal and to share.
I have an amazing and marvelous love."

You might want to write the Perfect Love Affirmation on beautiful note paper, attach it to your mirror, learn it off by heart (it's quite easy) and say it at least twice a day; once on arising and once more on retiring to bed. Deal with your resistance to deserving such a love and set out your personal preferences as to physical specifications; but whatever you do--be sure to include an unmarried clause. 'Recently separated' is usually not a good idea either - though I have seen some exceptions!

Also, if you *are* one of those unhappily marrieds (or stuck in some other less than delightful liaison) say the affirmation anyway and magical things could happen right where you are with the one you're with...or the problems and the person could move effortlessly out of your life. The words themselves are healing and you need to heal the pain in your heart.

Removing the Blocks to Receiving Love.

Unfortunately, it's not always so simple as reciting a daily affirmation to find the truly perfect companion. Many of us keep attracting painful and difficult mirrors of our own sexual and emotional blocks --which we will continue to manifest **without fail**, until we erase our own negative programming to mated happiness. And many of us have become so wounded and discouraged that we have retreated into the safety of our own celibate company. *The following combines two techniques that will definitely address the problem.*

Firstly, this technique does not work cold; "cold" meaning to repeat the affirmations entirely from the standpoint of intellect. Our large emotional boulders only budge when you're in the direct path of their negative power! In other words, you have to deliberately activate the old painful feelings -- much like a meditator practicing the Left Hand Path of Tibetan Mysticism (in which the negative passions are aroused in order to use their energies towards enlightenment). You must also stir up your memories of unfulfilled love, of sexual disappointments and compromises, of not being accepted by a mate for your true self.....and then, with your memory-induced angst fully felt.....
repeat the following several times:

"I....(say your name)....now un-create the blocks to receiving love in my life. I speak to my sub-selves as well as my outer self...

"A negative program for perfect love *(breath in)*
......is present within us. *(breath out)*
A negative program for **receiving** love *(breath in)*
......is present within me! *(breath out)*
We are not..*(breath in)*...this denial of love. *(breath out)*
I am not ...*(breath in)*...this rejection of love." *(breath out).*

Repeat the following twice:

"I am the Infinite Presence *(breath in)*
......of Perfect Love". *(breath out).*

Now continue in your chosen breathing pattern:

"Whatever I have created - between myself and perfect love,
I now accept - that I chose the experience,
I now forgive - myself, and those involved,
I now dissolve all painful emotions -
And release the energy into Love.
I am the Infinite Presence of Perfect Love."

Practice this Removing Blocks technique every day until you can remember your less than perfect past love experiences with acceptance and peace. Then begin to affirm **"I now draw to me..."** *and* **"I have an amazing and marvelous love"** *from the previous page.*
You, as the creator of your reactions to life - can also un-create and recreate.

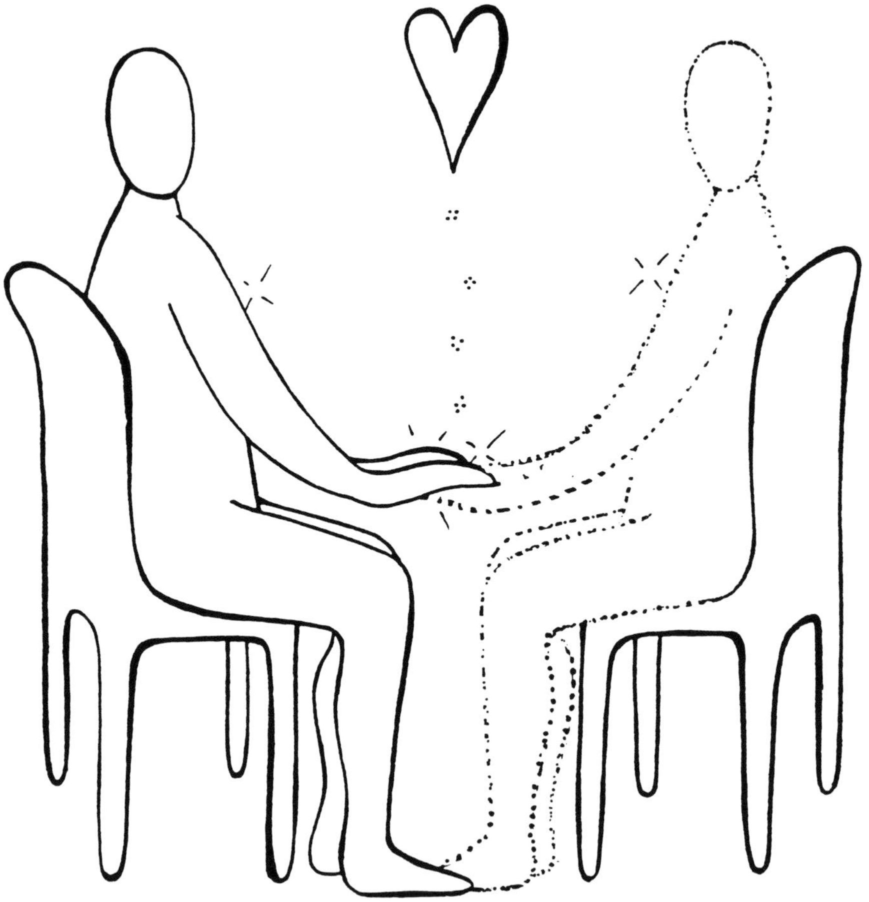

"Divine Belov
I receive thee
in my
heart."

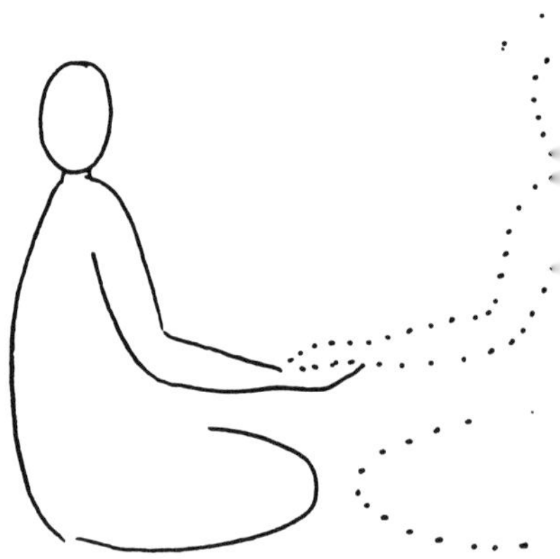

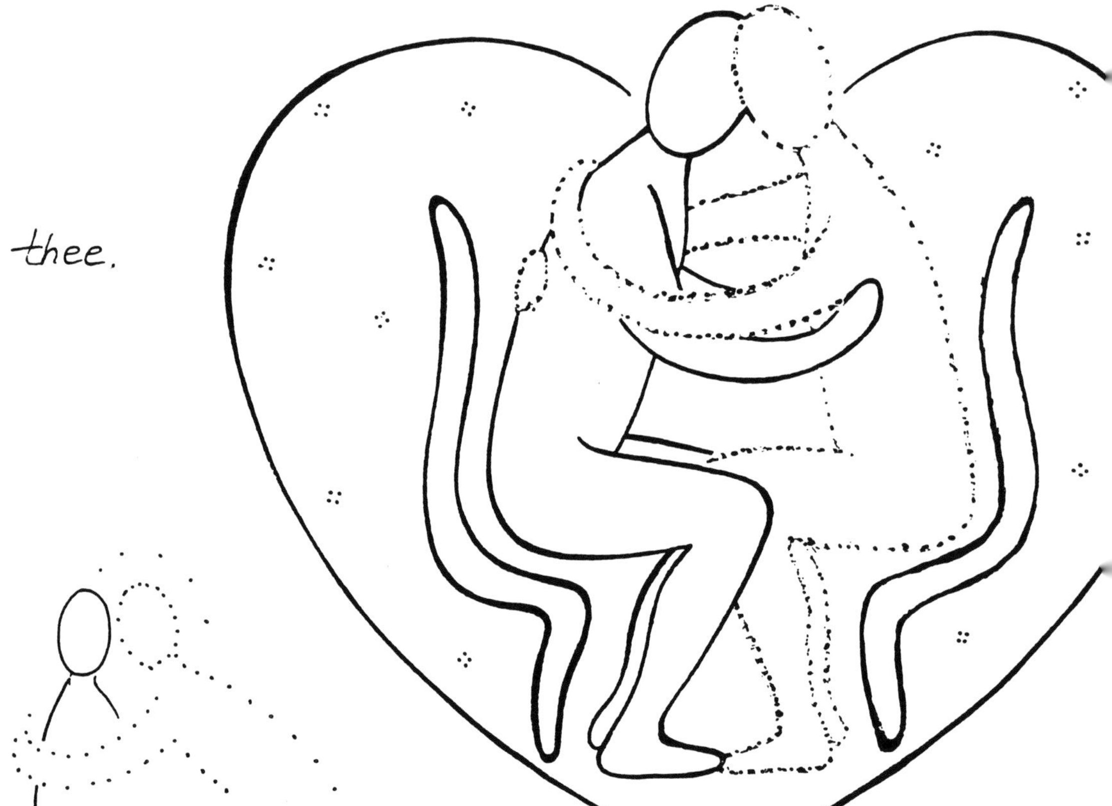

"Beloved,
I receive thee.
We are
joined
in
the
heart."

The final phase of opening the Heart Chakra follows. It encompasses **two** steps: the first, **Activating the Inner Beloved Archetype** completes the balancing of the emotional body; the second, **Activating the Cosmic Love Energy** connects the balanced Heart Chakra to the Energy body. **Do both.**

Activating the Inner Beloved Archetype .

First energize the hands. The energy channels for the heart begin in the hands. Ley lines (pathways) from the hands traverse the arms terminating in the heart; others ending in the feet discharge buildup and ground the heart electromagnetically to the earth. The hands are the organs of giving and receiving (healing or harming); what we **do** with the hands and how we **use** them, directly relates to the feelings we hold in the heart.

1) Sit comfortably, feet flat on the floor. Gently shake your hands (to loosen the wrists), rub them together until you feel warmth. Now separate and keep moving them a few inches in and out from each other until you sense tingling in both palms - you have now activated their magnetic poles.

2) Lay your hands, palms up, on your upper thighs (or if you're sitting on a lounge, you may decide to place them palms up, on the lounge *beside* your thighs - whichever feels right.) You'll start to note tingling in the hands. *Keep relaxed, but begin to 'breathe' in and out of your palms.*

3) Continue breathing in this way while you visualize an exquisite Being standing in front of you--who regards you with eyes of great tenderness and love. (Imagine your own, or choose Jesus, the primary Heart Avatar for the West, or Krishna for the East--there are others. All will activate the heart.)
Look into those eyes and repeat several times:

"Divine Beloved, I receive Thee." *(You may find yourself smiling.)*

4) This Being now sits directly in front of you, placing both his/her hands on top of yours. Imagine their gentle weight and warmth. (*You may prefer the reversed hand position with your palms facing* ***down*** *instead of up, in which case, feel your hands resting* ***on*** *the Beloved's.)*
Continue to receive the Divine Beloved's energy through your hands and keep repeating the above phrase for several breaths until you feel a slight movement in the heart (it can be a gentle or a leaping movement); also, there may be a change in your breath pattern.
Then affirm:

"Divine Beloved...." as you breathe in,

"I receive Thee in my heart.".... as you breath the out-breath ***into*** the heart.

By now a distinct energy and warmth will be flowing from your hands, through the arms and into your heart. **Repeat the above at least five times. If you desire to remain in this part of the meditation for several minutes, do so.**

5) Now see the Beloved lean forward and gently enfold you in his/her arms until you feel your heads resting cheek to cheek. This can be entirely mental or you may want to raise and hold up your arms in an imaginary embrace...keep your eyes closed.
While you rest in each other's embrace repeat the following for as long as you need to:

"Beloved, I receive Thee, we are joined in the heart."...or..

"Beloved...(name your Beloved)**, our hearts are One."**

6) With each repetition and with each breath, your Divine Beloved gradually melts into your breast, leaving you warmed, vibrating and aware of the Spiritual Heart. Finally, place your hands, one on top of the other in the center of your breast (you have joined the polarities in your hands), this will also activate the heart; or rest your elbows on your thighs and move the hands *out* from the breast (one in front of the other), about six to eight inches from the body and just hold them there. Eventually you may want to place your hands back in your lap. Make sure your eyes are 'soft,' and you feel an inner smile filling your heart and lifting the corners of your mouth.
Remain in this feeling of Love (with your chosen hand position) as you keep repeating:

"Beloved...(name your Beloved)**, our hearts are One." ....or..**

"Infinite Love, I rest in Thy Presence." [4]

---

4 When you feel the Presence in the heart, let go of the mind and enter the expansion through the senses--see Chapter 21 beginning on page 178.

NOTE: If during the Divine Beloved meditation, you notice unusual and subtle sensations arising in the heart - stop the formal practice of repeating the mantra and pay attention to the phenomena; allow them to increase while you surrender to the bliss and expansion. Also your breath pattern may vary (speed up or slow down), in response to the energy in the chest. When the feelings lessen return to the formal meditation. It can almost be like a wave, swelling and ebbing as the etheric heart rouses itself. Be sensitive to the flow, stopping and starting the mantras when necessary to allow the inner unfolding. If possible, try and cover all of the meditation procedure during which, you may notice a considerable build up of heat especially in the chest and arms. It's as though all your old emotions are being transformed into the Cosmic Fire of Love.

Throughout the day, use the following phrase as a continuing Mantra to keep the 'Love space' opening within you and the 'smile' within your heart:

" Infinite Love (or Divine Beloved), I rest in Thy Presence ."

For the Non Visual.

If you can't imagine a 'person' in your mind's eye try sensing a 'presence' close to you and conjure up a feeling of heaviness and tingling in your hands. A large, soft cuddly bear or other stuffed animal will help create the illusion. Just have it resting against your chest while you concentrate on the 'hands-touching' part; then, when it comes time for the embrace--hold the bear and imagine! And yes, although this is an illusion, a game, you are nonetheless creating an energy connection between the physical and the etheric-heart.

The underlying secret to opening the heart is relationship; that's the reason the Love Avatars gave us an object of sacred devotion--themselves! They only function as substitute Beloveds, however, for as long as it takes to awaken us into the love relationship they embody--that of the outer self with the Inner Self (the soul with the incandescent Source Awareness). Remember in the beginning of a relationship, how it feels to be deeply, passionately in love--when both of you *know* you're in love? Ah! - the euphoria of being in this world of love, of melting at the thought, the touch, the look of the other? Bring those old feelings back during the Inner Beloved meditation, then learn to sustain them--with *yourself* as the Beloved, the penultimate relationship that rejoins you to the ground of your being, the Source within all things. And remember the inner smile! The initial function of the meditation opens you to the continuing presence of the Inner Beloved. Eventually, when you begin to you know yourself as the Beloved. *You repeat it in the* **first** *person:*

"I am an amazing and marvelous Love,
A love beyond compare;
A mental, emotional, physical love,
A spiritual union fare;
Together, I'm One in the world,
To create, to play and to dare.
Together, I'm One in the word,
To restore, to heal and to share.
I am an amazing and marvelous Love.

The more self-complete you become, the more you will be able to say:

Love has
No expectations or demands;
Love has
No attachments.
Love is
Complete within itself.

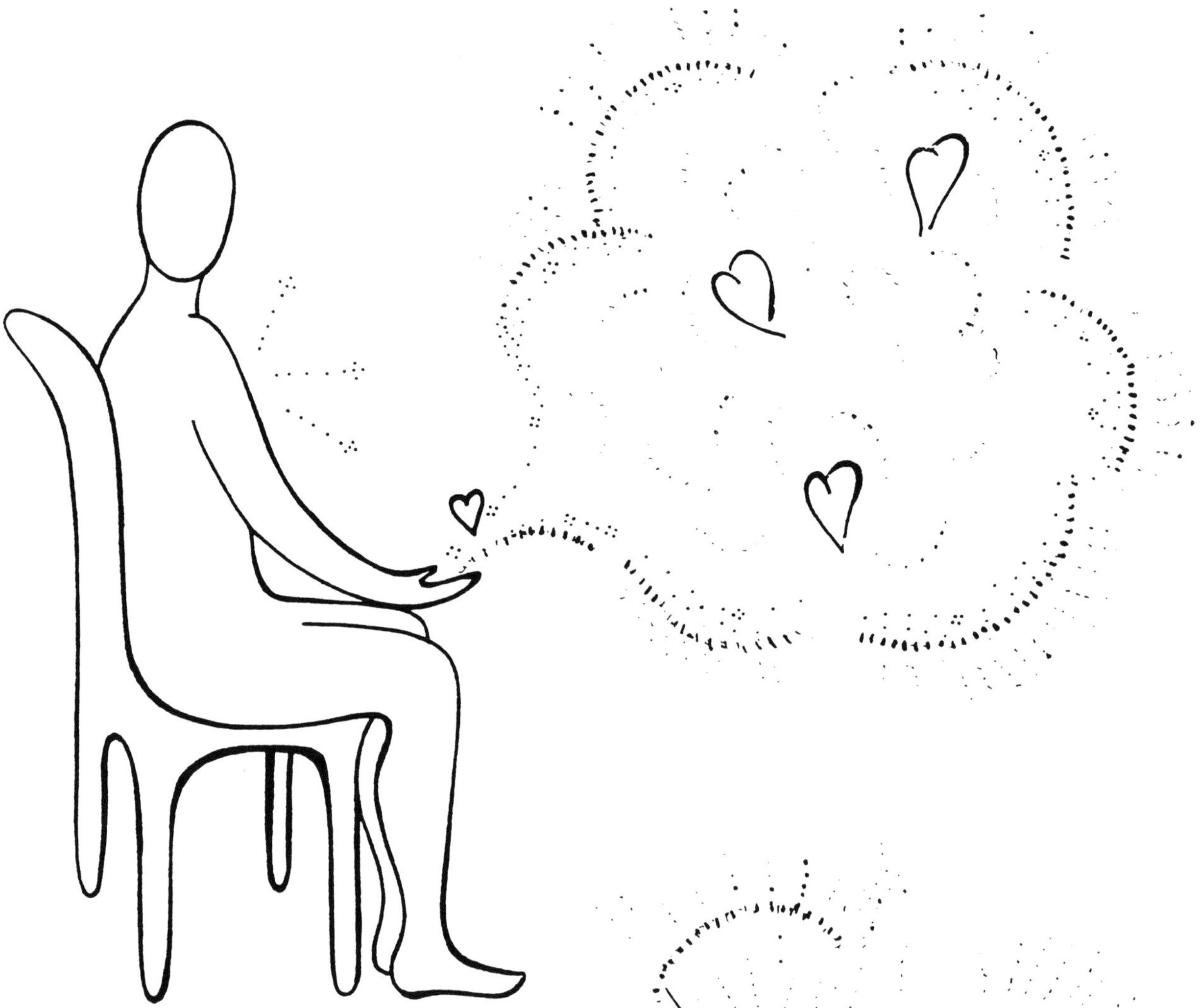

"I now receive
Cosmic Love
in my heart."

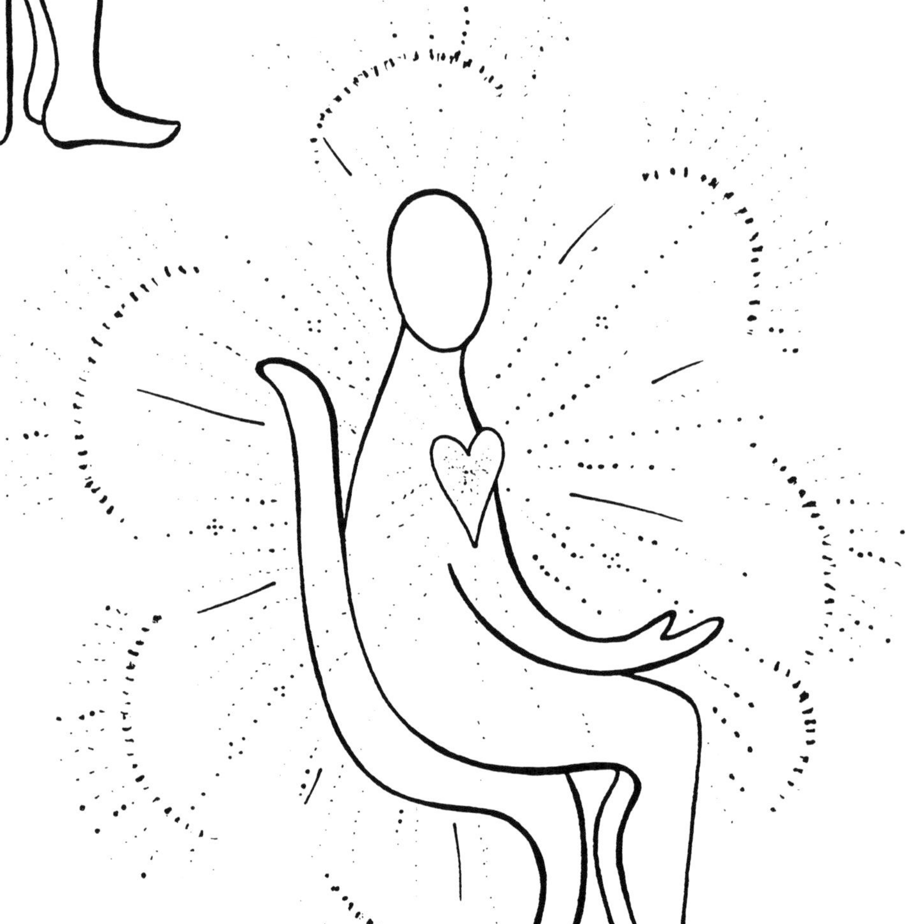

"I am the radiance
of Cosmic Love."

Activating the Cosmic Love Energy.

1) Sit comfortably, and instead of imagining a compassionate Being or Love Avatar in front of you visualize instead a large, radiant, rose pink cloud of energy. To help you see the color find something (a scarf, a piece of material, anything that looks rose pink and appeals to you), and gaze at it before closing your eyes; you will soon translate it into your dazzling pink cloud.

2) Begin to breathe the pink cloud in and out of your hands as you repeat:

"I now receive.... (breath in)
"The Cosmic Love energy".... (breath out)

Feel this in the hands as warm tingling energy. Repeat the affirmation until the energy in the hands increases.

3) Begin to draw the energy up your arms and into your heart as you affirm:

"I now receive..." as you breathe in,
"Cosmic Love in my heart"...as you breathe out ***into*** the heart.

By now you will experience the energy and warmth flowing from your hands, through your arms and into your heart. *Repeat the above affirmation at least five times, or remain in the meditation for several minutes until you feel an energy reaction in the heart.*

4) Now imagine that with each breath, the entire pink cloud draws closer and closer until it totally enfolds you; then you become so interpenetrated, that your heart along with every cell of your body fills with the radiance of Cosmic Love. You then breathe the energy in and out of your heart to others, to the neighborhood--to the rest of the world--to the Universe.

Repeat the following affirmations for as long as you desire:

"I am filled with the radiance...(breath in) **of Cosmic Love."** (out)

or...

"I am the radiance... (breath in) **of Cosmic Love."** (out)

And remember:

Love has
No expectations or demands;

Love has
No attachments.

Love is
Complete within itself.

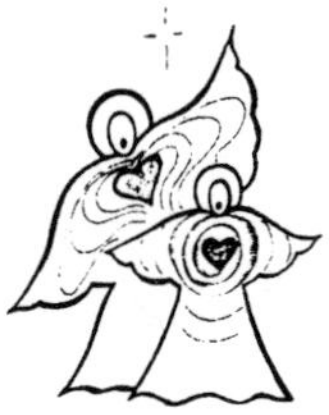

4.... MEDITATIONS ON THE FIVE SENSES

TASTE - Eat something *very* slowly and mindfully; savor the taste - don't talk! Discover the delights of dry bread or crackers held in the mouth meditatively. Buy some special food to experience; try something daring that you have never eaten before - like escargot, or something equally exotic, at least deviate from your usual diet. Receive food with reverence, it nourishes Spirit's outer body. Be very aware of tasting and enjoying, blessing and receiving the Life Force in the form of food.[5]

SMELL - If you have a fireplace, light a small wood fire, then sit, close your eyes and enjoy the smell of the burning wood. Later, add a few drops of perfumed oil to the fire. In the absence of a real fire, light some delightful incense and be very conscious of the aroma. Apply your favorite perfume, or buy and enjoy a new one. Go for a walk and tune in to all of the different smells around you, both sweet and pungent; receive them willingly. Do the same (smelling meditation) inside your house or room. Smudge[6] your house and yourself, then sit in the midst and meditate on releasing all the old outmoded things in your life - make a list. Let the lingering smell of the smudge remind you of your resolutions for change. The most basic survival and life renewal sense is smell.

HEARING - Turn off the inner mental chatter and become aware of the sounds around you. Initially, try to identify each one and listen intently for extra sounds. Discover the 'sound of silence.' Listen to soothing music, relax and receive it with your whole self not just your ears; feel where the different tones vibrate in your body. Better still, play your own music if you have an instrument; improvise and allow the music to 'play' you, rather than repeating familiar or set forms. Whether listening or playing become one with the music. Imagine that you can breathe the sounds in and up to the top of your head, then out and down through your feet. Do several of these complete music-breaths. Receive and fill your being with sound.

SIGHT - Remove all your clothes and in front of a large mirror gaze at your naked image very lovingly. Carefully accept everything you see without judgment. Then dress and fully clothed again - look at yourself just as carefully and lovingly. See everything about you in this moment as perfect; receive and smile at your reflection. Go to an Art Gallery or Museum and with one-pointed focus observe everything as a meditation; allow Spirit to draw you towards the things you need to explore in more detail. See the sun set and once in a while watch it rise - compare the rising with the setting. Sit alongside moving water and engage your eyes in the play of light upon the ripples. Repose yourself beside still water and marvel at reflections. Study a plant; try and draw it. Delight in the joy of seeing. Take your eyes on a meditative walk, preferably in nature - a park, a large garden: loosen any tension in your shoulders and neck, relax and soften your eyes. Now begin to observe the plants, bushes, branches, bark, pebbles and flowers. Begin to watch and focus on the spaces *between* the forms, rather than on the forms themselves. Keep doing this until you enter an altered state--explore that state. Return to wonder!

TOUCH - Be mindful of how you invite or reject touch from others. Sit or lie very still and experience your clothes touching the different parts of your body, then feel how your body (through your clothes), rests on the bed or chair; feel the bottoms of your feet in your shoes. BREATHE IN and feel the cool touch of the air inside your nostrils before it fills your lungs. BREATHE OUT and feel the blood-warmed air as it breezes out through your nostrils to complete its cycle. Do this breath for several minutes until **you** are no longer breathing--but instead, the breath 'breathes' you. Very slowly touch, caress, pat and stroke yourself all over; finish by holding your face very tenderly in your hands. Rest a moment with your face in your hands. You have traced the reachable limits of your solid physical form. Extend that awareness outwards by touching receptively the objects around you; feel their textures, *their* forms. Touch-explore all around your garden or yard--close your eyes while you feel/touch. Wash dishes without rubber gloves and let your hands *experience* sloshing around in the water and suds. Receive a massage or give a massage; enjoy a hot-tub, Jacuzzi, sauna or a swim. Know the difference between touching and being touched.

---

[5] Refer to Appendix 1. Food Meditation.

[6] A purification ceremony in which wild sage and sweet grass is burned.

COMBINING ALL THE FIVE SENSES

Put on the stereo. light candles and incense. Take a long hot bath perfumed with salts or oils. While you relax in the fragrant warmth sip some delicious drink and savor a premium confection--like Dutch licorice or Belgian chocolate...or whatever your heart desires. Luxuriate and pay attention to each of the senses in turn. To complete your bath rub yourself with a loofa, followed by a bracing cold shower (if you dare!) and finally massage yourself with scented lotion or oil (or have someone else massage you). Later - cook a wonderful meal, attending to all the details of preparation and noting the texture and taste of every ingredient as you flow with the rhythm of your movements. Notice and enjoy the cooking smells. Arrange and serve the food attractively. And finally, eat by candlelight accompanied by soothing music. *You may say that you do all of these things on occasion and "What's the difference?" The difference is your awareness--being mindful of your actions and your sensory input.* Make the entire experience a conscious meditation of all the senses. Still your thoughts and become the tasting, the touching, the hearing, the seeing, the smelling. If you sense-meditate with someone else keep talking to a minimum....better still, try and experience it all in silence. "Speak" with your eyes and your hearts! *The outer senses are the doorways to the more refined and expanded inner senses.*[7]

SENSING

Feel the flow,
Feel the flow,
        of being in the body.

Smell perfume,
Smell perfume.
        and every scent between.

Touch and feel,
Touch and feel,
        Textures rough to smooth.

Colors - colors,
Light and shade,
        See without - within.

Listen, listen,
Hearing, hearing,
        Silence - soft to roar.

Tasting flavor,
Savor, savor,
        Ask the tongue for more.

---

[7] Refer to "Time Shifting - Creating More Time to Enjoy Your Life" by Stephan Rechtschaffen, M.D.

5....HEALING MEDITATIONS & INVOCATIONS

EMOTIONAL HEALING - RELATIONSHIPS

Version One.

This is all done mentally for the purpose of releasing someone you love who has died--or someone with whom your relationship has ended and to whom you are still connected emotionally.

Visualize them sitting in front of you, then you say:

> **"I accept that in my essence, I am the Infinite Presence of Light and Love and - (say their name......), I accept that in *your* essence, you are the Infinite Presence of Light and Love. I am grateful for all the wonderful times we spent together and all the precious things you taught me. These I retain with love. I now release all grief and regret at your leaving and speed you on to your next adventure in the Light......**
>
> **I release you to your original Spirit and the Source of All that is."**

You then imagine yourself leaning forward and embracing the other person and in that instant, you both dissolve into each other and become the Infinite Light.

This is a very powerful technique but you may have to do it several times (perhaps every day from one to two weeks or longer) for a total release from emotional pain.

Version Two.

Version two helps us with the problem people in our lives--old friends, lovers or relatives who have become enemies, or just enemies - past or present.

You do the same visualization of imagining yourself sitting in front of the person, however, the affirmation is not exactly the same:

> **"I accept that in my essence, I am the Infinite Presence of Light and Love and - (say their name.......), I accept that in *your* essence, you are also the Infinite Presence of Light and Love. Whatever we have created between us in our separated selves (separated from our essence), I now accept.**
>
> **I now forgive (I forgive you and I forgive myself)....and**
> **I now release all that has happened between us - into the Light.**
> **I also release all negative thoughts, influences and entities that may be connected to us because of the past and I now send you forth in peace (or if the person is no longer alive), I send you to your original Spirit and the Source of All that is."**

If the person is very much alive say:

"I now release you in peace to your own path."

You then do the imaginary embrace as in Version One and merge together into the Light.

Do this every day until you no longer feel enmity towards the person(s).

The following are further adaptations and combinations of releasing techniques contained in this Chapter; they give you an idea of how to create powerful tools to fit your own specific needs.

INVOCATION FOR THE UNBORN CHILD

Many mothers feel the relationship they have with their children is far from happenstance. It appears highly likely our offspring come through us by reason of karmic debt or by choice - rather than from some random birth-lottery. The idea of 'karmic debt' presupposes some form of past life relationship, which may or may not have been ideal! Whether you accept or reject such ideas, the fact remains - if you are pregnant - and reading these words, you're in an excellent position to invoke positive energy and Light into your unborn on a daily basis, thus clearing the way for a constructive relationship between you both in the future and whatever else the entity is returning to resolve or accomplish. Remember, the incoming child already has its own Life-field containing all its potential (which of course interpenetrates your own Field) - and which you can balance and influence with your good intent and words of power.

The Ritual :

1) If possible, choose the same time of day and place to perform this; make it your special "Quiet Time" that cannot be disturbed.
2) Perhaps you would enjoy listening to a favorite CD or tape, light a rose-pink candle and burn some pleasant incense? Decide on your own ritual for connecting to your unborn.
3) Seat yourself comfortably with you hands resting gently on your belly.
4) Take several deep, calming breaths then send your 'breath' through your hands and into your baby. When you feel a distinct energy connection through your breath, imagine a radiant light above your head (that connects to the brilliance at the center of our galaxy) and begin to breathe this light down through your hands. Try several breaths.
5) Now speak directly to the baby within your womb. (If you haven't a specific name yet, just call it "Little One.") Close your eyes and picture your baby, ***then speak softly***:

"Oh Little One within,
I know that you have come
So I can be your mother.

Let me tell you now,
How much I dearly love you!
And if your distant past
Has not been kind or happy,
I clear that energy
And call your Angels to you.

I know that in your essence,
You are the Light of Love,
And I am the same.
Throughout the coming years,
let us always see
That essence shining through.

Be at peace my child and grow in strength within;
And until I hold you in my arms,
I love you and look forward to your coming."

Repeat any phrase as many times as you like, delete any of mine, or add your own special ones of encouragement and endearment.

GUILT REACTIONS

We have all experienced the intense pain of guilt, our guilt reaction to something we have done in innocence, ignorance or even (after the fact) with intent. There is almost nothing quite so excruciating or at times debilitating, especially if we find it impossible to forgive ourselves. This sensation of guilt can prevail in spite of reassurances and forgiveness from others. It grinds us to a halt and floods us with total and unequivocal self loathing and worthlessness. I am not referring to long standing suppressed feelings of guilt (that we only acknowledge intellectually), but those instantaneous, unforseen happenings that shame us in a moment...rendering us once more into a wounded-child being berated by a shadowy authority figure. *Agonizing as it may be,* **seize the feeling immediately** *and begin to heal the disempowered child within!*

Mentally repeat all of the following:

"I.......(say your name), **now un-create my guilt reactions."**

And in case you have some guilt-ridden sub-selves, repeat first:

"Painful guilt is present within us.
We are not the guilt."

Followed by:

"Painful guilt is present within me.
I am not the guilt." *Repeat.*

Then.....

"I forgive myself.
I am forgiven - (we are forgiven)."

Then.....

"We are the flawless and perfect Presence of Spirit."

Followed by:

"I am the flawless and perfect Presence of Spirit." *Repeat.*

Then finally repeat:

"All is well,"
All is as it should be.

I rest in the peaceful Presence of Spirit.
I rest in the joyful Presence of Spirit.

We are the perfect Presence."

You will find to your amazement, that all your guilt will dissolve in the matter of minutes!

AFFIRMATIONS FOR HEALING THE EYES

From a weekend workshop I did on "eyes" in the 80's, I learnt that the way you perceive out of the left eye is governed by your mother (and how she views life), and the way you perceive out of the right eye comes from how your father looks at life. This made total sense to me at the time (my right eye was weakest), but I did nothing about it! Naturally, parents usually impose their way of seeing the world upon their children. Then in the 90's when my right eye began to seriously fail, it forced me to investigate precisely just how I had bought-into my Dad's "views" on failure, success and fulfilling one's deepest dreams. He had inadvertently laid on me his own practical conditioning of..."This is feasible, but forget about that--that's totally unpractical and unattainable!!" So I learned to spend my life in compromise, doing 'half' of this and 'half' of that--never the whole thing. Even my husbands were only half the men they could have been! At a certain point in life the equivalent body symbol (the right eye) began to collapse - to draw my attention! *It got my attention!!*

Intellectually, I knew *why* my life had been the way it was and even *how* I should be changing it...but tell that to the cells of the eye! In the end, that's precisely what I did do. It figured, that if I was actually "eyeing" the world according to my father, I had to be willing to accept the fact--and the fact that he was essentially..**in that eye!** His first name was "Vernon," so I began touching my (closed) right eye firmly and sounding the key letters in his name, the first letter (**"V"**) and the two middle Focus letters (**"R** and **N**," which I sounded separately). Because all three letters were also Resonators (and have such a powerful effect on the brain), I decided to 'resonate' instead of sound them.[8] So I began to accept and transforming the energy that my right eye represented; as I sounded, beneath my fingers, the pain left my eye. I was elated. I also used the affirmation: **"Dad, I no longer see with your eyes, I have my own perception."**

But the next morning I awoke to puzzling pain in my *left* eye--the mother! Even though it was my 'best' eye, I still needed to acknowledge the perceptions I was holding in it--from her; perhaps the strongest was my attitude of passive resignation. In relation to my impossible first marriage, she once told me - "You have made your bed--now you have to lie in it....make the best of it." *(Note: this was my mother 45 years ago--not the sweet, wise lady I know today!)*

I began working on the "good" eye and sounding the first and middle letters from my mother's name. I also said the affirmation: **"Mother, I no longer see with your eyes, I have my own perception."** It took much longer for that eye to stop hurting. Finally, I sounded my own name letters (first and middle) into both my eyes (with my hands resting on them.) My eyes are now an ongoing project, I have 65 years to decondition!

The above is something you might like to think about and try - if you have a great variance between your left and right eyes. Look at the dominant perceptions of your parents--and see if you haven't borrowed them for your own eyes! Below is a general meditation for eye problems.

Imagine sending a very delicate violet/lavender light to the eyes, breathe it in and out of eyes as you say the affirmation.

The Power of my Wholeness Heals me.

I, ...(say your name)......hereby take full responsibility for the way I see my life.

I now recreate perfect sight in my eyes.
And whatsoever I have created between myself and perfect sight
In this and other lifetimes,
I now accept as a choice I have made,
I now forgive myself and any others involved.
I dissolve and return this condition to the Infinite Source.

---

[8] See Chapter 18, Power Tools for the Brain.

I charge the Life Force in my body to reinstate the pattern of perfect sight in the eyes.

I call upon the healing Angels of Sight to assist in this restoration.

I am the Infinite Presence of Perfect Sight.

So It is.

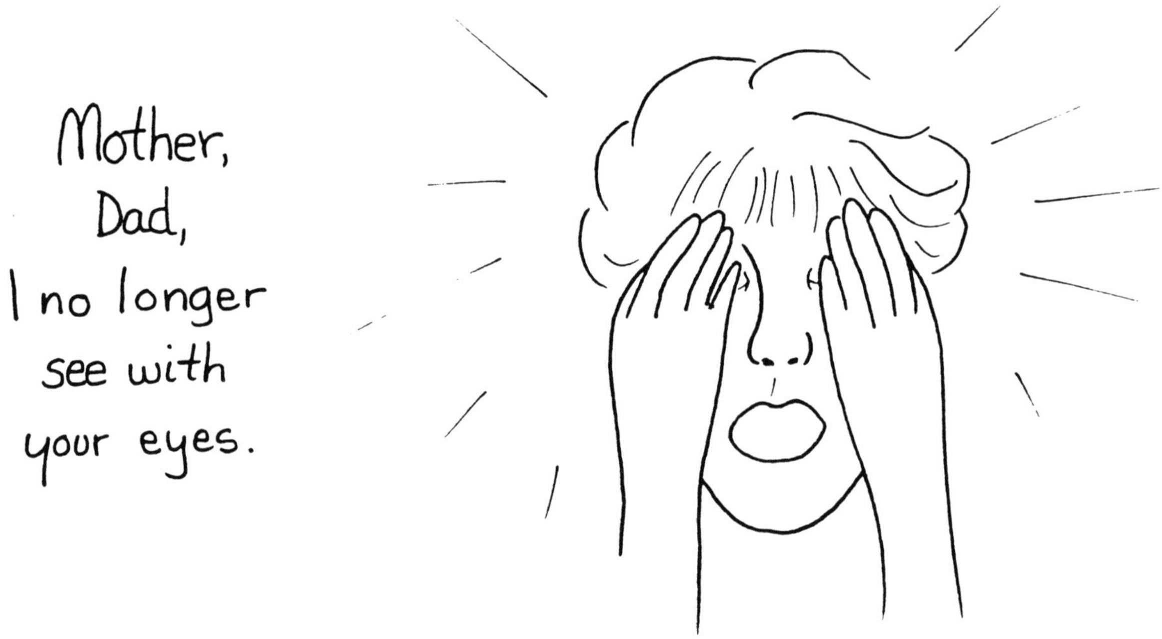

Note: Elsewhere in this book, the expiration and inspiration of the breath has been presented as an aid to activating affirmations. We will now take it a step further and use the power of ***deliberate rhythm*** as used in poetry and song. When practicing any affirmation you can always combine a breath pattern *along with* a deliberate beat--either way, you'll be able to entrain to the energy field of the condition (or the object) you're trying to invoke...thus magnetizing its presence within your **own** field and eventually drawing it to you.

The next page of affirmations are arranged in an exaggerated, rhythmical sequence. It is important to accentuate the rhythm of the stressed syllables (or words), because in doing so, you create a new powerful patterning (re-programming) for the brain. I have also listed the number of strong beats per line - so you will get the idea of how to discover the accents within phrases of your own creation and with the other meditations in this book. Affirmation and invocation becomes twice as effective with this method.

DENTAL TRAUMA

*Repeat three times daily a week before - and **between** dental visits when you're wearing temporary bridges or crowns. Also, continue for at least twice a day for a week **after** a dental visit that involves stress to the mouth or gums.*

Don't just 'rattle' this off while you're occupied with some other task - and expect it to work! Sit down with your back straight, feet flat on the floor (to ground the energy-discharge) and pay close attention to the words while you repeat and meditate on the phrases. As a preliminary, massage and slap the bottoms of your feet. You'll know the release has begun when you feel your feet starting to tingle.

"I......(your name)....now un-create my karma with teeth and dentists and I include my sub-selves from past and parallel lives.

"*Re*-**sis**-*tence to* **den**-*tal* **work** *is* **pres**-*ent with*-**in** *us.* (5 beats)
We are **not** *the re*-**sis**-*tence to* **den**-*tal* **work.** (4 beats)
I am **not** *the re*-**sis**-*tence to* **den**-*tal* **work;** (4 beats)

We **are** *the* **In**-*finite* **Pres**-*ence of* **heal**-*ing,* ((4 beats)
We **are** *the* **In**-*finite* **res**-*tor*-**ati**-*on.* (4 beats)

I **now** *re*-**lease** *all my* **bit**-*ter*-**ness,** ((4 beats)
I **let** *go* **all** *my com*-**plain**-*ing* **now!** (4 beats)
What **ev**-*er has* **par**-*ted my* **teeth** *from* **me,** (4 beats)
In **this** *and* **oth**-*er* **lives** *gone* **by** -- (4 beats)

I ac-**cept** *the re*-**spons**-*i*-**bil**-*i*-**ty,** (4 beats)
I for-**give** *my*-**self** *for* **loss** *of* **teeth.** (4 beats)
I **end** *my re*-**sis**-*tence to* **den**-*tal* **work.** ((4 beats)
And to **all** *the* **mon**-*ey it's* **cos**-*ting* **me.** (4 beats)

I **now** *ful*-**fill** *my* **des**-*ti*-**ny,** (4 beats)
To be **rad**-*iant and* **power**-*ful, suc*-**cess**-*ful and* **lov**-*ing.* (4 beats)
I am **Rad**-*iant and* **Power**-*ful, Suc*-**cess**-*ful and* **Loved."** (4 beats) **So be it.**

FOR MANIFESTING WORK

"*I* **have** *the* **per**-*fect* **job** *for* **me,** (all have 4 beats to the line)
Ex-**act**-*ly* **where** *I* **need** *to* **be.**
I **now** *full*-**fill** *my* **des**-*ti*-**ny.**
And **streams** *of* **mon**-*ey* **flow** *through* **me.**

(These simple and effective affirmations have all their accents in place, now you try and figure out your own breath pattern.)

17.....ENERGY EXERCISES

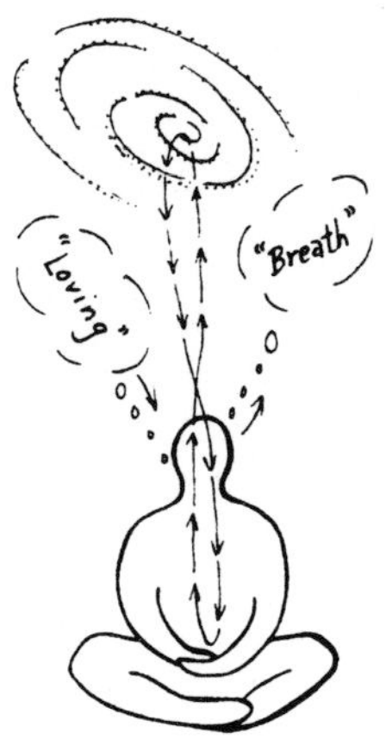

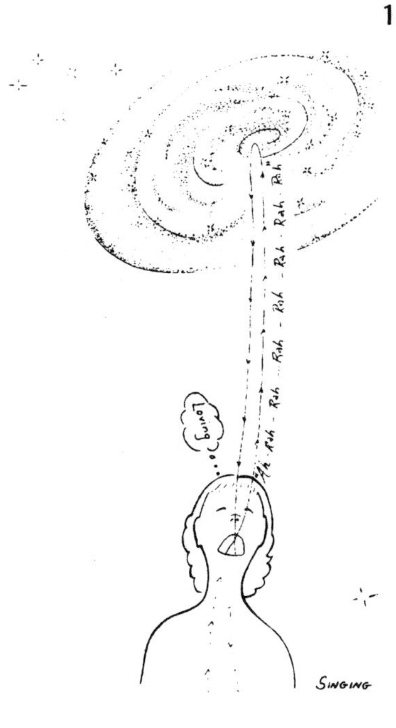

1....CLEARING THE AURA

For this, your hands (with their magnetic poles in the palms), become a balancing tool. You will use them to discharge uncomfortable or negative energy and to re-balance your own Life Field.

(a) Clearing the Inner Field.

1) Sit down, remove shoes; rub, knead and slap your feet thoroughly. This aids in grounding and discharging through the soles of the feet. Now stand up with your feet shoulder width apart and concentrate on the body sensations.

Eventually, do all of the following exercises with your eyes closed.

2) Cover your face completely with the palms of both hands. Slowly brush your hands down your face until the tips of your fingers touch your chin. *Then flick your hands out to the sides.* ***Repeat three times.***

3) Place both hands on the top of your head and firmly pull them from the front hairline backwards to the nape of your neck. Use enough pressure in your hands to feel the shape of your skull through your hair. *Flick hands out to the sides.* ***Repeat three times.***

4) Lift both hands to the forehead (as though shading your eyes), now raise your hands forward - then overhead and then backward, in a big semi-circle from the brows to the nape of the neck, as though you're wearing one of those astronaut's space helmets - and you're tracing its shape in the air with your hands. *Flick hands out to sides.* ***Repeat three times.***

5) Cross your arms over the chest and firmly grasp each shoulder with the opposite hand. Use your hands to press and squeeze the arm muscles and continue doing this massaging, squeezing movement down the entire length of each arm - to the wrists...then slide hands (palm across palm) and *flick out to the sides.* ***Repeat twice.***

Third repetition for 5): Again grasp the shoulders, but instead of kneading and squeezing, take a firm grip and with a 'stripping' motion, pull the hands down the arms to the wrists and then *flick the hands outwards.*

6) Place your hands flat on the upper chest, fingers touching the collarbone, then firmly pull the hands down over the breasts, belly and thighs - and as far down the thighs as you can reach without bending forward. *Flick hands out to sides.* ***Repeat three times.***

7) Stand now with hands on hips; as you grip your waist, your thumbs rest on the **belly** side with the fingers fanning out behind onto your back. (*This is the beginning stance.*)

7a) Still with your thumbs resting at the waist, move your fingers backward and upward slightly until they dig into the strong vertical muscles that run each side down the spine. Keep digging in to those muscles with the fingers, while you inch your hands up your back as far as you can reach.

7b) When you can't get your hands up any higher, press and sweep them firmly **down** the back across the buttocks and down the backs of the thighs as far you can reach. *Flick hands out to sides.* ***Repeat from 7 to 7b three times.***

8) (Keep your eyes open for this one.) With both hands grasp the left leg as high up the thigh as possible. Now with a stripping motion, pull both hands simultaneously down the leg until they reach the calf. At the calf, kneed and squeeze the muscles for a few moments before completing the sweep down to the ankle. When you reach the ankle, *keep your hands there* - but lift the leg up and pull your foot through your hands. Replace the foot on the ground and complete the movement with an *outward flick of the hands.* (If you can't balance, sit down to do this; it can even be done lying on a bed.) ***Repeat three times with each leg.***

After completing these eight steps, stand with your body relaxed and eyes closed. Take two or three deep breaths. Still with your eyes closed make several mini-circles to the right (as though circling tightly around your spinal column), then change direction and circle several turns to the left. Open your eyes. You should now be feeling much 'lighter.'

You have just cleared and rebalanced your inner Field (Aura), but before clearing the outer Field - a very important instruction: the Perineal/Yoni Contraction.

Clearing the Aura

Clearing the Inner Field

▷ Step #2

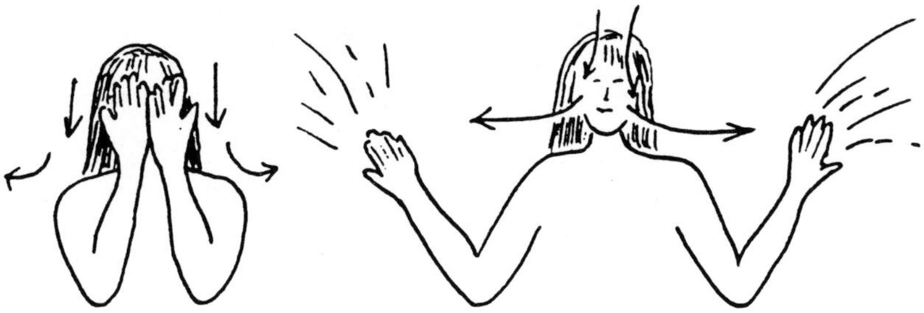

▷ Step #3

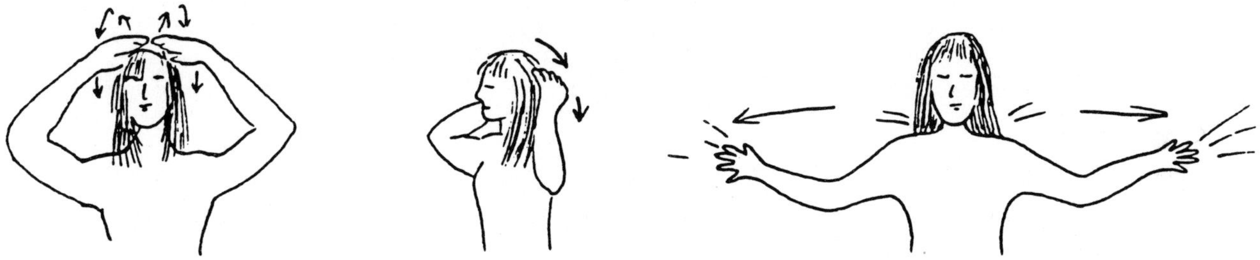

▷ Step #4

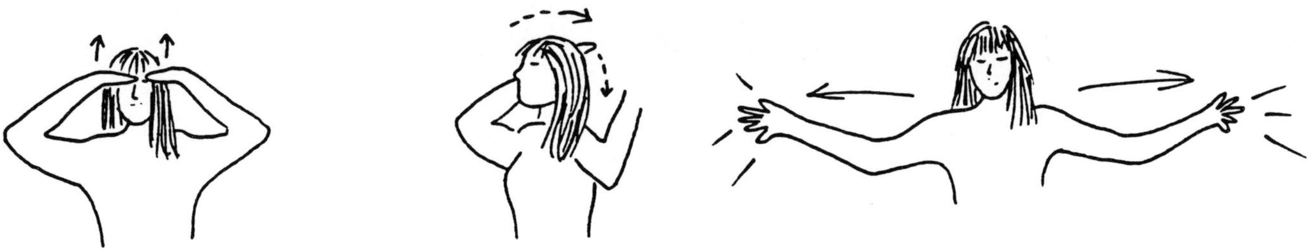

Clearing the Inner Field

▷ Step # 5

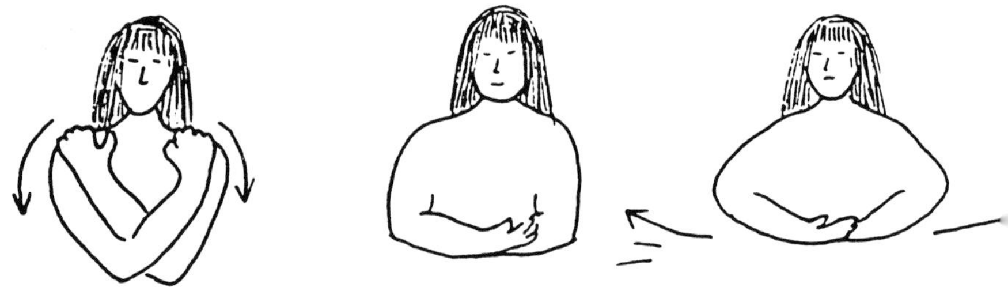

▷ Step # 6

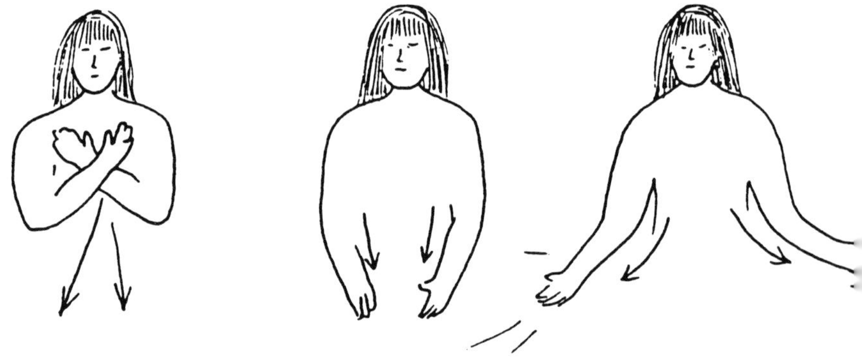

▷ Step # 7

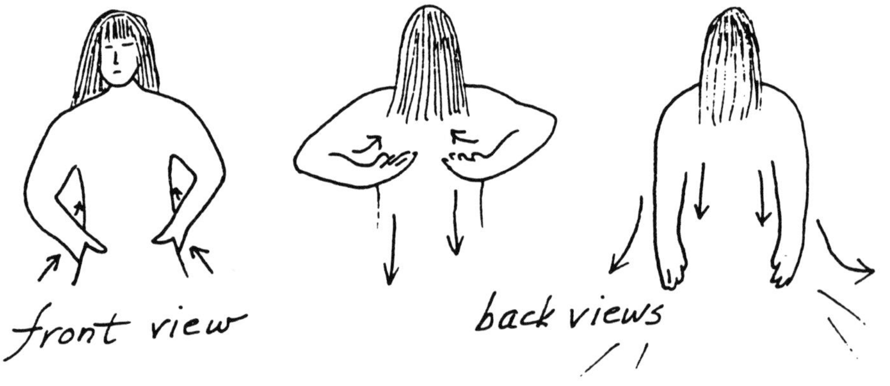

Clearing the Outer Field

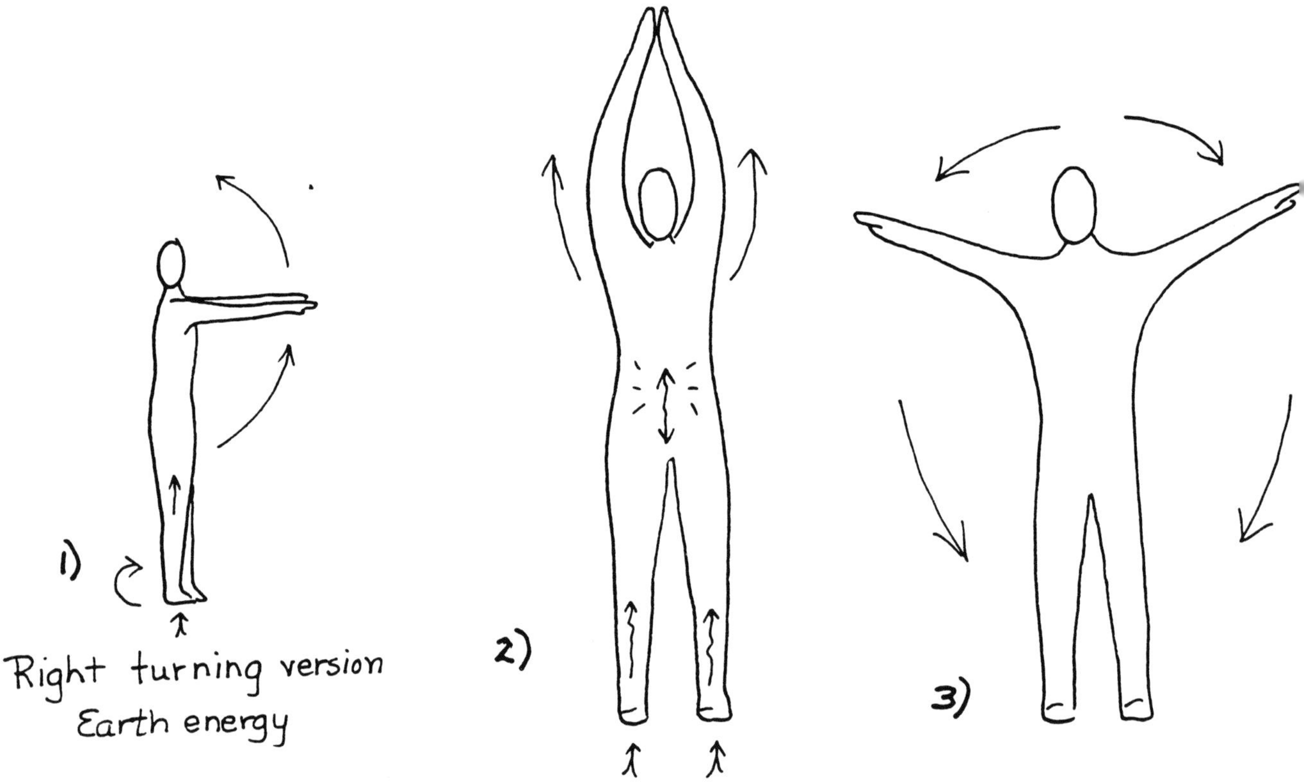

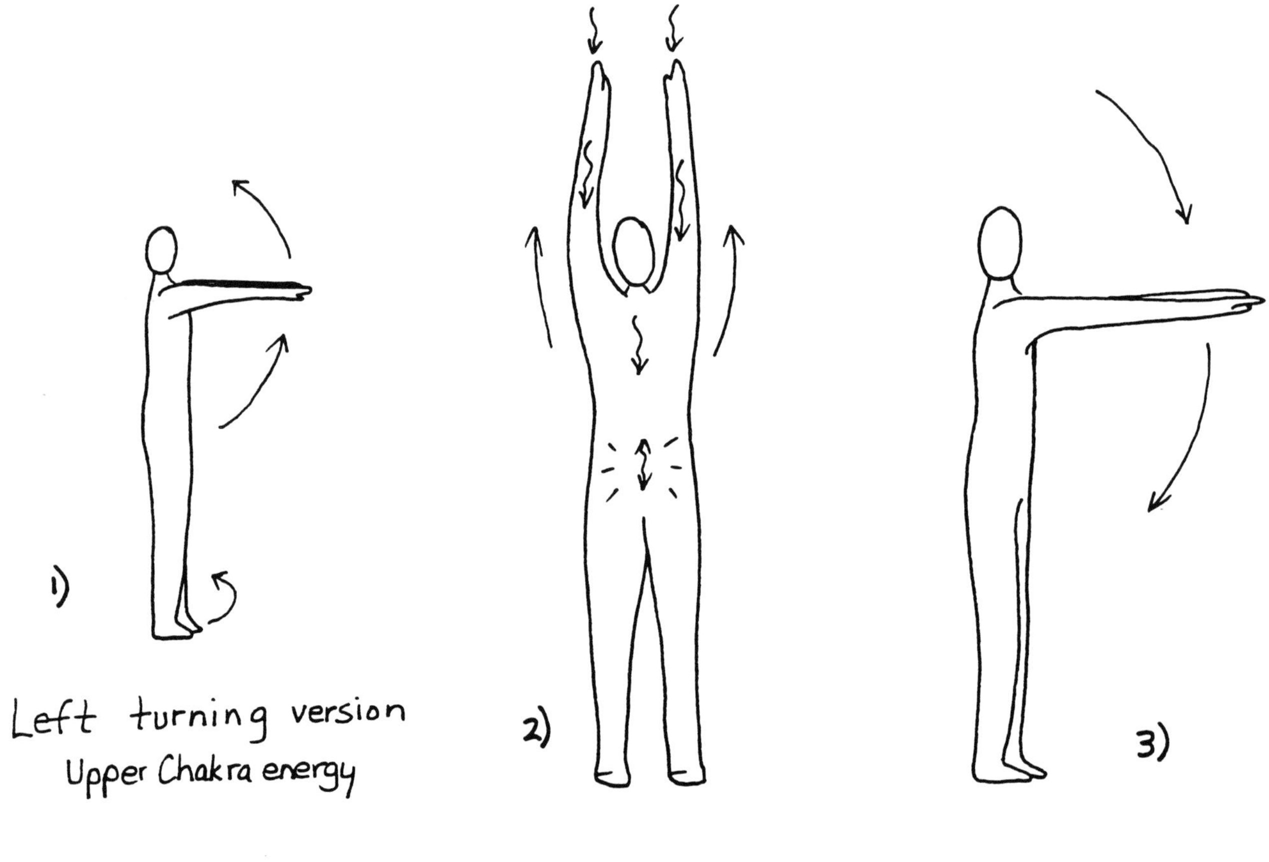

THE PERINEAL/YONI CONTRACTION.

Called "The Aswini Mudra" in Hatha Yoga, the contraction is used to put pressure on and activate the Kundalini energy at the base of the spine. Combined with intention, it can direct energy anywhere in the body--up or down. It is also one of the key movements for awakening the psychic-/physical blisses present in every one of the Chakric energy centers. Western medicine knows it as the Kegel exercise; named after gynecologist Arnold Kegel, who in the 40's reinvented it as a method for female bladder control. Subsequently, it proved a boon for improving sexual performance, increasing sexual enjoyment and enhancing reproductive organ health for both males and females. The Kegel method is described on pages **110 -11** in the excellent book by herbalist James Green, entitled "The Male Herbal" (also providing useful ideas for couples), published by the Crossing Press.

For our purposes, we will use it to *direct* energy in the body and will refer to it as the perineal/yoni contraction (or the P/Y). The perineum is the muscle on the floor of the pelvis separating the penis from the scrotum, and the anus from the vagina; yoni is the Sanskrit term for vagina. **The action is a strong upward contraction of the perineum/anus or anus/vagina, followed by a relaxation.**

c) Clearing the Outer Field.

This much simpler exercise is done in four directions. If you want to, you can elect to face the actual four directions of North, South, East and West, but it isn't essential. ***Also, try it with closed eyes.***

1) First, slap the soles of the feet; then stand tall, spine straight, head erect, arms to your sides.

2) Breathe in as you raise both arms **forward** and up, until you're standing with your arms high above your head, palms together.

3) Hold this position and **hold the in-breath** while you "pulse" the perineum/yoni muscles up and down for five to eight strong pulses as you draw the earth energy into feet and legs.

4) Relax P/Y and breathe out as you lower your arms **outwards** and down to your sides.

Complete these movements by taking a deep breath.

a) Now make a right-angled turn to your right and repeat the 1 to 4 sequence.

b) After one deep breath, take another right-angle turn and repeat the sequence again.

c) Repeat b) and you have returned to your starting-point direction.

Take a final deep breath, you've just made a square (four-directional) pattern.

When following this 'right-handed' direction you're receiving earth-energy in through the feet. Now to draw energy down from the upper Chakras, you reverse the direction and somewhat change arm and hand positions. Repeat the entire sequence, but turn **left** instead of right--and when you raise both arms forward to above the head, this time **do <u>not</u> bring the palms together.** Next, "pulse" the P/Y contraction (with the breath held) while drawing energy **down** through the hands, arms and spine **into** the Perineum/yoni area. Then, **do not** lower the arms outwards to the sides as before--instead, keep the hands facing each other and lower the arms to the sides in the same manner as they were raised - a very powerful recharging exercise!

To Complete both left and right versions of the Exercise:

1) Continue to stand as before. Close your eyes and imagine that instead of a spinal cord, you have a thin steel rod that extends from your tailbone and into the ground between your feet. (If you're doing this in a tenth floor apartment, your steel rod is going to be *very* long!!) Should this image of a rod make you feel uncomfortable, visualize instead your own pink and white spinal cord; this feeds into the sciatic nerves of the legs and forms your primary electrical grounding system.

2) With your body, make several **<u>very</u>** tiny circles around the imaginary rod (or spinal cord). Circle first to the right, then to the left--keep the circles tiny, you're barely moving, and try to do the same amount of turns in each direction.

3) Take three deep breaths. Stand quietly and note how different your body feels after the exercise. Are your toes and the soles of your feet tingling gently? If so, that means you are discharging and grounding. This doesn't always happen the first time, but when your energy channels open and the blocked areas release, you will begin to feel many sensations such as energy rushes, tinglings, and even hot and cold chills. Your Light Body is coming alive!

2.....DISIDENTIFYING (disassociation) TECHNIQUE

On occasion we get totally off guard and find ourselves 'awfulizing' over some actual or imagined transgression, or our worst fears surface and race like stampeding cattle through our brains. Our head aches, we can't think of anything else, we can't sleep, we are in total torment. For this painful condition a very simple remedy exists - **disidentify**!

Disidentifying is based on a basic Buddhist premise:

you are **not** your body,
you are **not** your mind,
you are **not** your emotions.

But you can *think* about all of these as 'parts' of yourself. The question then is "Who are you?" -- "Who is doing the thinking *about* the thinking?" Some would say Higher Mind, or Soul, Infinite Spirit, Essence--it depends on which cultural bias you're speaking through.

In a crisis, we tend to identify ourselves with the part of us that is suffering, instead of disassociating and looking at the symbolic message it contains for our illumination. Body parts and their psychological equivalents are well documented, Louise Hay's "You Can Heal Your Life" is a good example, as are certain dream interpretation books.[1] (What happens in the waking state is the "Waking Dream" and can be analyzed in the same way as sleeping dreams.) The disidentifying technique particularly lends itself to dissolving troublesome thoughts and emotions.

To Begin: *Name the emotion or emotions that are dominating your compulsive thought cycle.* It could be fear, anger, resentment, addictive love, self-pity, etc. Let's take "fear" as an example.

***Repeat mentally*:**

"Fear is present, I am not the fear, I am the Infinite Presence of courage and strength," or "Light and Love"......***you*** formulate your own most appropriate antidote.

For this to work and be successful, it must be done *with the destructive emotion strongly present;* you feel it, you acknowledge it - but **not** as part of your Spiritual Self or Essence. In the beginning it might take up to five minutes of inner recitation before the destructive or self-defeating emotions and thoughts vanish. You're opening the pathway to your higher Spirit by naming yourself as such--you're making an actual connection through the power of words. Eventually you will be able to dissolve the separation with one or two repetitions of your chosen affirmation.

If your sub-selves are particularly doubtful and resistant, change the tense to "we" - **"We are not the fear, we are the Infinite Presence..."** *Call their bluff, educate them as to who they really are and always have been, the higher Spirit! Better still, talk to your hurting parts from the viewpoint of your higher Mind--from* **that** *consciousness say "You," - "You are not the fear!"*

When I first introduced this concept to my second son Ricky, he was only five years old and prone to painful and debilitating tantrums. One day, when he had paused in mid-tantrum exhausted for breath, I told him I knew a way he could control his rages...if he wanted to! Dark hair disheveled and damp with sweat, he regarded me wearily but with definite interest. So I reminded him of his *real* identity--a Spirit inhabiting a physical body that had thoughts and emotions. He believed me. I told him to repeat over and over in his head, "Anger is present, I am not the anger, I am a Spirit of Light and Love," and the rage would eventually vanish. He sat perfectly still for two minutes frowning with concentration and mouthing the words. Finally he muttered in a terse voice, "It's not working, I'm still angry!" "Keep repeating it," I said firmly as I walked away - and he did. Another five minutes went by and he called me, surprised and a little puzzled. "It's all gone!" Then he asked, "Where did it go to??" **That was his last tantrum.**

There were other occasions for Ricky involving other emotions, the most memorable happened when he was in Junior High and had contracted a painful plantar wart on the sole of his foot. Referred by our regular doctor, we ended up at the office of a specialist in the 'wart field' whom neither of us had ever set eyes on before. Ushered into an examination room, we waited and we waited! I sat on a chair while my totally stressed-out son sat on the edge of the dreaded examination

---

[1] See Bibliography.

table swinging his legs and arms spastically in an effort to release the tension. Then the speculating began: his school friends had fed him horror stories and he just knew the wart was going to be dug out on the spot with a sharp scalpel. Finally he flung an arm in the air and gasped, "Gosh, I wish I could relax!!" Fortunately I remembered "disidentifying" and on the spot we worked out a suitable affirmation...something like, *"Terror is present, I am not the terror, I am the Infinite Presence of Peace and Calmness."* He settled down almost immediately reciting the phrase earnestly under his breath. The biggest suprise came ten minutes later when the Doctor finally walked in. A more gentle, smiling, reassuring old man you could not imagine--with an equally charming elderly nurse assistant, who also happened to be his wife. The cure for the wart was not the knife, but a magical prescription potion. "One of my patients," the doctor said with a twinkle in his eye, "not only cured her own wart, but everyone else's warts on the street where she lived!" We carried on the tradition! **Disidentifying really works, and you can apply it to any situation.**

3.....FINDING THE POWER OF THE MOTHER-FATHER GOD-GODDESS

This technique invokes ancient archetypal powers that correspond to energy centers and pathways in the body bringing them to life within us, namely, the polarized Root and Crown.

Part One: Activating the Universal Goddess Energy.

Practice twice a day. *To begin - first masssage or slap bottoms of feet.*

1) Sit on a comfortable lounge or straight backed chair, with feet flat on the floor but not touching each other.
2) Imagine a large sphere of radiant green light several inches below your feet. Green is the Earth Mother color for nourishment and abundance. Close your eyes, concentrate on your feet and the radiant green light below them.
3) Now breathe the green energy in and out of your feet with each breath.

As you breathe, mentally repeat:

"Beloved Earth Mother..... breathe **in** to the soles of the feet.

I receive thee"........ breathe **out** of the soles of the feet.

*Repeat the above **5-8** times or until the feet begin to vibrate, tingle or even get hot - the sign that the energy centers in your feet have been opened.*

Activating the Feminine Polarity (Root Chakra).

Whether in a male or female body, your Goddess (feminine) energy resides at the base of your spine in the Root Chakra. Honoring and receiving the universal Earth Goddess activates your own feminine power - the inner Goddess energy.

1) Continue to sit breathing the green light in and out of your feet.
2) You will now begin to breathe it all the way *through* the feet, up the legs and into the base of the spine.

Breathe **in** *through the feet and up the legs as you mentally repeat:*

"Beloved Earth Mother.....

Then as you breathe **out** *into the base of the spine, repeat:*

I am nourished and sustained by thee."

*Directed by the breath, 'see' the green light flowing continuously through the feet and into the tailbone. Repeat **5-8** times or until the flow establishes itself --you should eventually feel heat in your lower spine (tailbone) and belly.* ***Practice twice a day.***

The Abundance Breath.

As you continue to feel the energy flowing through your feet and legs, you will now direct the green energy so that it fills your entire body.

Breathe **in** *through the feet to the base of the spine as you repeat:*

"Beloved Earth Mother......

Then as you breathe **out** *and fill the rest of your body with green light, say:*

I rest in your abundance."

Continue the breath and the affirmation until the green of abundance not only fills you, but extends out into the room, the house, the neighborhood.

Part Two: Activating the Masculine Polarity (Crown Chakra).

The masculine energy or "Sky-Father Archetype," polarizes at the Crown Chakra on the top of your head, again, regardless of gender. Remember, you are exhorting archetypal energies corresponding to counterpart polarities within your own energy system. Belief in literal Gods and Goddesses ***is not the point,*** *the invocation ritual becomes the tool that opens channels of subtle force connecting us to the upper centers above the head as well as the energy Chakras within the physical body.*

1) Begin by stimulating the skull centers: firmly massage your scalp for several seconds and complete the process by rapping gently all over the head with your knuckles.
2) Relax your eyes and feel as though they have become very soft and gentle. Enjoy the feeling while repeating inwardly "Soft eyes, gentle eyes," for several moments.
3) Imagine a large sphere of vibrant purple light suspended three or four inches above your head. (Purple in this case represents protection and wisdom.)
4) Now tap your fingers on the crown of your head to bring the focus there, you will soon be able to do this mentally and not need your fingers. As you breathe **in** - sweep *up* to this purple light, then as you breathe **out** - begin to move the light *down* around your head and shoulders like a cowled cape. Now that you have some sense of the movement, do the same breath with affirmations.

Repeat the following 3-5 times.

Breathe **in** *and sweep the breath from your Crown -* **up** *to the purple Light as you say:*

"Infinite Sky-Father......,

Breathe **out** *and draw the light -* **down** *around your head and shoulders as you say:*

I receive Thee."

Repeat the following 3-5 times.

(Be certain your eyes remain very relaxed in the "soft-eyes" mode.)

5) Again, focus on your crown (now within the purple radiance); this time you will completely surround the body with purple light by drawing it even further down from the head and shoulders and flowing it around your body like a long protective cape. *Proceed as follows:*

With your awareness at the top of your head, breathe **in** *and say mentally:*

"Infinite Sky-Father.....,

Breathe **out** *and surround your body with purple light as you say:*

I am guided and protected by Thee."

Part Three: **Joining the Polarities - the Inner Marriage.**
You will now sweep the Crown polarity **down** *to the Root Chakra at the base of the spine, thus merging the masculine and feminine polarites within the physical body.*

Pretend you are breathing **in** *through the top of your head as you say:*

"Infinite Sky-Father.....,

Now do a strong P/Y contraction[2] *and hold it as you breathe the energy* **out and down** *the outside of the spine to the tailbone saying:*

I bring Thee to the Mother."

Repeat 3 times. *(You have just consciously connected your inner/outer Archetypes, your masculine and feminine polarities.....three times for good measure!!)*

The God-Goddess Union Meditation.

Relax and be aware of the energy now pulsing in your Crown and vibrating in your feet, then repeat mentally:

"Mother-Father, God-Goddess," *(as you breathe* **in** *feel the energy concurrently in both the Crown and feet Chakras)*

"I rest in Thy abundance and protection." *(as you breathe* **out** *simultaneously draw the energy from the Crown* **and** *the feet* **into** *the Root Chakra with the P/Y contraction.)*

Make **three** *P/Y pulse-contractions, one as you say each of the above underlined words.)* **Practice this last affirmation with the P/Y "pulses" by itself till you get used to contracting with the words.**
Finally, you may also like to visualize your core-self radiating green light for abundance (the Earth Mother Goddess) surrounded by a purple aura for protection-wisdom (the Sky-Father Archetype).

AFFIRMATIONS FOR THE ROOT CHAKRA *(the Base of spine energy center.)*

To be said before or after the God-Goddess Union Meditation or used as separate affirmations when needed.

"My life is peaceful and perfect,
I am always safe and secure,

I have the perfect place to live,
Exactly where I need to be.

I have abundant money,
For everything I want to do,

All my wants are satisfied
And everything I need is here.
My life is peaceful and perfect."

---

[2]Refer to the Perineal/Yoni Contraction instructions from "Clearing the Aura."

Figure Eight Breath

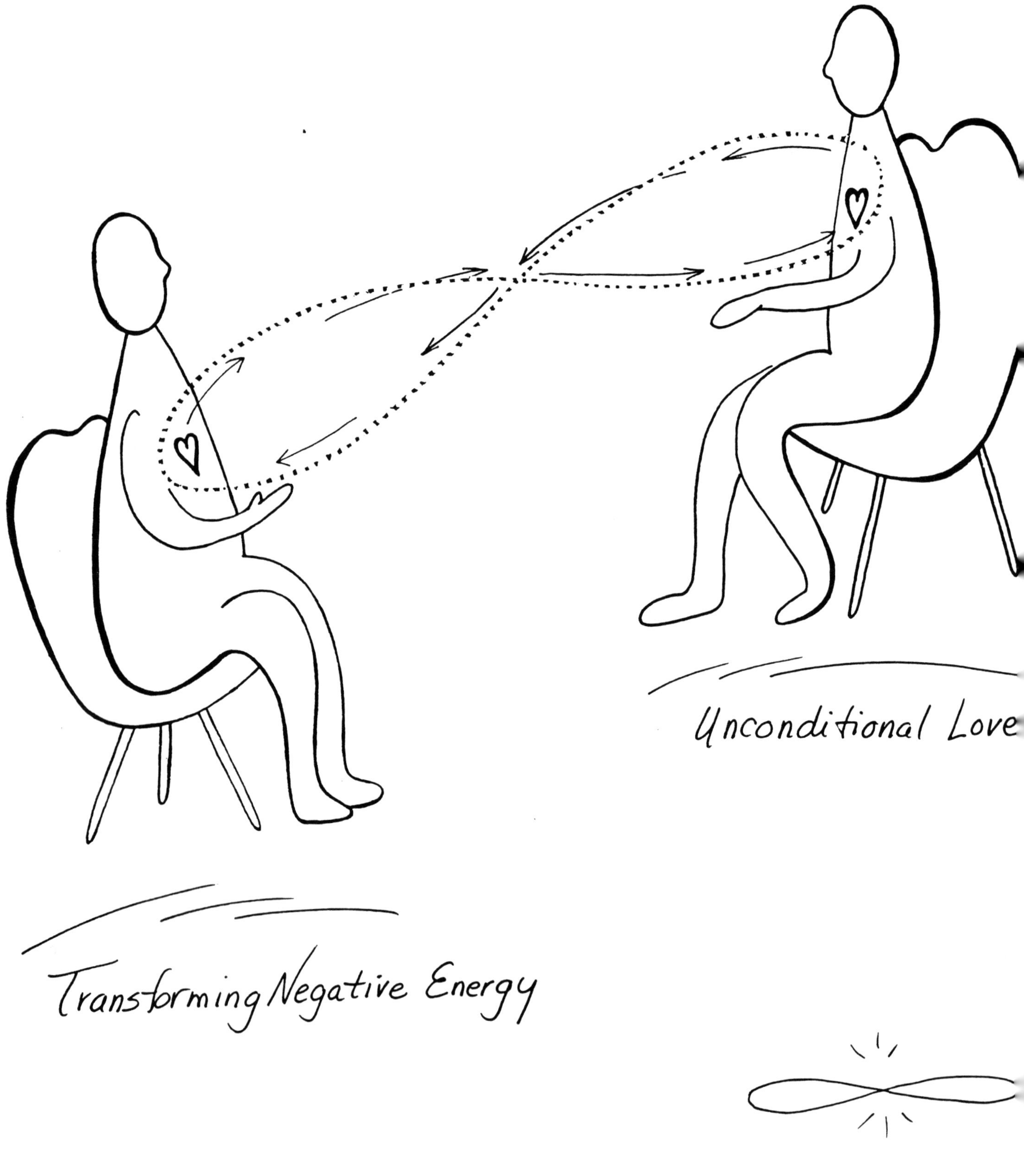

4.....THE FIGURE 8 (Unconditional love) BREATH

This technique uses intention (along with the breath) to transform problem energies into the power of Love and healing. The figure 8 is another symbol for the ancient ouroborus, the dragon eating its own tail, an icon of great power with many meanings. For the early Greeks, it meant 'All is one,' for the Egyptians, 'Immortality.' We will use it in the sense of connectedness, to trace the path of the transformation breath from one person to another.

Imagine yourself having a confrontation. It happens to all of us. You're sitting across from someone who's in the process of delivering you a personal lecture or just bawling you out. Not a pleasant prospect by any means and one in which your reactions could include fear, resentment, anger...even attack! By all intentions, you would more than likely be on the defensive.
*Such encounters are perfect opportunities to practice the Figure **8** unconditional love breath.*

The Technique:

1) Size up the situation; recognize calmly that the person sitting opposite has decided to blast you with very uncomfortable vibes.

2) Don't judge, close-down, stiffen-up or cross your arms.

3) Relax completely and allow yourself to open to the energy--because that's all it is, **energy** generated by emotion.

4) Go one step further and take responsibility for attracting the situation, for you *do* have the power to transform it literally before your eyes; make this an opportunity to change the energy from being negative and destructive to positive and constructive.....if only from your standpoint.

The secret to changing the frequency involves receiving it, turning it within you and breathing it back again as acceptance and love.

5) Begin to *breathe in* the unpleasantness. As you breathe and receive the energy, visualize your breath in the form of a figure **8**. Circle one part of the **8** *into* you as you breathe in, then turn it around and send it back again (as love and acceptance) when you breathe out--continually receiving, transforming and sending through the figure **8** breath.

6) As you practice the breath, ask for the right words to say to further heal the situation.
Such breathing brings you into an altered state; you are no longer in the separated outer mind, you have made the connection to your higher Self. Remember, intention and breath alter the nature of emotional energy....then the appropriate sounds (words) will modify it even further.

In addition to one-on-one encounters, the Figure 8 breath can be used unobtrusively in group or crowd situations to change negative energy into positive. Intersperse the Figure 8 breathing with serveral Galactic (loving) breaths.

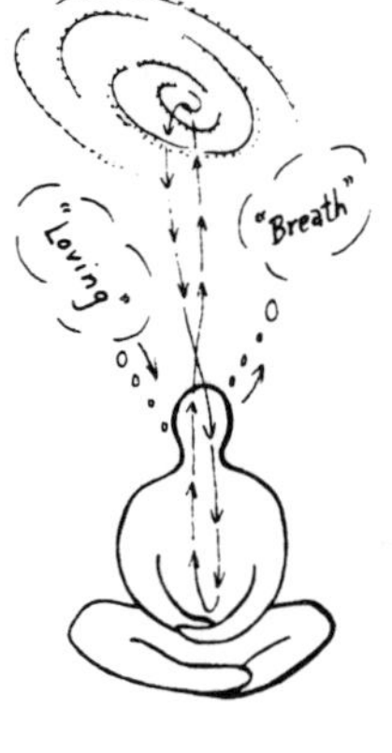

The Goddess Energy Breath

"Vase" Breath

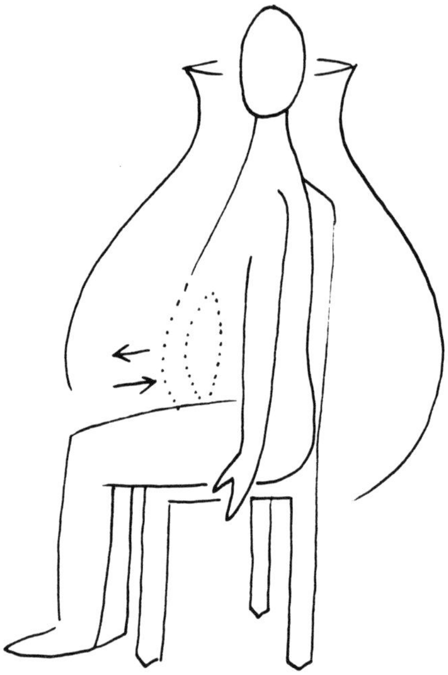

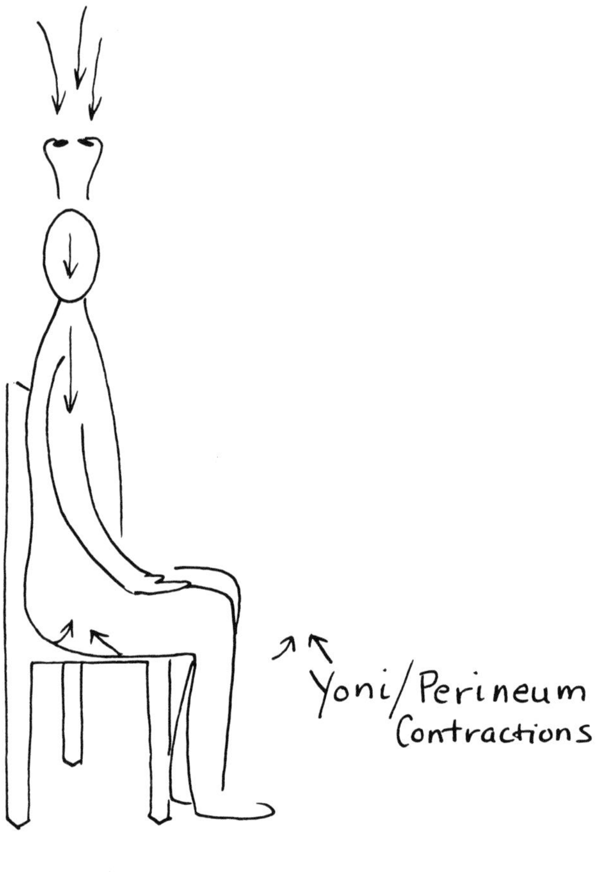

Crown Sniffing Breath

5.....ACCESSING INSTANT ENERGY

The following three methods can be used separately, or in sequence, building into a powerful culmination with the Bliss Breath. However, the last exercise, The Energy Sea, is a completely independent practice. As to the promise of 'instant energy' - you will not be disappointed!

a) The Goddess Energy Breath - "The Vase."

1) Sit on a straight backed comfortable chair with feet flat on the floor.

2) Breathe in and draw the green Earth Mother energy up through your feet and into your stomach. Now the next time you breathe in, make your belly as round as possible, as though it's a spherical vase filled with green energy. Do this two or three times, to get used to the feeling.

3) Having established the feeling of breathing into the belly, next turn your attention to the expiration. Breathe in and 'round' the stomach (as you've been doing), now breathe out very slowly, all the while squeezing the lower belly tighter and tighter as though expelling the air with your stomach muscles--while at the same time, making a very slow Perineal/Yoni contraction--until all the air has been discharged. This leads naturally to a strong inspiration with a nicely rounded belly again. Try this breath sequence several times until it becomes effortless.

4) Next, when you breathe out and squeeze the belly flat, you are to 'empty' the contents of the vase (the green energy) into the upper body.

Here's the total sequence in a nutshell:

a) You breathe the green energy **in** through the feet and up into the vase-belly.

b) Then breathe **out** squeezing the green energy (from the filled vase) into the upper body while you contract the belly and draw up the perinium/vagina.

Do ten vase breaths in a row, ***then one very deep rest-breath****, followed immediately by The Crown Sniffing Breath.*

b) The Crown Sniffing Breath.

The intention is to sniff energy in through your crown and down the spine to the perineum area (between the sexual organs in the male and ***at*** *the yoni/vagina in the female). Although this can be done lying down, it becomes most effective when sitting with the spine upright and feet grounded flat on the floor, as in the vase breath above.*

1) Concentrate on the very top of your head and imagine you have a pair of nostrils up there.

2) Take strong rapid sniffs while simultaneously contracting the perineum/Yoni area - for each sniff you do a tiny contraction/relaxation, as fast as you can.

You don't pull the stomach in with this, just contract (pull up) the perineum.

Do at least 20 or more sniff/contractions. You'll find it's somewhat like winding up a spring, eventually it gets harder and harder to sniff.....that means you have done enough, the energy is 'wound up' and ready to go! This build-up can then be used for instant energy or it can be discharged into the body as bliss (through the Bliss Breath), which of course is very vitalizing - and quite surprising, if you haven't done it before!

c) The Bliss Breath.

Although undoubtedly a bliss-inducing procedure, I sometimes call this the 'mixing breath' because it mixes together the activated energies from both the Crown and Root Chakras, bringing about another inner "marriage" of the polarities in the human energy system.

To continue on from the prior Sniffing exercise:

1) You are already sitting with spine erect, feet flat on the floor and you have just completed a series of Sniffing Breaths--in fact, you're so full of energy, you can't possibly fit in another sniff! At this point relax and take a rest-breath, a deep breath **in** from the bottoms of your feet up to your crown and **out** down to your feet again.

2) Then begin to sniff very lightly and rapidly through your nose, or (if it's more comfortable) pant with your mouth open; **at the same time as you are sniffing or panting,** slowly and steadily begin pulling in and tightening the lower belly while simultaneously contracting the Perineum/Yoni.

You'll notice that towards the end of the rapid sniffing or panting, these mini breaths will become slower and slower and more powerful as the bliss becomes more intense. At the same time, you should experience a wave of bliss (which can be mildly pleasant to sexual) beginning in the pelvis, moving up your spine and penetrating the various body centers There may be several waves of bliss and you should perform the panting (or rapid nostril breathing) for as long as it takes the "charge" to disseminate into the cells. **Sometimes you may need to take a slow breath and then go back to the panting in order to release all of the charge.**

3) Following the Bliss Breath, take two more very deep rest-breaths **in** from your toes and up to the crown, then direct the **out** breath from the Crown back down to the toes.

To repeat the cycle.

Do another ten Vase breaths **a)***, then -*
One rest-breath, then -
Twenty or more Sniffing from the Crown breaths **b)***, then -*
One more rest-breath, then -
A final series of Bliss pantings **c)***, followed by two or three final rest-breaths.*

You will *not* **generate the same amount of energy if you only do one cycle!**
These incorporate the three bodies (physical, Chi and Light) and result in greatly increased energy; they can be performed morning and evening....or when needed.

Both the Vase and Crown Sniffing breaths can be used independently to generate physical energy *without* the bliss. **The Vase Breath:** when practiced out of the bliss cycle, needs twenty repetit-ions to gather a sufficient charge. If you find twenty in a row too much to tackle, try ten - then a rest-breath, followed by another ten; then two rest-breaths to finish up. The resulting energy can last for most of the day....then you can do a repeat if necessary. **The Crown Sniffing Breath:** used alone, gives an immediate boost when you find yourself suddenly exhausted or depleted after extreme exertion. Don't try and do twenty breaths in public, people will think you are hyperventilating and get alarmed - instead do short, quiet, *surreptitious* bursts of eight to ten sniffing breaths whenever required. I find crowded public places ideal, no one notices unless they happen to be sitting next to you on a bus..then you can say you're doing a breathing exerecise for energy!

(Vigorous bursts of the Sniffing Breath exercise gave me miraculous energy during some very heavy digging and earth removals when I was building my Sacred Earth-Mother/Sky-Father garden. I would just pause, lean on my shovel and do some rapid sniffs--explaining to my curious co-worker that it revived my strength--which he accepted because it obviously did!)

d) The Energy Sea.

Here at last, you have something to do lying flat on your back in bed, on a couch or even the floor. A good time to practice is at the end of the day for ten minutes before you fall asleep; if you take an afternoon siesta, try it as you drift off. However, be warned--along with restoring vim and vigor, it has a reputation for increasing the libido!

The technique has been adapted from an old Taoist meditation that consisted of a lengthy poem translated from the Chinese. On first reading the poem and the energy claims, I simply didn't believe they could be true. My curiosity won in the end and I experimented with the text, eventually shortening it and attained excellent results with less verbiage. In this exercise you will activate the lower energy circuits of the Chi-(energy) body.

1) Lie flat on your back with your legs out straight and arms beside you on the bed.
2) At first read silently and eventually commit to memory, the following:

"This energy Sea, *(breathe **IN** and up)*

This flowing Chi. (*breathe **OUT** and down*)

From the point below my navel, *(breathe **IN** and up)*

To the soles of my feet." (*breathe **OUT** and down*)

3) Keep repeating the above verse and breath pattern over and over for five to ten minutes before falling asleep. You may need up to ten days of practice before the energy kicks in.

The first sensations usually occur in the feet, which begin to get hot or tingle; then eventually you will notice a definite flow of energy going from the feet, up your legs and into the belly button. Later, try placing your hands gently on your midsection over the navel; this will intensify the energy and heat in the Power Center.

On feeling 'pooped' after a jog or any other sustained vigorous exercise, I often collapse on my back somewhere and recover by doing the Energy Sea technique. Also when I used to work out with weights in a gym, I would employ the Energy Sea to make a rapid recovery between sets.

Give this strange inert exercise a fair trial. Do it for ten days to get the energy channels operating, then it will work for you instantly whenever you need it--in situations and locations where you're not in a position to practice any vigorous sniffing or panting!!

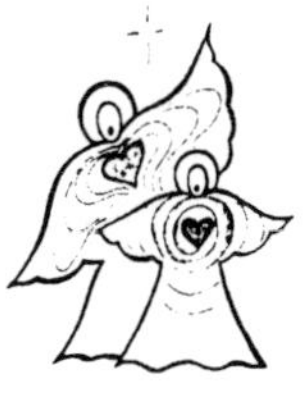

18....POWER TOOLS FOR THE BRAIN

Before presenting the 'power tools' for the brain, I want to comment on a 1996 Associated Press Release that appeared in our local newspaper. It contended that Americans were becoming musically brain-dead and that the majority of the present day population were growing up incapable of carrying a tune--unless born with a lyrical ear and destined to become a musician like my youngest son Ricky (who sang happily in the cradle). Before he could speak he hummed at meal-times--which was always a sign that he liked the food! It didn't matter *where* he was munching, he sang in the car, in restaurants, at picnics. We always anticipated 'musical' meals! Then again, he *was* born into a musically inclined environment, and this, according to the newspaper article, appears to be the exception these days.

Educators say the tonal-dearth trend has developed in America over the last 100 years. At the beginning of the century (without radios or TV), people made their own music and usually learnt to warble on their mother's knee. In the evenings, the family sang around the living room piano and when at social gatherings (apart from everyone singing lustily together to some kind of musical instrument), it was quite normal to be asked to get up and sing a solo. Not so today. Most people would be appalled by such a request! The belief is, that when left unstimulated from an early age, the neurological pathways enabling us to feel comfortable with our singing voices close down and never develop. Fortunately, those pathways can be re-activated. At any age, we can train ourselves to feel confident in carrying a tune--without everyone around us blocking their ears! The "musically brain dead" newspaper story only concerned itself with remedies for school children, whereas my work primarily targets adults, but there's no reason why you can't get your kids to join in with you for some rousing, family voice-releasing!

Part of my solution uses the power of Resonators--these are the 'power tools' to re-activate the brain. In addition to the traditional ones, **"M," "N,"** and **"NG"** (discussed fully in Chapter 4), you have the less obvious and more curious **"B," "P," "J," "L," "R," "V," "W,"** and **"Z."** All of the Resonators re-calibrate brain patterns and more than that, some of the lesser known ones enable us to enter into altered states of consciousness.

Sounding The Extra Resonators:

You begin by resonating the chosen letter several times on one continuous tone (your lowest comfortable note is best) for as long as your breath can sustain the pitch. (Breathe deeply and relax between each note.) Then try sounding them through one octave of an arpeggio[1] and finally, remember to occasionally resonate with your hands over your ears to experience the enhanced richness of tone.

Letter B...

Although **"B"** can be 'rolled' much like letter **"R,"** its resonating sound is quite different. When you make the "rolled" sound for **"B"** (like **"Brrrrr"** when you're feeling the cold), the relaxed lips rest together while the air is buzzed through them setting up a rapid vibration. To *resonate* **"B"** alone, the lips are under more tension. You may have difficulty in arriving at the correct position at first, but there's no mistaking the strong resulting vibration when you get it right! It will almost tickle and remind you of blowing through tissue paper on a comb.

a) "Think" about pursing the lips, but don't quite do it. Instead, slightly tighten the tension in the top lip and lightly say **"Buh, buh, buh"** to get the feeling of the lip position.

b) Then leaving the lips slightly pursed and partly together "buzz" the air through them with a slight sensation of inflation on the inside of the upper lip. *The upper lip should vibrate the strongest.* Look at the image of **"B"** (from Chapter 21) while practicing, it will help focus the energy.
This can all be quite tricky to get the hang of at the beginning! Keep trying. Do several of the long continuous tones and also practice with your hands over your ears to fully feel the resonance.

---

[1]See "How to Sound an Arpeggio" from Chapter 12.

c) On the "**B**" buzz, choose a comfortable low note and take it up through an arpeggio. Make three repetitions of each note (of the arpeggio), before ascending to the next. *The hard palate in particular and certain bones in the skull will vibrate with this exercise.*

d) Remember to look at letter "**B**" and begin again on a comfortable low note; now *without* the repetitions take it slowly up an arpeggio in a series of long resonating buzzing tones; then try moving it higher into the *next* octave (above the one you began on). You'll find it's more difficult to maintain the buzz in the second octave.
Sometimes the vibration will simultaneously resonate the inner ear, the root of the tongue, the muscles under the chin, the cheek sinuses, the crown of the head and even tickle the tear ducts (at the nasal edges of the eyes). Remember to also sound and listen with your hands over your ears, it helps to maintain the tone, particularly over the second octave.

Finally, close you teeth firmly and challenge yourself by making the "rolled" sound for "**B**" (mentioned previously), but in a *controlled* manner by attempting to "**Brrrrrr**" through an arpeggio. It's easy to sound like a car revving it's engine, or a kid playing "airplane," but see how low you can sustain one "**Brrr**" and then 'arpeggio' it up through the three triad notes and into the next octave above. You'll notice they're easier to do the higher you sound, but because of the larger quantity of air needed to vibrate the lips, it's also much harder to sustain the note. Take it easy though, the effect on your brain will appear similar to playing a Pan pipe flute.....you'll get a space-y-ness due to an increase in oxygen.

Letter P...

The frustrating thing about resonating letter "**P**" is that it sounds practically the same as letter "**B.**" However, there *are* subtle differences between the two--and it still needs sounding in the context of it's own energy and meaning.....especially if you have it prominently in your own name! First *look* at the letter "**P**" establishing it *along with its meaning* in your mind, then begin much the same as you did for "**B.**"

a) Say "**Puh, puh, puh,**" to get the lip position. You'll notice that "**Puh,**" has a 'soft' soundless attack (the "**uh**" has sound, the "**P**" is silent) which you maintain throughout the resonating exercise, whereas "**B**" has a 'hard' sounded attack.

b) Then (as for "**B**"), leaving the lips almost together "buzz" the air through them with a slight sensation of inflation on the inside of the upper lip. Looking at the image of letter "**P**" from (Chapter 21) while practicing will help focus the energy. Do several of the long continuous tones.

Letter J...

Be prepared for a complete shift in sensation as the resonance receives its direction from the teeth rather than the lips. *The resonance will move from the back teeth to the front, the higher you sound.*

a) Look at the "**J**" letter and say "**juh, juh, juh**"....using the same sound as in the word "just." This gives you your basic mouth position.

b) Now keep you teeth together and with your lips pursed *and open* maintain the "**J**" resonance from against the clenched teeth, "**Jjjjjjjjjjjjjjjjjjjjjjjjjjjjj.**"
In addition to the sides of the lower jawbone, you'll immediately notice a vibrational shift to the upper sinuses (the bones of the forehead) and as you go higher, to areas on the top of the head. The facial bones in front of the ears can also vibrate.

Because of the rather intense brain stimulation, don't overdo on this one. After a couple of rounds, relax, and gently direct the breath to the newly vibrating areas in your head. Then rub your scalp vigorously and finish by gently tapping your head all over with your fingers....this has an equalizing effect.

Remember to relax between Resonators taking several deep breaths to integrate the aftermath of each sounding. If you begin to find yourself feeling slightly discombobulated, immediately balance the energy by sounding **"N."** *Don't attempt to go through all of the Resonators at one time and do no more than two new ones at each session. The combined effect can be too expansive and overwhelming for some people. It may be more prudent for them to incorporate just one new one (in addition to* **"M," "N"** *and* **"NG"**) *per week--to more gradually stimulate the brain.*

Letter L...

Again, a new and different experience. **"L"** is more subtle than the others and one of the easiest to resonate.

a) The teeth remain slightly open; place your tongue on the hard palate behind the top front teeth and produce a steady continuous **"L"** sound.

"L" will resonate the upper surface of the tongue to some degree, but most of the vibration originates from the root of the tongue, the soft palate and the pharynx (the cavity linking the throat, nose and mouth). The nasal cavities and bony septum also vibrate, with the resonance moving up the soft palate, the higher you take the tone .

Letter R...

With **"R,"** you can engage in three distinct methods and effects:

1) The rolled **"R"** as used in speaking Spanish and German.

2) The **"R"** resonated with the teeth clenched - a strangled growl!

3) The final one made with the teeth open and the tongue curved inside the mouth, to create the un-rolled or velar-**"Rrrrrrrrrrrrrrrr"** as used by most English speaking peoples. *(Other than the jaw and throat, this one vibrates the sides and back of the skull.)*

Letter V...

This feeling and sound might remind you of school days and blowing through a "paper-comb."

a) Begin by saying **"Vah, vah,"** a couple of times.

b) Then rest the top teeth on the lower lip and resonate a continuous **"Vvvvvvvvvvvvvvvvvv."** *The vibration begins under the chin, extends up through the jaw to the ears and finally at the back of the neck, close to the head.*

Letter W...

Here's the old 'dog barking' sound - **"Wuh, wuh,wuh."** Say it a few times slowly to get the placement and feel the strong resonance it produces.

a) Then maintain the lips in the **"W"** position and sustain a long **"Wwwwwwwwwww"** sound. *The strong vibration can be felt at the very back of the skull (where the neck begins) and seems to enter the brain (from that point) as you maintain the sound-intensity; also the lower jaw will begin to register. Experience this for yourself and discover the different areas you can vibrate with this sound.*

Letter Z...

Where I was born, this letter was pronounced **"Zed"** and not **"Zee"** - it took me some years to get used to the change; now, I rather enjoy it!

a) Simply clench the teeth and resonate a continuous **"Zzzzzzzzzzzzz"** sound. *You will be immediately aware of vibration on the top of your skull. Place a hand up there and your hand will begin to feel it. You'll also feel the sound strongly in the lower jaw and throat.*

Try and keep the meanings of the letters in mind while you are resonating them...or those specific meanings that hold the greatest emotional 'charge' for you.

In order to make sense of these analyses, be sure you have first read Chapter 5, "Your Name" and in particular, the summary at the end. Here follows a random list of interesting people - some you may know of - some you may not. In these names, I don't always give a full analysis, but you will be able to follow and understand the most dominant energies.

Some hints for trying to quickly analyze a name:

1) Most important energy (if not the Drive (**first** letter), is frequently the Focus (**center** letter(s).

2) The next important energy lies in the letters immediately *surrounding* the Focus Letter(s).

3) Look for a (several-times) repeated letter throughout the *entire* name.

4) Pay attention to the Aim (**last**) letter and the one directly in front of it.

5) A vital clue to an outer strength or problem may lie in the seldom used middle name.

6) If you find out the person was adopted, you may discover not one, but two birth certificates and usually the very first one (made out by the birth mother), contains vital missing information about the personality not found in the adopted-name.

Don't forget to note if any letters have supplanting-sounds (such as: the "E" instead of "Y" at the end of "Mary" and "J" instead of "G" in the middle of "Roger") and take those into consideration.

We begin with a great communicator....

Elie Wiesel; passionate social visionary; 1986 Nobel Peace Prize Laureate, Holocaust survivor, accomplished, prolific author (35 books) and lecturer. The four **"E 's"** and two **"L's"** allow both the "power of the word" and a voice (**"E"**) to the people (**"L"**). The **"W"** Drive fires up enthusiasm and the motivating force to show off his vision. Focus letters **"ES"** in the center of Wiesel (his work-environment name), compel him to 'focus' on communication and mutual understanding (**"E"**), and to work for a better world society (**"S"**). The compassionate visionary aspect of **"S"** enables him to foresee this ideal society in spite of the world's racial patterns of fear, suspicion and hate.

Operating through the transformed level of the **"L"** energy, his vision goes beyond racial confines into a profound respect for the intrinsic value of individual life. *"We are all responsible to another."* The two **"I's"** (and his many books) have rendered him very visible as he persists in drawing attention to all levels of social injustice - also aided by the **"W"** Drive of **W**iesel. The indomitable staying power of both **"S"** and **"W"** can be summarized in his own words: *"It is almost forbidden to give up."* He is described by his peers as a "beacon of conscience to the Western World."

And now, another person famous for his words....

James Earl Jones; accomplished and seasoned actor of many outstanding films who reigns even more rich and famous because of his unique and sonorous voice (Darth Vader in *Star Wars,* King Mufasa in *Lion King,* the CNN spots we associated with the Persian Gulf War, plus other familiar voice-over TV commercials.) This name is especially unusual in that James is *not* known as "James Jones," but "James **Earl** Jones." A special stress has been placed on "Earl" and to uncover a primary life purpose we'll begin by discussing this middle name. The first letter **"E"** not only governs self-expression but communication, speech and the voice. The **"E"** Drive letter of **"Earl"** presents a hidden agenda--to use the voice (or communication), in a physically and mentally powerful way, reinforced by the middle **"AR"** - the Focus/Challenge letters. The last letter of Ear**l**, the (**"L"** Aim letter) represents his powerful speaking and communication before the public...*part of his life's aim.* In relation to this, notice how the Aim and qualifying letters in both Jam**es** and Jon**es** are identical. **"S"** can compel one to seek distinction, money and social acceptance and with *this* name, distinction came to James Earl Jones through developing the voice-power aspect of **"E."** You may well ask: **"How does this all fit in with the two "J" Drive letters ..??"** Letter **"J,"** especially when repeated, may indicate a physical challenge or problem that the person was born to master--and yes, he *did* have one! And this physical challenge *happened* to connect powerfully to the voice - during his childhood James Earl Jones overcame a serious speech impediment - stuttering! As possibly the most famous and glorious speaking voice in the world, he has inspired us with his determination to conquer a daunting physical obstacle (Letter **"J"**).

Next, someone whose life is dedicated to 'death'.....

Dr. Jack Kevorkian; "The Suicide Doctor," famous for his many assisted suicides around the country and his legal battles against what he sees as his 'responsibility to the world' (**"V"**), to help end the prolonged suffering of the terminally ill. His name contains three **"K,s"**.....the letter concerned with matters of life and death or rejuvenation. In Kevorkian, the central Focus comes from the letter **"R"** - the power of ideas--or challenging the fixed ideas of others. But *which* fixed ideas? The answer rests in the letters *either side* of the **"R"** in Kevorkian, the **"O"** on the left and the **"K"** on the right. His personal mission through his work, challenges the accepted ideas on what constitutes compassionate care-giving (**"O"**) for those in the process of dying (**"K"**). The preceding letters **"EV"** initiate the social vision he's determined to communicate, and the **"KI"** gives the nature of the vision--to call attention (**"I"**) to the manner of 'death-from-disease' (**"K"**) - and also to his part in attempting to shorten suffering through assisted suicide. The **"AN"** (the Aim (of life) letters at the end of Kevork**ian**), represent his wish to be identified with and remembered for (**"A"**)--*his desire to bring a new critical analysis and balance (**"N"**) into the process of dying with dignity.*

The **"J"** that drives the first name embraces the "justice" aspect of the letter, which in Dr. Kevorkian's case brings a preoccupation with justice for the dying...and of course, he's always stirring up controversy (and getting into trouble with the law) because of his actions and beliefs!

An interesting contrast in the ***polarized*** *application of letter* **"K"** *is Pro-Lifer* **Rita Marker** *(with the* **"RK"** *Focus in the middle of her 'work-in-the-world' name); she opposes the work and ideas of Dr. Kevorkian with her Anti-Euthanasia Task Force.*

The two following names show how the letter energy can become inverted and polarized in destructive and disturbed people....

Adolf Hitler: the Master Mind of the 3rd Reich; the instigator or World War 2; the leader (**"A"**) of the Fatherland (the traditional name for Germany). Letter **"D"** governs "the father." Driving force for the **"D"** is letter **"A"** (at the beginning of **A**dolf); **"A"** potentiates supreme leadership, which Hitler finally attained. The question one asks is - what *kind* of leadership? Apart from indicating "the father" energy, letter **"D"** *can* foster total authority and possible domination. Adolf Hitler not only became the total (Godlike) authority and father-figure for Germany at that time, but he also planned to impose his authority over all of Europe and the British Isles...for starters!

The **"O"** Focus/Challenge in the middle of Adolf, however, became the true key to Hitler's driven and destructive personality. Turn now to Chapter 8 and study this letter to receive a full understanding of the energy in its general, balanced and unbalanced aspects. In the light of **"O"** normally characterizing nourishment and "the mother"--when this energy is reversed *and* found adjacent to letter **"D,"** the **"O"** can result in a need to *control* women. Under Hitler's regime, during the late 30's and early 40's, an organization called "Germany the Father-land" used selected women (who epitomized Aryan qualifications - tall, blonde, blue eyes), as breeding stock to birth a new Master Race. Of course, they were inseminated by their perfect Aryan male counterparts! The women chosen for this breeding stock, considered it a great honor to be part of the Grand-Plan. **The Grand-Plan was set in motion....** *to produce a Master Race containing pure cultural blood that would take over the world and annihilate all inferior races, or subjugate them into slaves.* The beginning of this plan took effect with the breeding program and the Jewish Holocaust.

Look now at the central *three* letters in A**dol**f, - you have **"D"** on one side, **"O"** in the middle and **"L"** on the other; the two flanking letters are the energies that most influence the **"O"** Focus. The father authority in **"D"** (remember, Hitler was then the supreme ruler of the land), not only controlled the women, but also designated which of the population (letter **"L"** governs 'the public'), were fit to live, die, be free or enslaved. Jewish people (considered inferior by the Nazi Party), from all of the conquered European countries as well as those in Germany, were systematically rounded up, interned, starved and worked to death or killed in gas chambers; their body fat made into soap, their skins into lamp shades and other objects of interest to the "master race." Finally, with the **"F"** in Adolf as the Aim letter, Hitler's Aim was to be proud of everything he had done and to set an example for his people!! **An interesting exercise for you to try:** look for someone else with the name of Adolf and compare how they have used the same letters. The name "Hitler" - I leave for *you* to analyze, but before *truly* understanding how the letters fit, you may first have to study a biography of his life and times.

And followed by....

Timothy McVeigh; convicted Oklahoma bomber and mass murderer, referred to in the press as "America's Most Hated Man." In this name, the two **"M's"** and the **"V"** stand out, together they mean **family and social idealism**--and as publicly revealed about his life, McVeigh has intense ideals and comes from a very supportive family background (unlike Hitler who did not always enjoy a happy childhood because of his father). In the light of Hitler who destroyed millions, McVeigh's crimes pale by comparison...but only in measure of degree! Whether you believe McVeigh to be a fanatical, heartless monster or the scapegoat for some unfathomable, behind the scenes shenanigan, the two men do share that unmistakable **"O"** Focus in their personality names (Tim**o**thy and Ad**o**lf), which in both cases became polarized from nourishing and preserving life--to the opposite--destroying and rending family and community...all to uphold their passionate beliefs.

Returning to Timothy McVeigh: two **"T's,"** can bring emotional sensitivity, personal disappointments and perceived injustices; the injustices were national/social issues governed by letter **"V"** (his stated feelings about the Government-instigated Waco family/community massacre that took place exactly a year before the Oklahoma bombing). The **"E"** and two **"I's"** certainly brought a need to express and draw attention to these injustices. However, his personal vision of making a difference in the world (also letter **"V"**) seems to have reversed itself in the choice of destruction and revenge ("An eye for an eye"), and the attention he drew created yet another kind of social injustice--because his act disrupted and destroyed countless family units including mothers and children (**"M"** and **"O"** inverted). Letter **"H"** (the Aim letter of the last name, McVeig**h**), also means, purposeful plans, will power, discipline and what you would like to be famous or remembered for--should you fulfill your vision! Once the dedicated soldier, his personal vision seemed to go sour after an Army career disappointment...now he will be remembered for a singular act of infamy--not of honor.

Contrast the above with the following profiles of benign international mother and father figures:

Mother Teresa; saintly Roman Catholic nun, universal mother-figure; bastion of the sick, dying and poverty-ridden (especially in India but now world-wide). The sensitive, spiritual **"T"** in Teresa formed the impetus for her life of religious devotion and commitment; the two **"E's"** gave her a strong 'voice' to express and speak her needs to those who would help her establish and further her organization for the poor; the **"RE"** (double Focus in Te**re**sa) resulted in mental power to forcefully present her ideas; the **"S"** eventually brought enormous success for her cause--with prestige and money (she also won the Nobel Peace Prize); and the **"A"** Aim letter enabled her to end her life as an outstanding world leader in a normally disdained occupation. *Mother Teresa is the assumed Spiritual Name and the filter for the birth name of* **Agnes Gonxha Bojaxhiu**. Looking at her original name, we receive the definitive energy of this remarkable and dedicated woman: the **"O's"** and **"B"** provided selfless empathy and 'mothering' compassion; the two **"H's"** brought vision, hard work, self discipline, willpower and also eventual fame; the two **"N's"** resulted in an almost martyred obligation to others through her belief in God; the two **"G's"** gave an unrelenting energy for physical labor; the **"A"** Drive (from Agnes) propelled her into leadership. *Most unusual of all* are the twin Focus letters from the middle and last names containing **"X's"** -- **"NX** and **"AX."** These powerful Challenge letters underscored her long life of devotion and service, with the **"X"** power to call in and focus a multitude of scattered energies...with considerable mental brilliance! On a *transformed* level, **"N"** takes responsibility to heal and balance and **"X"** maintains an intense spiritual center; finally, with the "**A**" **combined with** "**X**" (from Boj**ax**hiu), it made her a world leader with formidable abilities to focus on the issues at hand. *From the above, you can observe the importance of the original given name - even when not in active use, its energy still sets the tone and pattern of the life.*

And there is the inimitable...

Danny Kaye: this greatly loved, joyous, actor, comedian, dancer and singer entertained the world in the middle of the 20th century through a great many films, theater, Broadway, radio and TV shows and world tours; he also conducted symphony orchestras and spent the final 30 years of his life as ambassador-at-large for UNICEF. Knowing of his marvelous exploits and then looking at "Danny Kaye," the name that went with the public man--*it did not add up!* And it doesn't. His real name holds the secret - **David Daniel Kaminski**. To study a biography of this charming and charismatic being, every single letter in his much longer birth-name *does* make sense and adds up to the extremely complex and talented man known in public as Danny Kaye. (This almost nick-name version of the original has two "**Y's**" added for good measure; thus making sure he could do things in his own inimitable way!) We will not attempt to discuss David Daniel Kaminski in its entirety, but we'll look at some of the outstanding energies. Four "**I's**" throughout the name created someone born to perform who was truly happiest on the stage before a live audience, in fact, his magical interaction and love affair with an audience became legendary (two "**K's**" together with all those "**I's**"). He brought joy and laughter, yet at the same time, had the power to deeply touch and move people (the transforming level of "**K**"), and releasing his own inner intensity (the "**K**" again), he could show the world his heart under the cloak of comedy. In Danny (a picture of health and vitality), we also have the life-enhancing aspect of "**K,**" - it gave him his great interest in health and medical matters.

Keep in mind, an assumed name becomes a focused filter for the birth name: the "**D**" Drive retained in "**D**anny" reflected the unusual *three* "**D's**" from **D**avid and **D**aniel. Danny Kaye embodied the *positive* Father Image (loving guide, protector, exemplar) and as his life unfolded, he more and more assumed this role (note his film, "Pennies from Heaven"). He especially adored and enchanted children, becoming 'father' to the world's children through his long involvement with UNICEF - which evolved into his personal world mission (the "**V**" Focus letter in Da**v**id). *If we stopped right here, we would only be touching a part of this remarkable name energy, but we'll turn our attention back the 'filter' name:* The "**N**" doubled in Danny, gave him his intense desire to serve and heal (through the medium of laughter) and with "**E**" as the Aim letter in Kaye...he gained the "last-word" on how he wanted to express himself - and also fired up his "golden double-talking tongue" to uproariously mimic other languages! *Rent some old Danny Kaye movies (The Secret Life of Walter Mitty; The Inspector General; Hans Christian Andersen) - and enter another world!*

The Time-line Aspect of Names....and Christopher Reeve.

It's obvious that all names have a time-line and certain energies don't fully kick-in until after specific life-changing events. For most of us this process moves smoothly, almost imperceptibly; for others, it strikes suddenly and changes everything forever! For successful actor **Christopher Reeve**, his personal world-changing event occurred when the riding accident he suffered left him an instant quadriplegic. Initially, the three "**E's**" in **Reeve** (the work name) predisposed him to an occupation that used vocal skills (acting), but frequently when the "**E**"s" are doubled *and* enclosed by consonants, they imply a challenge to free expression - or in this case, a challenge to the *usual* expression of talent! Up until his near fatal fall from the horse, Reeve *did* enjoy unrestrained self expression (the last "**E**" of Reev**e** is open and not limited); but after the accident (the serious time-line event), the limiting double "**E's**" kicked in...he is still the same talented, creative actor, but without a mobile physical body to express himself through! Yet, several months after his fall, he emerged as a powerful, charismatic inspiration to others, as though enriched and transformed by his ordeal...and he began doing some amazing things: attending functions in his life-support wheelchair, giving talks and interviews and now directing films!

When a big time-line event occurs in a life, it will directly relate to the central Focus name energy.

As to *why* he has been able to transform such a devastating life-blow?--much of the answer lies in his first name, Christopher, with a sensitive, intuitive "**T**" Focus in the middle. *Letter* "**T**" *always challenges us to seek spiritual answers, or to search out inner strength in times of stress.* (The physical restrictions have opened Christopher Reeve to the power of his indomitable Spirit.) Once established, the inner support from the "**T**" suffuses outward from the center of the name in both directions. On the right, the "**O**" developed emotional maturity plus support from family and loved ones; then the "**P** eventually resulted in a sense of peace and tranquillity that now extends to everyone observing and listening to him; "**H**;" brought (and continues to elicit) enormous public support for his future vision of recovery for himself and others suffering a similar misfortune; finally "**ER**" as the Aim energy at the end of Christoph**er** - enabling him to powerfully communicate his ideas about the need for spinal injury research. *Now return to the "T" Focus in Christopher and look to the left:* letter "**S**;" after the accident, the effect of the more sensitive and spiritual focus changed his attitude to success along with his public image (a different *kind* of respect and acceptance now exists), along with how he makes and spends money (there's a tremendous financial drain for medical expenses!); next in line comes "**I**" - he no longer *draws attention* to his abilities as an actor, but to the staggering needs of a quadriplegic--which also has opened him to the intuitive, spiritual and creative resources of the letter; in addition, "**I**" also governs the breath. The accident unfortunately altered his manner of breathing--it's now through a machine instead of his own lungs--although he is able to breathe for longer and longer periods without the respirator; next comes the powerful and compelling "**R**" releasing new mental powers and ideas - which further intensifies the "**R**" Drive at the beginning of **R**eeve....his "work-in-the-world" name.

From the central "**T**" Focus, we've almost moved in both directions through the entire letter energy of Christopher and we're up to "**CH**," the very front of the name and the driving-force of the personality. The powerful "**K**" *sound* of "CH" (in **Ch**ristopher the "**H**" is silent), *can* predispose some to a physical challenge and in this case, the body indeed encountered an especially crippling challenge. Most frequently, the combination energy of "**CH**" instills a private or public passion for helping others. *Christopher Reeve's way of helping others now drives every part of his personality.*

The above gives you ideas for how to analyze a complex name like "Christopher" and to see how it specifically applies to that remarkable person - Christopher Reeve...a true "Superman."

Observe your own "time-lines" and notice how these events changed you--and how you then accessed new and different levels of meaning within the letters of your names.

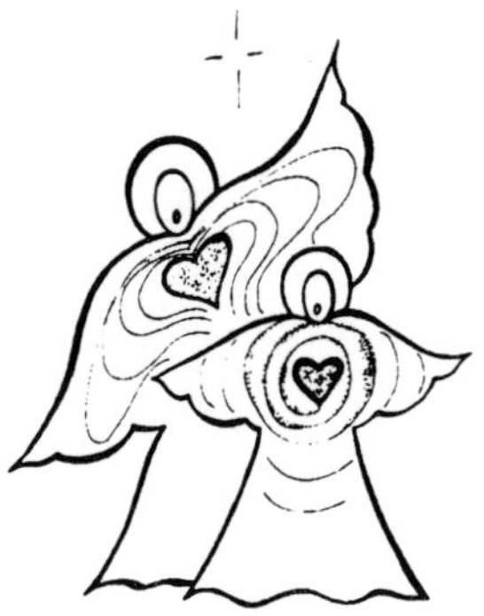

Instead of sounding all the vowels daily, take a six day break and concentrate on just one vowel a day. I mentioned six, because we will add an extra "vowel." Several years ago, when researching semantics, I found that some speech experts regard the letter **"Y"** as a vowel, and (with the exception of **"Ow,ow,ow"** and **"Ah,ra,ra,rah"**), it's already the secondary letter when we repeatedly sound vowels **"A,yae,yae...E,ye,ye...I,yi,yi...and U,yu,yu..."**

Here are the vowels with their corresponding body placements:

A -- The middle of the chest (Heart Chakra), the Inner Beloved, sense of touch.

E -- The lower throat (Throat Chakra), the power of speech and song, sense of hearing.

I -- Between the eyes and also in the Forehead (Ajna and Third Eye Chakras), opening to higher Spirit (the Sacred Breath), inner vision, inspiration.

Y -- The Navel (The Fire Chakra), will power, independence, energy, heat, sense of sight.

O -- The Mid-belly (Water Chakra), the inner child, nurturing, pleasure, bliss, sense of taste.

U -- The tailbone/perineum (Root Chakra), sense of smell, the foundation, security, the state of stillness.

The above meanings are based on traditional Eastern understandings[1] which I have directly experienced physically and emotionally through my personal practice.

In General:

As you sound, visualize the **"A"** in the heart on the first day; the **"E"** in the throat on the second day and the **"I"** in the forehead on the third day (which prepares the head centers to receive the Presence of Spirit). Returning to the middle of the body--on the fourth day you sound and visualize the **"Y"** at the navel for a strong and powerful will; on the fifth day--the **"O"** in the belly for emotional balance and on the sixth day--the **"U"** at the base of the spine for security and abundance in the united God-Goddess. *Mentally repeat and visualize the letter you're working on (in its bodily location) just before you go to sleep. It's also possible to practice this exercise silently while 'singing' the letters mentally.*
The letters "Y, O, and U" designate your *embodied* consciousness; the vowels "A, E, and I," indicate your heart, voice and mind connections to Spirit through self expression, creativity and inspiration.

The Advanced Vowel Exercises:

1) Visualize the chosen vowel in the appropriate body part during the day, place it there when you wake up (while you're doing your humming) and see it there as you fall asleep at night.

2) Find your base-note and chord for the day; sound the separate notes of the arpeggio through one to three octaves with the chosen vowel, while being aware of its place in your body.

3) Speak and sing the chosen vowel while moving the head, face and body.

4) Find your range and instead of using **"Kah,kah,kah"** to swoop up to the top note, try it with the vowel instead. Your low and high range will be modified by the particular vowel you work with.

5) Read all the meanings of the selected vowel and contemplate on how it can expand your awareness and improve your daily actions.

---

[1] Read "Wheels of Life, a User's Guide to the Chakra System" by Anodea Judith, Llewellyn Press.

6) Regardless of whether you *think* you have any needs connected to the particular vowel, develop the empowered range of the vowel by practicing all the different sounds for it suggested in Chapter 9, "Sounding for Specific Needs."

Meditation on the Vowel Placed in the Body.

1) Settle yourself in a comfortable place until you feel calm and peaceful. Have in front of you the image of the letter[2] you plan to contemplate, or draw your own.

2) Take the fingers of one hand and tap them gently and repeatedly over the corresponding place in the body where you will visualize the letter, ending with a circular motion.

3) Relax, look at the printed image of the vowel while you softly repeat it mentally, (use the **"Ah"** sound if using **"A"**); close your eyes, see the letter in your mind's eye first, then 'see' it in the appropriate body part, where you will not only visualize, but *feel* its energy-presence. If you have trouble picturing it in the body, look at the letter, close your eyes and "draw" it on a mental slate board.

4) For a few minutes of tranquillity, feel and observe the letter within you as you breathe in and out - repeating the name of the letter mentally on each inspiration and expiration. *Imagine your breath flowing through the letter (at its body location).*

The colors of the letters when visualizing:

In my own experience when I try to see a luminous white **"A"** *in my chest, the best I can manage is a very pale white color, and in spite of turquoise being the empowering shade (in Tibetan mystical practice) for the throat, my* **"E"** *persists in showing itself as a deep clear yellow-gold (the color of Amber - the* **emotional** *specific for the throat and the color for the center of the galaxy); I very much wanted a white* **"I"** *in my forehead, but it insists on remaining a deep purple. The* **"Y"** *in my navel appeared instantly as a deep black--understandable, as black denotes the will, but so far both the* **"O"** *of the belly and the* **"U"** *of the Root also remain adamantly black...possibly because emotions and self-support must also involve willlpower!! These colors may change of course and for you who read this book, the colors* **you** *see could be entirely different!*

Galactic Breath Vowel Meditation.

The next phase calls for you to envision our own spiral Milky Way galaxy,[3] with it's brilliant center containing billions of blazing suns. As you breathe IN, imagine you're taking a Light-breath from the radiant core of the galaxy - down *into* the body at the point where you have placed the chosen vowel (drawing the breath through the letter itself). Then, as you breathe OUT direct the breath (and the vowel), UP to the galactic center again.

Another Version: when you breathe IN mentally **say**-and-see the letter in its body location; when you breathe OUT direct the letter back to the galactic source, *while you mentally say:*

"Breath."

For example:

a) Breathe IN to letter **"E"** in the throat. "Pulse" it several times (while holding the IN-breath) *by mentally repeating:* **"Eee, Eee, Eee, Eee."**

b) Breathe OUT and direct a whole stream of **"E's"** out the top of your head to the radiance of the galactic center *as you mentally repeat:*

"Breath."

---

[2]from Chapter 21 "The Sacred Symbols."

[3] Compare with the 'Galactic Breath' described in Chapter 4, "Releasing the Voice."

Practice this deep sweeping breath, with affirmations and visualizations four or five times--or more if you feel the intuitive need. Practice the same direction of breath and affirmation/visualization for each of the five vowels.

Please don't overdo this one, particularly with the letter "I" in the forehead. It can open up the entire gamut of head-receptors; you might end up receiving too much energy and enter (far too rapidly for your own comfort), into an expanded state. Should this happen, immediately stop the meditation and do the following procedures:

Begin to hum the grounding Resonator **"Mmmmm, mum, mum, mum, maaaaaaah"** *and the balancing Resonator* **"Nnnnnnnnnnnnnnnnnnnnnnnnnnn"** *several times, followed by* **"Ssss-ah, ssss-ah, sssss--aaaaaaaaaaaaaaah"** *directing the breath to your feet. If you continue to feel hazy, discombobulated and detached, your 3rd eye is still far too open and you're probably receiving more energy than you can handle.* <u>*For this, there are four remedies*</u> *-- try them all if necessary:*

1) *Speak and sing the vowel* **"Aee, ay,yay"** *and* **"Ah,"** *also* **"Ah, rahrah,"** *as when you do your daily releasing technique with the vowels. The sounds will* physically *stabilize the identity energy in the body.*

2) *The second remedy uses the 'energy transformer' in the spleen (a little used center about four inches to the left and on a line with the Fire center in the navel), place both hands on top of the spleen and breathe the energy down through the head and into the spleen center, where you can visualize it as a golden light (from the center of the galaxy) flooding the body.*

3) *Take a small pinch of salt on your tongue and drink some cold water.*

4) *A personal trampoline makes another instant stabilizing and grounding tool.*

St Paul wrote in his New Testament Epistles, "It is not yet known what we are to become." Our becoming would appear to entail an evolution into an expanded form of life able to comfortably access more than one dimension. We seem to possess non-physical 'muscles' that need careful and gradual development. Until we can encompass our full power of being in an integrated body, each small expansion needs to be gradual and balanced. The descent of Spirit into our corporeal form could well begin our ultimate destiny. For more indepth information read the next Chapter, "The Sacred Symbols."

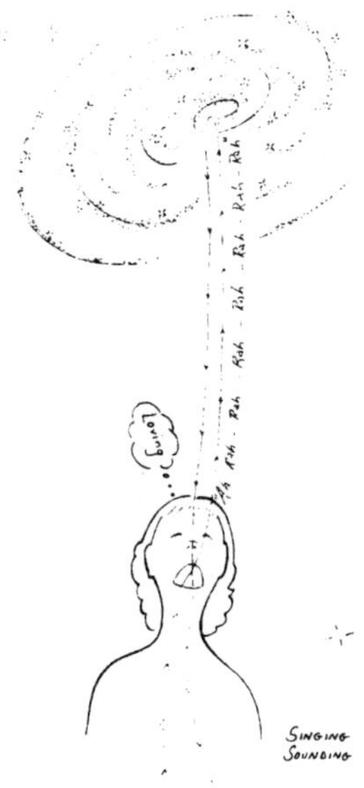

Many ancient cultures regarded their alphabets as holy, their language symbols representing Divine Sound in visible form--the Sacred Word. Sanskrit, Pali, Tibetan, Hebrew and Arabic are some of the traditional sacred languages. In Tibet, prior to the invasion by the Chinese Republic in the 50's, each monastery had special "book-burial" rooms where undisturbed old manuscripts lay returning to dust on the shelves. No matter how decrepit or worn, the holy texts were never destroyed or permitted to rot on the ground; each letter image possessed--no **was**, the essence of its meaning! Whereas here in the West, our speech symbols are based on the Imperial Roman alphabet (itself, borrowed from the Greek) and contain a strictly utilitarian function--for control, communication and commerce. So on the surface, Western language has its origins in the doctrine of a dominating culture with an all-too-well-known ethic: subdue lesser races and make them dependent on our own, so we can exploit them and their natural resources. The more educated (or lucky), tend to "follow the donkey" - trotting after more and bigger successes--and often, excesses!...(evident in some of the more mundane letters meanings). The less fortunate fall under a different imperative: be good, dutiful, unquestioning worker/slaves within the consumer goods mind-set....so you can continue to be exploited by the financial powers controlling you behind the government and the media. *Crass materialism apart, another deeper meaning does hide within our alphabet, and all language (because it symbolizes the essence and sound of Spirit), remains sacred--whether acknowledged as such or not.*

Beginning in duality and progressing to oneness, the alphabet *when used in names* embraces five levels of meaning:

1) The **outer** - this particular soul-life.
2) The **inner** - the additional presence of past soul-lives (sub-selves).
3) The **balance** - union of the **outer** soul *with* the **inner** sub-selves.
4) The **transformation**--union of higher Spirit with the **balanced** soul and sub-selves.
5) The **interdimensional Super Being** (to come) - the united Spirit, soul and sub-selves within an integrated physical, Chi (energy) *and* Light body.

Every one of the 26 alphabet images contains the potential for all these levels. Up till now, this workbook has given information and useful techniques to get you through to level **3** on the list, the **balance.** With this Chapter we approach **4**, the **transformation**--which always sounds somewhat unattainable and unrealistic. Let's face it, enlightened states are not understood or encouraged in Western society. Echoed by a friend only yesterday, most ask, "Of what use are they anyway??" And, "How can enlightenment be my *real* state of mind?" For instance: historically in Christianity, many of the mystics were either martyred or struggled to maintain their expanded vision in the face of a suspicious and hostile establishment. The appearance of Eastern teachings in the West over the past few decades has helped somewhat and today's cases of spontaneous 'awakenings' aren't usually disparaged as demon possession; none the less, they're often psychiatrized, medicated and institutionalized - in that order!

Non-duality, with all its interesting variations, has no evident practical function, especially in our mercenary culture--whereas in Eastern traditions and in those of most indigenous peoples, it's an accepted and natural part of the human psyche. The outer mind can't fathom expanded mental states (which can only be known through direct experience), and if you try and talk about them, no one will understand what has happened to you. Such 'mystical' lapses are dismissed as aberrant behavior, and as madness! And to the limited, dualistic mind **they are!** Also, being "awake" is not *necessarily* the same for everyone who gets there--although in some instances it can be--all of which causes confusion for Western seekers. Enlightenment consists of not one, but many states of enlarged awareness which when fully explored, culminate in an all encompassing expansion. Make no mistake, the underlying quality of every mind **is already** transcendent (regardless of race and belief), but the basic bright-awareness remains veiled behind the outer-mind conditioning and chatter. This surface conditioning favors the outer-mind at the expense of the universal and interdimensional consciousness. Some people (through various "openings" and disciplines), *have* partially regained their essence-nature, however, their new awareness is not necessarily complete if deeper personality factors have not yet come to light and been integrated. We are much more than our apparent selves; various past-life influences (hovering in the subliminal background), also need prodding awake--that's why we brought them with us in the first place and that's also why we keep having to come back into a physical body. *Integration is the name of the game!* Until dealt with directly, our sub-selves harbor and act-out the deeper emotional failings and cravings within us. Now and then, glaring examples surface in the so-called "spiritually advanced," even those who have gone beyond ordinary identity into no-self and no-mind still fall prey to the old "nasties" of irrational fear, greed, unresolved anger and sexual compulsions. The full expansion goes beyond emotion, self, mind and body. For instance, someone can enter no-self (without identity), but their limited mind and messed up emotions remain fully intact - or they can become no-mind (with expanded clarity and all pervading emptiness), yet still know the pain of ego separation and erratic emotions. Then there's the most totally terrifying experiencing of all.....no-body (in one, or more of its many variations), which often leaves the "normal" outer-self in total chaos! *Eventually we must integrate all of our sharded and scattered holographic parts, then what we have known as self, mind, emotions and body will enter the next stage of human evolution - or, will we actually return to what we really have been all along??*

The intrinsic key to understanding our complex nature issues daily from our own throats! The language we speak conceals the resplendent glory of the sacred vowels. Superficially, these vowels represent man in the five modes of duality--as a body/ego **(A)**, a mind **(E)**, a higher Spirit **(I)**, with emotions **(O)** exploring an external environment **(U)**.

The Vowels as the "Dual-Self."

A - *ego and body :* **"I am me - a self - in a container."**
E - *mind, intellect:* **"I am me - thinking and knowing."**
I - *inspiration:* **"I am me - discerning, creating."**
O - *emotions:* **"I am me - feeling and wanting."**
U - *expansion:* **"I am me - giving and taking."**

Another Way of Grouping Vowels:

The Mundane:

Vowels **A, E** and **O** = **Body/ego, Mind, Emotions.**

The Transformative:

Vowel **I,** the pure creative flame of Spirit igniting **A, E** and **O** with inspiration and Life Force.
Vowel **U,** the *balanced* intake and outflow of the Infinite Presence, **as - A, E, I** and **O.**

In full potential, ALL of the vowels become the non-dual nature of transcendent existence.[1]

The Vowels as "Transcendent-Self."

Sacred A - *becomes the underlying Ground-of-Being, the Source, the Primal Essence through which.....*
the separate ego (as such) vanishes and dissolves into....
the non-existent, no-self, the all within the All, the NO-Thing that is everything.

The Realization:
"I am that I am." "I do not exist." "All bodies are the One Body." "There is only One Self."

---

1 For the difference between vowels and consonants refer to page 25.

Sacred E - *becomes the ever-present, underlying, radiant consciousness through which.....*
the intellect/mind of incessant thought dissolves into....
the no-mind, no-thought, boundless and limitless within the clear awareness; the Universal Mind-Matrix.

The Realization:
"The ocean of awareness flows within me." "I am the clear, fountain of bright awareness." "Thoughts are the enemy." "Within this One Mind, and beyond words, all beings everywhere contain themselves." "We all exist as fundamental incandescent light which remains ever present, ever translucent within us - there are no distinctions." "There is only One Mind."

Sacred I - *becomes the immortal Life Force/Spirit, the Breath, the primal fire of bliss through which.....*
the manipulative need for attention transforms into...
the conducting rod of creative Spirit - the Life Force flame of pure inspiration.

The Realization:
"Doing takes place without 'doing,' yet everything gets done." "Life Force bliss flows without ceasing." "The conscious breath directs the energy." "I am the ecstasy of creation."

Sacred O - *becomes dispassionate-compassion; joy beyond joy; awareness as wonder through which....*
the nurturing and emotional demands dissolve into....
the non-emotion of clear, calm dispassion; the expanded unnamable feeling-sense; the transformer of painful emotions; the generator of Infinite Love.

The Realization:
"I am without emotion, yet I encompass all emotions." "I play and explore with an open awareness." ("Unless ye become as a little child, ye cannot enter the kingdom.") "The kingdom was never a place; it remains always - as a state of being." "Love is not an emotion - it is a radiant field of energy."

Sacred U - *becomes the expanded reality behind the multi-level experience of the fully awakened super-being through which.....*
the usual perception of external reality as form dissolves into....
a limitless, effortless and non-discriminate expansion both within and beyond the physical, Chi and Light bodies.

The Realization:
"Underlying all forms is the One (form)." "All forms are the Infinite Presence." "I am all forms, I am the Infinite Presence." ("Ye, must be born again, to enter the Kingdom of heaven") "I am reborn where I have always been and where I exist as Light-body-Spirit." "In union with Spirit my body is limitless."

These states of being and realizations probably only scratch the tip of the iceberg. Who we really are and what we're destined to become - is in the making! My own expanded states (a great variety), have occurred sporadically throughout my life. A constant experience of "brightness" and oneness-with-all marked my earliest childhood. Until I was four and a half, my family existed on a remote wheat and sheep farm in northern West Australia. The climate, noted for it's low rainfall, just met the bare requirements for growing wheat. Most of the year we lived in a grayed-out, arid, bush-land; but with the first rains of spring, the earth exploded briefly into lushness and color. First came a faint velvet of green which gradually swelled into carpets of grass, then wild flowers graced the land with yellow, white and pink straw-flowers stretching as far as the eyes could gaze; scarlet and green kangaroo-paws (a furry flower) brightened the scrub along with delicate orchids; the gum trees (boughs heavy with honeyed blossoms) gathered bees and sticky, insect-trapping sun-dews grew close to the ground and had to be inspected on hands and knees. A magical time for a dust-urchin like me! I also had my special hiding places filled with soft ferns, mosses, glinting rocks and the sense of enfolding "presence." But the magic soon faded! By age four, the awareness of "presence" and the oneness had gone--as though I'd lost the key to a secret garden. A different atmosphere of despair, fear and failure replaced the bright awareness. Hit with the hard times of the Great Depression in the 30's, my Dad abandoned the farm and we went to live in the large city of Perth, five hundred miles to the south.

Most of my earlier mystical episodes (not all of them pleasant) were evoked by nature or unusual changes in the quality of ordinary sounds. The one I hated the most would happen in my bed when I was trying to sleep; a dripping faucet or other rhythmic noise would sometimes set up a peculiar sound pattern in my head, which then proceeded to remove all sense of physical boundary (*a terror beyond words to a tiny child*). My body would gradually balloon to an immense size--at first filling every space in the house, then extending to the fields outside and finally, filling the sky; all that remained of "me" was a paralyzed "pin-prick" of awareness engulfed by the universe. Eventually, I **was** everything--every pulsing atom! After an agonizing period of time--the sensations receded and my exhausted little body would reappear on the bed, with my usual mind (somewhat numbed) once more in my head. I never complained about it to my parents (some inner sense warned me to keep quiet) and I was deeply grateful it didn't visit me every night, but when it did, the physical "swelling" always followed the same sequence--a patterned sound from the outer to the inner ear expanding into a whirling, all-encompassing energy. *As I grew to adulthood, it followed me intermittently and by the time I discovered it to be a much sought-after phenomenon of Buddhist Vipassana meditation--and I wanted the experience--it had ceased altogether! Short of doing a Vipassana retreat (which I debated a number of years), I did not know how to bring it back.*

Another more tolerable "altered-body" state arrived during my pre-Buddhist years in a crowded Pentecostal prayer meeting. On this particular night we were all on our knees in front of our chairs (elbows on the seats), to begin the ritual of bringing down the higher Spirit. Our hearts and voices lifted in spontaneous exultation and soon the room was charged with psychic energy--but then we always went 'electric' in those lively meetings! After five minutes of boisterous devotion, a strange body sensation silenced me; I didn't swell up thank heaven! - but energy, heat and vibration began expanding (*and* expanding) from a point in the middle of my chest until every physical structure had vanished--including my bones; I became a white, intensely glowing "body" of light, barely contained in a paper-thin covering of skin! This mercifully lasted only a short time, perhaps fifteen minutes at most. When I could finally speak and relate the somewhat alarming phenomena, no one in the room could decide what had happened to me--except, that "Spirit had blessed me greatly!" *With three* **"A's"** *in my original birth name (***"A"** *governs the body as well as the ego), I now realize such physical transcendence is a valid aspect of* **"A's"** *sacred energy.*

After moving to Canada in the 60's, and becoming a Hatha Yoga teacher, I periodically spent time at the Sivananda Yoga Camp in Val Morin, Quebec. During one such visit, a large group of us had just finished an asana class with a new teacher and to complete the session, he "talked" us through the usual deep relaxation. Like the rest of the class, I lay flat on my back on a folded blanked, but when I had finished relaxing everything from the tip of my big toes to my eyebrows--the part that I call "me" was nowhere to be found! There was no "self," no personal identity of any kind--just a vast emptiness! My body still lay flat on the floor, my mind in confusion, my emotions in shock, while the rest of the class filed out of the room. Eventually, the instructor and his assistant came over and knelt beside my (by then) weeping form. I explained with some terror, that I had ceased to exist as a self. He laughed and said "Hasn't this happened to you before--haven't you ever gone into no-self?" I wailed "No-oh" and went back to sobbing. They took me, still wracked with grief, for a walk in the tranquil forest above the ashram and sat me down on a large rock overlooking a pool. I cried non-stop for the next three hours. Needless to say, my old crappy self eventually returned and I became "normal" again!

Four years after my Yoga Camp experience and as part of an intense sojourn with Tibetan Buddhist practice, I found myself living and meditating alone in Vancouver, Canada. A phrase from an ancient Buddhist text (a borrowed book) had begun to implode my mind--I found myself reading and writing it, pondering its meaning....and as well, keeping up with my usual hours of formal meditation. Within days, this led to three presageful dreams. The first dream: in the near distance, a vast ocean of immeasurable brightness stretched before me. The second dream: a small very white elephant walked along a trail towards the ocean (white elephants are sacred in India and symbolize enlightenment); then in the last dream I was inside a ridged, shadowy passageway that lead to a distant point of light. A week later, during a powerful massage, I entered the 'passageway' (of my dream) and at the other end emerged into the light of the brilliant ocean--the massage had triggered my own birth experience and in remembering it, I was "reborn" into the brightness of my original childhood awareness. I sat up from the body-work and must have looked strange. My friend Phyllis, stared at me intently and said "What's happening?" The full impact of the awareness hit me; I flung my arms in the air and screamed **"I do not exist!"** I had once more returned to the "Secret Garden" of my infancy and childhood. For the next three weeks, I wandered Vancouver's lush garden-parks uniting with daffodils, tulips, tree trunks, nature. People were different and *un*-natural compared to everything else around me. I had access to their thoughts, their separations and their pains; but from my position--that of a thirty-nine year old 'enlightened' *infant*--I had not been given the chance (*none of us get the chance*), to grow and mature within the radiant consciousness...so it too faded, leaving me with yet another memory of unsustainable transcendence. Two subsequent dreams at the time comforted me. In the first, I was an enormous infant being wheeled in a giant perambulator by two large and benign guardians (a well protected baby--with a lot of growing up to do!); in the second dream, I felt myself sinking deeply into rich, brown soil, a soil that rested, warmed and nourished me--as though I was a freshly planted "seed" and needed to rest and germinate. All the parts of the puzzle were not yet assembled!

Since then, I've had 26 more years of growing up and been prodded with several more notable awakenings--reminders of the inner radiance; they would descend on me when alone, or startle me in group situations--but none ever remained. My experiences with the five senses showed that each of them--sight, smell, taste, touch and hearing, formed its own pathway to this underlying "ground of being" and also opened portals into other dimensions; and although many of my experiences had come through seeing,[2] hearing (along with speech and song), promised to unlock a vastly different and profoundly integrating energy....*which I have detailed for you in this workbook.*

When we communicate with each other, we're really voicing our sense-gathered impressions, along with our thoughts and feelings *about* the information we've sensed. Our infant babblings begin the process of communication; we use voiced sounds to respond to an outer world that we touch, taste, hear and smell--providing we've got all our faculties! The inner sounds are another matter, they arise with or without the help of our ordinary ears and connect us to sub-selves, higher Spirit, Devic realms and other dimensions and time warps.

In 1980 I began my research into people's names and the letters of the alphabet. During these observations, a startling discovery emerged--the letters comprising a name represent the *sounded form* of Spirit *within that particular person* and also reveal the life potential (from the mundane to the mystical) *of* that person. **As already noted, the most important letters in a name are the vowels, they stand out as the vital core-energy of Spirit and a "code" for the enlightenment process.** This book now culminates with the 'profound' aspect of the vowels and the human evolutionary possibilities they reveal.

Please understand, the awakened experience is not a static state, but one of constant movement and change, change that propels you towards a fully expanded self. Your outer habits and thoughts will constantly pull you back from expansion, and until you're 'awake' all the time, you almost *have* to surrender yourself to a moment-by-moment practice. The choices abound! Saint Paul exhorts in the Bible, "Bringing every thought into subjection to the Christ within." If you're a New Ager, you might release those pesky thoughts into the Light - or into the "Christos"...or if a Buddhist, you might dissolve them into Buddha nature...or if a Taoist--see them as part of the Tao. A traditional method - just watch them flitting through the mind and let them "flit," or gently dissolve them with the breath. *You'll find an exquisite interim behavioral practice from Christian mysticism in a tiny volume called "The Practice of the Presence of God" by Brother Lawrence. (Ask for it at any Catholic or*

---

[2] Read further on in this Chapter under the heading, "A Few Transformation Notes."

Episcopalian book store.), or for other ideas read therapist Nancy Napier's book "Sacred Practices for Conscious Living."

In each moment, it all depends on which awareness happens to be present--that's what you work with; you can flow with what's there, or change it--you *are* in charge. Finally, should the longed-for "brightness" fountain up through the heart, choose to remain in the fountain and increase its flow with the breath. All thought gradually vanishes in the cascade of light...and along with it go doubts and emotional fears. In the future, more and more of humanity will enter the all encompassing bright-awareness (more and more frequently) and when we get used to being there--we'll act as a body of *deliberately* functioning transcendent people!

NOTES ON THE TRANSFORMATION OF THE SENSES:

A spatial shift into transcendence can happen through any one of the five senses. **Take seeing for example:** when "seeing" with another person - without wavering, allow your eyes to relax into their eyes--while at the same time, release all resistance, self-judgment, fear and finally--thoughts. *The energy leap into transcendence may happen very rapidly!* You may both go through together, or one person might merely catalyze the other...and then observe. My most recent experience of eye-contact expansion happened with a very aware person whose first name also began with letters **"Ri"** *and* we shared **"E's"** in our last names (mine, from my maiden name). Within seconds, the energy running through our bodies (and in the three feet of space between us), quickly became incandescent. Together, we entered the majestic, all-Mind, no-boundaries brightness, and we both stood motionless, enfolded in that awareness, for almost an hour.

Begin to notice the interactions you have with other aware people, and how the conjunction of your name energies enhances your ability to amplify consciousness together.

The following walking meditation includes several simultaneous mind-body modes and works equally well if you are alone or part of a group-intention. It expands the senses of sight, smell and touch (body boundaries). Practice with extreme care.

Begin your walk; unfocus the eyes slightly, relax your mind and look only at the spaces *between* the solid forms as you slowly walk past them. Bushes and plants in parks and gardens are great for this. *Try not to make mental judgments on your observations - just observe the form (or space) without distinctions.* Gradually the "seeing" opens you internally, first to the reverie state (all while you are awake and walking), passing quickly through several memory flashes from life, then on to old familiar dreams (that could also be images from past lives), culminating in an augmented sense of space. It's hard to explain, but your physical boundaries will have changed. This is the dangerous stage, because in your new mind state, the body no longer matters *(that's when people think they can fly out of windows, or walk across streets through on-coming traffic!).* At this point, **you must listen** to your witness-self which will warn you internally to watch out for the vulnerable (and valuable) outer body--so only *note* the feelings of a limitless form, you can enjoy--but don't act on them! Having circum-vented that phase, you'll soon begin to smell (never before detected) extra-sensory fragrances exuding strongly from the surrounding plants, bushes and trees....as though the Nature Devas are welcoming you to their domain. Finally, you'll start seeing all objects in their essence without distinctions, as wonderful shapes and colors devoid of their language-labels. Even discarded garbage appears vibrantly beautiful to the extended sight. This multi-sensing meditation always follows the same unfolding pattern; your witness-self will note the signs and comment..."Ah yes, *that's* happening now, and oh!--now we're passing through this phase." *All of the above listed phenomena should be present in each session - who knows? you may develop your own unique sequence, but you should always see the same signposts on the journey.*

Warning: Do not use the previous meditation as an escape from your outer reality; use it to inves-tigate the expanded and interdimensional capacity of your own senses. For physical safety reasons during such sensory enrichment, the outer mind still needs to be present and in charge. This is the "witness self" and always remains to one side within the expanded mind---***it is the Guardian of the Inner Threshold (to other dimensions) and your way back to what you know as external reality.*** Much

as you may not *like* your ordinary three dimensional reality, it's what you have to function in--unless you want them to lock you away!!
Although these other dimensions interpenetrate our own, you need to be aware of ***when*** *you are traveling through the inner-landscape, and where you are within it - in relation to the 'normal' one!*

The sense of touch often sets off the other senses--it interrupts the intellect and says, "Pay attention!" Did you know that feet electromagnetically ground us to the earth and also function like direction-finding antennae? Naturally we ignore them when they 'call' us, unless we've opened up their mini-Chakras.[3] Next time you're at a large public gathering, picnic, party, dance, seminar, try letting your feet guide you instead of your head! (Although some of us do have a head-radar as well!) You'll feel the feet and sometimes the legs gently pulling you in certain directions; mostly the feet will react by vibrating and tingling...and it's not athlete's foot! They're the little known sensing part of us just waiting to be used! In another type of walking meditation you focus on the soles of the feet and what the earth communicates through them while you're walking. At first (to sensitize the feet) they need to be bare - later on you'll feel them guiding you even through your shoes and boots.

Choose a large area of grass in a park, meadow or other expansive natural area - preferably free of broken glass and other sharp debris. Prepare your feet by slapping and briefly massaging them on the bottoms--then sit still for a few moments while you breathe energy in and out of the soles. Now start to walk with all of your sensing down in your feet--you'll be amazed at what you'll discover. Your feet will take you to the hot-spots--areas where more energy and even heat seem to issue from the ground. They'll also 'walk' you to the power areas connected to trees and other natural objects. You can tune into the energy - receive it, augment it--or both. Respectful communication with Devic nature spirits is also a possibility.

Look down at your hands for a moment. *How we take them for granted!* Such amazing, complex and incredibly sensitive organs! They receive and send, bring in higher energies from above the body[4] and move and focus healing energy. Sometimes when a healing *needs* to happen...and your outer mind is blithely unaware...your hands will begin to tingle, become hot, and assume a mottled pink and white appearance (as they pull in extra blood) - or all of the above--these signal you that Spirit wants to work through your hands. *Then it's time to listen inwardly for where you're supposed to lay them!* Hands also become energy antennae in the case of distant healings (and balancings) - not just for people, but locations as well. In distant work you might use maps, photographs and newspaper cuttings; place your hands slightly above them and concentrate the energy downwards through the palms; they will tingle and you may also sense a color to project through the hands with the breath. Both the feet and hands contain mini-Chakras (they're actually left and right magnetic poles). Feet will activate when you slap and massage them; hands, when you rub them together. After a vigorous rubbing, hold your hands several inches apart, palms facing each other....you'll soon feel a charge of energy running between the left and right magnetic poles in the center of each palm. *I have often sat in the bus on my way into town, palms resting on my knees (and facing each other) running the energy between my hands. This action opens the channels for the upper Chakra energies to come down and flow through the hands--so do it often.*

A general sensory phenomena begins when a strong overriding physical or mental signal interrupts what you're doing or saying. Providing you understand the signal when it calls (so you can stop other mental distractions), it will initiate a series of subtle body sensations--sometimes in the small of the back, chest or crown of the head. I'm always intrigued by the summons and when these signals begin, I've learnt to give them my undivided attention, or at least enough attention (when I'm with others), to allow them to unfold. The rule: let your awareness follow the feeling and allow yourself to progressively receive and go further into the sensations--no matter how strange. Eventually, an inward 'shift' happens, taking your outer awareness with it. You'll find yourself literally in two dimensions and in two mind-modes simultaneously. (Don't forget, the witness-self must remain in charge of the vehicle!) In this altered state you may feel the presence of your guides, guardians or higher Spirit (or those

---

[3] To open the feet, see Chapter 17 "Energy Exercises" page 155.
[4] See "Clearing the Inner Field" from Chapter 17 (page 153) and Chapter 14 "Opening the Throat Chakra."

belonging to the person you're talking to) - *felt as a lightness and opening at the back of the head, tinglings and chills from the Crown down through the shoulders and chest, a gentle pressure (almost like a hand) on the upper back...those with expanded sight will also see them!* The full experience may bring direct insight, with pictures, words and emotions about a present situation (or a past life) - any number of things make themselves known when the inner lines of communication are open in this manner! The summoning signals don't arrive willy-nilly, they always have a reason! You learn to trust the journey and *allow* yourself to expand into it.

Sight and Light. On rare occasions, reflected light will strangely increase its intensity and begin to glow. Consider this ą "light-summons." My last light-summons took me through a profound self encounter; I went on a microscopic journey within my body, where I observed and integrated the male and female archetypes of my own duality--and for about a week I returned to the bright awareness! Each morning my witness-self would awake, suprised and delighted to find I was still 'there' in the brightness, and that sleep had not erased the expansion! A precious week!!

A few comments on **seeing** in reference to color-frequency (actually another form of sound). Sometimes, a specific color may suddenly become evocative and intense, leaping out at you for an entire day--or two! Your eyes seem to select that particular hue--and only that, from out of its normal milieu. A pair of red shorts will walk by, then a red hat, now a scarlet backpack leaps out of the crowd, nothing but red cars seem to be on the road--and as though disembodied, a red book jogs down the street!! Whatever color has intensified will keep up this brilliant bombardment until its work has finished! You may even ask: "Why am I seeing this color so much today?" *A part of you needs the nourishment of that special shade and your eyes pull in the frequency.* Then sometimes **all** colors begin to radiate a kind of luminosity beckoning you to receive their energy. *And no--you don't need new glasses--there's nothing the matter with your eyes--they've just extended their perception momentarily.* In the final aspect, everything you see becomes the sparkling colors of the Sacred Form and this, strangely enough, links through to taste--when you can choose to "feed" upon and be nourished by that particular shade...the Source Essence--as color![5]
Each sense has its own unique super-acceleration moving you into greater and greater transcendence. Pay attention when the senses call you in unusual and unbidden ways...and it has to be unusual to break the spell of the outer mind! Remember, you are much more than you think you are....allow yourself to become.

The Superconscious Mind connects everyone to the Universal Mind-Matrix, a many layered tapestry of group knowledge and experience from this and other dimensions. Most of humanity remains unaware of the superconscious Mind--let alone the Universal Mind-Matrix! You will greatly augment your life when you can tap into this source of knowledge at will. The actual access happens through your outer mental channels; the ordinary mind merges with the superconscious, then both function simultaneously to access the higher knowledge--the outer intellect remains fully present--though somewhat to one side! To begin the process: simply **know** that you can receive all the information you are ready to use. When posing a question, *do* your research--read, ask, assemble your data--then **relax** (you have done everything possible with the outer mind). Now expect your higher faculty to supply integrative and inductive insights over and beyond what you have so far discovered.....which often arrive at unexpected times--even in the bath! Always carry a notebook and keep one by your bed. It's exactly like linking to a computer-information highway via your brain! Disbelief, doubt and impatience block the door to the insight..*outlaw all such thoughts - forever!* To relax your mind during the process practice the "Nostril Breath" from the Tranquillity Meditations in Chapter 16. Eventually, with only a slight shift in consciousness, you'll be able to ask any question and immediately call in the Superconscious Mind. *There is a saying: "If you can ask the question, the answer is waiting in the wings."*

---

5 See Appendix 1.

Practicing the Expanded Senses.

These suggestions are addressed to the 'awakening householder.' They work best when you are alone, outside, walking the streets, or otherwise interacting with nature and the world - not when you are shut serenely in your room with your eyes closed, or moving in the routine familiarity of your home--or surrounded by demanding people (those all require different techniques!). Some of my most dynamic expansions begin when I walk down my back steps and take the delightful half mile walk to the bus; twenty minutes on Public Transport (a meditation on its own!) and I am in town, moving all over the place, doing my errands and all the while experiencing a great variety of expanded states. At home, I tend to lock into writing, gardening, painting or composing music, interspersed with an occasional client...all of which have their own expansions!

O.K....so you're outside about to embark on this adventure, but before you detect which of your senses will draw you in and expand your awareness, begin with "Soft Eyes, Inner Smile" from page 177 adding your intention to enter a no-mind state. This initiates the process. Within the next several minutes, take note of your most dominant sense--that's the one to follow, it will intensify and pull you more than the others. If it's hearing, all sounds will change subtly; the voices on the bus or the traffic noises may appear louder...as though someone turned up the volume; they will also sound *different and at times muffled.* Instead of resisting, align yourself, enter and *become* each sound, then simply become "sound." Stay relaxed, open, listening and discover where it will take you in your awareness; often other senses go into accelerated expansion after the first one takes you "in." I've already said a great deal about sight, so you know where to go with that. Touch usually expands physical boundaries, so be careful, remain in charge of the body; but if Spirit wants to take that route, you might feel drawn to briefly rub and caress textured things with your hands as you walk past them. Receive the feelings and allow the sensations to expand you. Smell may be a challenge--the bad ones (stale tobacco, body odors, garbage, etc.) have a habit of vanishing when you lovingly accept them as Essence Source. Temperature, an aspect of touch and body boundaries, could attract your attention. If it's summer and you're heating to a crisp, or winter and it's chilling your bones and numbing your feet...align with the heat or the cold. Relax and open--don't fight it; this summons the Chi body which is impervious to temperature extremes.

I don't want to give the impression that only *one* sense will augment and remain dominant for a long period of time (although it *can*); usually--as I've said--you begin with the one that takes you through; it will swell to a peak then gradually recede to be followed by another sense. Remember, you have five senses and they can enhance concurrently or one at a time. Also, let your feet and legs move you in various directions - you'll connect with, or avoid certain people without even trying. Your plans for the day may change during this adventure (it's called "going with the flow"), but everything that needs to happen and get done - will, and you'll have a delightful time in the process. Should you stop somewhere to eat, forget Mom's voice in your head and for once eat exactly what you really want. Either practice the eating awareness meditation from Appendix 4, or allow the sense of taste to expand you through pleasure.[6] Focus entirely on the food, admire and appreciate it, savor each bite and feel the hard-soft textures on your tongue and as your teeth chew. Think of nothing but the exquisite taste and touch of the food and like a baby at the breast wrapped in the sensual pleasure of eating, *become* your mouth, tongue, lips and teeth. Feel, taste, enjoy....feel....taste...enjoy! If you can maintain this interactive meditation throughout the day you'll be in a constantly changing flux of experiences that pulse from outer mind, no-mind, outer mind, interspersed with the intermittent ebb and flow of sense expansion and sensual pleasure. You "think" when thinking is appropriate or necessary, the rest of the time you abide in awareness. And in the face of all the external stimulation, you constantly choose what to allow and what to let go of. One part of you orchestrates, while another surrenders to the greater flow beneath the surface phenomena. In the beginning, practice this alone. Naturally, during your expedition you will interact with a great variety of other people - then you watch how readily you can move from outer mind back to the inner expansion...or even maintain both mind-modes at the same time! After any encounter, immediately return inward with "Soft eyes, inner Smile." It's hard to describe being both "in" and "out" simultaneously--but you will know when you get there! Later on test

---

[6] Be <u>certain</u> to read Part Four of the excellent book by Sondra Ray, "The Only Diet There Is." Celestial Arts.

your mastery by taking a day trip with an acquaintance - who may *not* be aware! *Let all of your days become remarkable.*

SOME LETTER TRANSFORMATIONS and TECHNIQUES:

Transformed "A." We all think our identity (our sense of "self"), resides in the head - especially in the face or behind the eyes, and in duality-mode, this is the case. However, with the arising of bright awareness and universal oneness, the **"A"** as ego-self transforms into higher Spirit and sinks into the heart (the usual domain of letter **"W"**). The heart/chest then becomes the new seat of awareness for **"A"**--and from the heart arises the fountain of brightness.

Letter "D" in particular and some "Y's." Transformation begins when you can look hard at the role "duty" plays in your life. Are you 'duty-bound' to live out the expectations and demands of others? What do the authority voices in your head say you <u>must</u> do to fill a community slot or a family expectation? These "put-upon's" that you carry around may not serve your life's true pattern. At some point soon, the **"D"** (or **"Y"**) in your name may demand you listen to your *own* inner "warrior" - follow *your* drum, *your* desires--and with total determination embody *your* authority! And that is the *least* you can do for yourself, it's just the beginning--your true authority lies within your higher Spirit. When this arises, you'll experience a magical inner 'clearing,' like opening a window and taking a deep breath of fresh air; then instead of feeling the usual intensity, seriousness (and perhaps despair of fulfillment), you'll find yourself strangely lightened. Nothing has changed, yet everything is different. Any need to protect your position and hold your ground has vanished. Suddenly you're open, generous, receptive--and filled with a confidence and power you have never known before, let alone even imagined! *You* are not doing anything, *you* are not struggling and striving....you're spontaneously in the authority of your higher Spirit.

Letter "E" in particular plus ALL the mental letters in general "C," "I," "N," "R," "Q," and "X." *Those with these letters in their names will most readily awaken to non-duality through transcending mind.* (This also applies to those with the *sound* of **"E"** in their names, such as Ricky, Marty, Mary etc.) When the awakening occurs, the power of the intellect, the wealth of learned knowledge, the persistence of thoughts will all vanish into the emptiness of no-mind/All-Mind. In the initial "witness" stage, the realization dawns that this boundless, bright awareness *comprises the basic natural state of all beings....*you then know with certainty--that it exists everywhere--effulgent behind all conditioned awareness. The individual mind, as such, dissolves into the ground-of-being, where there is only ONE mind embracing everyone. To the average and even super-clever intelligence (locked in duality), the above statements will rightly appear incomprehensible - they do not relate in any way to the experience of conditioned-mind and can only be validated through direct experience. *The process of mental awakening returns you to where you are in essence.*

Crowds of babbling people can actually precipitate a type of mental opening. Next time you find yourself in a very peopled, noisy situation - restaurant, conference, bus, airport etc., instead of tensing to protect yourself from the cacophony, or becoming irritated, begin to perceive the "noise" as Infinite Sound. This involves relaxing *into* it, opening *to* it and fully *receiving* it. Then within seconds, it's as though you have entered a sound-sanctuary; the din around you retreats to a softened buzz. I liken it to an invisible, encapsulating shield, or bubble of awareness. The breathing deepens and something within the brain opens like a flower, bringing a marvelous, yet gentle, expansion of consciousness. From then on, you'll sail through your engagement (or commitment) in a state of virtual tranquillity. It's an example of the Buddhist "Left Hand Path" where you convert potentially destructive or debilitating energies into tools to further your awakening.

The power of **"E"** can even generate a mental "Shape shifting." Whereas **"B"** (and sometimes **"T"**) permits the actual physical-emotional shape shifting (as does **"O"**), letter **"E"** brings direct mind-to-mind entrainment. You suddenly become conscious that the thought patterns in your head no longer belong to you and then startle to realize they're coming from the person sitting opposite (or next to) you! Then, if **"B"** and/or **"O"** are also in your name (and I strongly suspect **"N's"** also play a part in this), you will directly register the actual physical and emotional "body" of the other person. *And not to forget the name energy of the person you're dealing with - their energy also amplifies the process!* To give more detail: I automatically enter this mode if I need a particular understanding of some one else; usually I'm in the middle of a private consultation with a client who has a very unique way of thinking and feeling. It usually happens when I'm face to face (although mental and emotional states can leap over the phone). During the expansion, my own mind alters drastically--it seems to shrink itself and retreat to one side, while the empty space it leaves fills up with an assortment of strange and foreign thoughts, thoughts and ideas totally different to the way I usually think...then, I remember the "shrinking" sign, and realize I'm "inside" the thoughts of the other person....*or they're inside me!* I can then tell them exactly how they view the world and in what way they feel themselves set apart from everyone else. *These detailed observations have never been denied!* A further enfoldment brings the illusion of physical change. (My original name has **"B's,"** an **"O"** and an **"N"** - all empathetic letters.) I begin to feel my bones, muscles and skin reshaping themselves, my body re-formatting to *the other person's* body! Eventually, I'm looking at them through their eye sockets, feeling *their* physical structure, *their* emotions and thinking patterns--I exist simultaneously, as both myself and them!

The experience will last for as long as you need to understand (and in some cases) comfort and encourage the other person. Such profound interactions expand one's mental, emotional and physical boundaries and bring compassionate understanding. A notable occasion happened to me while living in Canada. It was the late 60's in London, Ontario and one of my very special and unique Yoga students had driven me home after class. She came up to the apartment for a brief visit and modestly gave me some of her quiet wisdom before she departed. Then for some unaccountable reason, an entrainment shift began in my doorway as she said her "Good-by's;" I rapidly 'became' her and remained within her strong bones and calm mind for the next two hours. She had left me the gift of her essence without diminishing herself.....you see, we really **are** One Body!

Another level of expanded **"E"** (and of all mental letters) happens without warning during ordinary conversations with other people; *but usually only after your Throat Chakra has been opened.* In this case, you are **not** channeling an entity, nor are you speaking through one of your sub-selves--it is your *own* augmented voice and might eventually be how you'd speak (all the time) when you're completely awakened. And just as after the Throat Chakra opens, you can deliberately connect to the inner-voices--and sing like an angel, the same apparently happens to ordinary speech....except that in ordinary speech you are *not* turning inward! In fact, during a normal chat, or even a formal presentation, the inner-voices are usually furthermost from your mind! In this case there's no prior warning, the speech-expansion arrives in a split-second, often in mid-sentence. You go on speaking, but in a different, greatly augmented, super-charged voice and you're just as astonished as your audience...as if... "Wow--what's happening, where did *that* come from?" The sudden power of the words can actually be *felt.* Everyone around you reacts to the energy, including you! The enlarged voice is not so much about volume (though that may be part of it), but has everything to do with incredible richness of tone and quality of expression. In addition, your perceptive and analytical powers increase, often accompanied by refining information appropriate to the subject under discussion! This speech phenomenon also appears in situations requiring sudden and super-normal authority--with only two or three words needing to be spoken. That's all it takes! This commanding effect can also be quite startling. *Outer-mind concedes to higher Mind in response to the needs of those present.* For all the mental letters, (**"E," "C," "I," "N," "R," "Q,"** and **"X"**), the higher Mind waits patiently on the other side of ordinary thought--to expand you back into that part of yourself. The super-conscious connects our external minds to the abiding no-mind brightness. It's time to become the pathway through.

Letter "J" in particular. When some **"J's"** become open to Spirit, they may leave their outer bodies and minds behind when they meditate and 'journey' deeply into other dimensions, beginning with the etheric, and often return with phenomenal knowledge. During this state, they're usually in deep trance and take some time to regain their sense of ordinary reality. This also occurs when **"G"** *sounds* like **"J"** as in "Marge" and "Roger." These profound meditative experiences vary greatly with the individual.

Letter "K" in passing. On the *practical* level, "K" maintains, enhances and honors the Life Force in the body. As to its power to bring **in** the Life Force - a friend of one of my associates legally changed his first name so that it now begins with a "K" and immediately thereafter his wife conceived--they had been trying to have a child for years!!

Letters "O," "B," "K," "N" and "M" in particular and *all* the other letters in general, for each has its unique emotional color. More compelling than dialogue (and the bottom line in relationships), emotion forms the glue connecting human beings together--but sometimes it's more like "Silly-Putty;" it can pull away in opposite directions at the drop of a hat---or an insult! One of my teachers once said, "There are only four permissible emotions, love, joy, peace and a passionate curiosity for life."

How can emotions be balanced and even transcended? The process of transcending the body begins with the melting of physical boundaries and ends in the experience of no-body; the realization of no-self can happen in an expanded, boundless body--or your old familiar one! When emotions begin to transcend, they may vanish entirely...the good along with the bad! Many of these opening experiences are equally uncomfortable and sometimes downright terrifying to the witness-self (when present). My very first entry into unfathomable "no-emotion" reminded me of a scene from the film version of Frank Herbert's classic epic "Dune:" The young hero, now under the effect of the mind altering drug melange (and having just lost everything to war - including his beloved father), finds himself and his mother marooned on a rock outcrop in a vast desert of sand. In an altered state of consciousness (while his mother weeps), he surveys the desolate scene and from his new and strange dispassion ponders, *"Where are my feelings?"* Then moments later, he lifts his head to the night sky and shouts to his dead father, "Father--the sleeper <u>must</u> awaken!"

And we too must awaken from our long sleep, though not through dependence on some external substance, but by freeing ourselves from all external crutches.

The intense connections we form with each other create emotional crutches and when these crutches slip from us, we feel strange, cold and bereft of belonging. How can the contradiction of "compassion-less compassion" make any sense? I puzzled this question deeply once, while giving a three day intensive in Canada that included a Sound workshop and several private consultations. My abilities as an empath enable me to receive and understand the emotions of others--it's my key to helping them. Midway through this weekend, all my emotions evaporated and instead of my usual connectedness, I found myself 'floating' through a detached and expanded awareness. My witness-self thought of it as "coldness," but it wasn't really--I was just absolutely empty of any kind of feeling. Yet from that emptiness a great wisdom seemingly flowed through me to everyone. All their emotional needs and questions were met and answered; words of sympathy, understanding and commiseration were spoken by me - to the satisfaction of all (I know, because I asked questions later), but I myself (totally without emotion)--***felt nothing!*** *I had ministered to emotional needs from the place of no-emotion!* It had never happened before. After returning home, the dispassion remained and my witness-self grieved for my missing emotions. I felt remiss...somehow inhuman! it took the better part of a week to regain my usual empathy and connectedness with people. A great many years earlier in Australia I had known seven remarkable days of effortless detachment in response to a dramatic change of heart, mine, towards a visiting mother-in-law! However, that occasion was not entirely devoid of feeling, my usual reactions of judgment and pain were replaced by a serene joy.

But think about this! - why do we insist on being hooked up, or hooked *into* other people - enduring their burdens in addition to our own, intensifying our pain by allowing ourselves to be emotionally "dumped" upon, or actually enjoying being miserable? In this instance, emotions cloud the mind...and make the body ill. A strong and basic part of us yearns to be emotionally attached (but happily) to friends, family and lovers, yet in most spiritual disciplines, emotions are not encouraged and in the enlightened expansion, they vanish entirely! *But wait!....there is a solution to all of this!*

You first begin by allowing yourself only constructive emotions and if plagued by negative ones, practice the "Disidentifying Exercise" from Chapter 17.[7] **It is vital to realize that you are**

---

[7] Turn to page 154.

essentially *not* a body, *not* a mind and *not* your emotions, you are Spirit inhabiting those multiple containers; therefor, it stands to reason that those are the *very factors* that utterly vanish when you expand into your enlightened reality; you become no-body, no-mind and no-emotions...you enter the potent reality of your Spirit Self. The "no" in the previous statement refers to "absence of" - absence of the *limited* conditioned body, the *limited* conditioned mind and the *limited* conditioned emotions. We are here to learn to function within a multidimensional reality with an integrated and multidimensional form. The function of enlightened emotions is not *always* to remain in detached dispassion, the mind and body awarenesses have many modes, so has the emotional awareness. Although we all must learn this as part of waking up, **"O,"** **"B"** and **"N"** in particular (when awakened) can function either in the highest expansion--fully detached from ordinary emotions, or, when the occasion calls for it, as recorders and transformers of any intense emotional energy around them--including, what they observe on TV, read in the news, or hear over the radio. Empowered to be in the world, yet not affected by it, they become conscious and precise emotional 'vacuum cleaners' using the transformative power of emotions to heal, change and recreate. And part of their enlightened role in life is to teach others how to do the same.

Transforming External Emotional Energy.

Firstly, how do you know when you're *supposed* to do something with the energy...I assure you--there will be absolutely no doubt! If a really bad occurrence comes up like a dreadful accident, murder, kidnapping or international incident--or a very heart-warming and inspiring event and you're reading about it in the paper or casually watching it on the TV news....suddenly, in an instant, a tsunami of deep anguish, understanding and compassion will utterly fill and overwhelm you--you become an ocean of intense and deep emotions--you're fully recording the emotion connected to the situation and may have to fight back wrenching tears and grief! *All this in about three seconds flat after taking-in the situation.....*the very opposite experience to the dispassionate, non-emotional expansion that I had in my workshop in Canada--but just as transcending! Spirit is calling you to work by filling you with the emotional energy. And the work must take place immediately--while you are fully under the influence of the feelings--then, and only then--does the most powerful transformation of the energy takes place. **At that moment** you transform it within you and breathe it back again--to the photograph, the news report--as a positive healing emotion.

The Basic Technique:

As soon as the emotion has gripped you, shift into disassociation-mode ("the emotion is present, I am not the emotion"), then say mentally:-

"**......**(name the emotion)**...is present,**
I now transform this ...(emotion)**...... into....**(love, peace, forgiveness etc.)**....**
And return it to bless, heal and enlighten this situation, person, etc."

Keep saying and doing this until the intense feeling has depleted itself. During the process, those of you who "see" will in addition project color through your hands as you're breathing out; those who do not - can also use the hands and breath to project the changed emotional energy - and finally, sound to the situation with the inner-voices. When Spirit calls you (as described above), you have no choice in the matter--the energy overwhelms--you transmute it into an antidote on the spot and return it back as healing. At other times, when *you* select and choose what to work on, you're more dispassionate, and usually without intense emotions. Specific situations will also summon you and for these you'll use maps, photographs or visual memory; perhaps you'll even set-up a group of like-minded associates and meet on a regular basis. Additionally (on a much smaller and less dramatic scale), you can continually transform the emotional residues left in the world around you - while you're out walking, commuting, shopping, doing your regular 9-5 job. The business hustle and bustle world throws some sensitives and empaths into a tailspin and many retreat into a protective shell for fear of being overwhelmed. For those of us who've learned to cope in mundane situations, the healing work is all mental, even the sounding. I'm sure you'll develop your own techniques and I hope, greatly expand on mine. At times I receive the energy into myself and then breathe it out to the Galactic Milky Way center, particularly if it's to balance earth energies, but for peoples and events I do a "reverse," I charge it with Love and return it to the situation.

Letters "T," "U," "V," "W," "X" and "Y." With these, we've almost completed the Ladder of Transformation, and the last four are linked in shape as well as function.

In summary:

"T" connects the outer sensing with the expanded faculties of intuitive awarenes. It challenges us to mentally balance the extremes of light and dark within our souls.

"U" transcends the boundaries imposed by duality. The traditional final vowel, it holds the blueprint for the integrated super-being--the progenitor for "sacred humanity."

"V" begins with inner vision--of the self as sacred, and humanity as one Being, one Essence.

"W" has two visionary **"V's"** side by side yet also meeting in the middle--in the heart of man. *Love just doesn't happen, love is something you choose and when you no longer need to reflect yourself "off" others*--you reflect the love from within.

"X" shows the **"V's"** on top of each other yet joined in the middle, **in the form of man**. Our feet and legs (the bottom "V"), our arms and hands (the upper "V"), and where they meet is the cross-over point between earth and sky energies. Idealy, **"X"** shows the dual nature of man empowered and in balance, with all the supra-normal faculties functioning.

"Y" the "extra" vowel takes the **"V"**-vision and establishes it in a fully empowered integrated physical body, bringing enormous focus and willpower to heal and balance the world. *Refer to Chapter 20 and the position of the sacred vowels in the physical body -* **"Y"** *sits in the power-in-action center at the navel,* **"A"** *joins* **"W"** *in the heart and* **"U"** *remains the foundation-energy for the "new man/woman" at the base of the spine.*

And with More Detail:

Letter "T." In many ways **"T"** is a terrifying letter. It summarizes the heights and depths of the human soul. Its shape suggests a fork in the road: on one side, an arm points to the heights of spiritual development, sensitivity, gentleness, kindness and intuition; on the other, the arm points to the depths of spiritual denial, degredation, violence, cruelty, bestiality and craving. Most **"T's"** find themselves drawn in either one or the other direction (towards Spirit or away from Spirit), but once in a while, a well-meaning **"T"** endures the full awareness of both extremes--inspite of reaching for love and light, they're horrified when darkness and rage overtake them--and they usually become violently furious for "good" and noble reasons!! - or they're periodically overwhelmed by cravings and compulsions. Those *choosing* the darker side of **"T"** mirror the beast within us all. To find the balance, remain aware of both extremes within yourself as well as in others, then accept that these violent polarities will remain so long as we choose duality over integration. Another interesting **"T"** thought: at the physical cross-bar of the arms sits the thymus, the gland in the upper chest below the throat believed to augment the immune system and considered in mystical lore as the seat of a new energy center (Chakra). **"T" also marks the Vivaxis point**, the point from which you grounded to the magnetic core of the earth when you took your very first breath at birth *and* the point in place and time (where and when) you began your life's journey. You can re-activate this important connection with special breathing.

The "T" Breath. Picture the gorilla thumping on his chest and announcing his power....but go about it a little more gently when *you* thump your chest! When you feel you've woken up your thymus lie flat on your back, feet together, arms out straight in the form of a **"T."** Next, breathe in through your hands and into the thymus, as you hold your breath, pulse several beats into the thymus (it will begin to tingle), then breathe out through the feet and visualize the energy going to the center of the earth. Eventually, you will have a tingly, vibrating pathway between all these points. Breathe the **"T"** breath for as long as you desire.

Letter "U." The basic blueprint for human transformation--the underlying potential and reality--of not only the balanced intake and outflow of Infinite Presence, as integrated **A, E, I** and **O** energy *within* the physical form, but also that potent reality in relationship with others, with nature and with interdimensional realms. **The "U" Breath:** see Chapter 20, Advanced Vowel Sounding.

Letter "V." The mystical symbol of united vision. Regard your left and right eyes as the upper points of the "V", and their intersecting point at the bottom--as your 3rd. eye (or pineal gland in the brain). The mystic "V" can also represent the left and right frontal lobes of the brain.

The "V" Breath. When breathing concurrently **in** through both eyes and **out into** the 3rd eye-pineal, you develop the capacity to bring in other frequencies beyond the normal range of light; Yogis call it "bringing in Prana, the Life Force, believed to trigger dormant brain functions and activate the transformation process. *At first, perform the breath with open eyes.*

Letter "W." *Reverse your tendency to be the center of attention; take time out, retreat from public view and interaction for a while. When you do find yourself in company, watch yourself. Watch how you speak and draw attention to yourself in front of others--even total strangers. For a change, do things for* ***you*** *(there's no one you have to impress). Clean house, paint, garden, fish, go to the office; do your thing, but not with the thought of anyone else seeing it--do it just for you alone--for your satisfaction and pleasure. Stop constantly seeking someone else to notice and admire you and your efforts. YOU admire the fruits of your efforts--praise yourself! Be giving and enthusiastic to* ***you****, feel enriched and self-complete within your aloneness.* "W" governs the chest and heart (both the physical and the etheric); the etheric heart houses the inner Beloved--should you choose to reunite with that part of yourself and activate your heart-breath.[8] Discover yourself as the Spirit of Love, complete and content...then from that detached yet totally encompassing place, you will become a worthy leader - in whatever capacity your higher Self compels you to be once more visible in the world.

The "W" Breath: Say the affirmation and mantra and visualize rose pink in the heart /chest:

> **"All that I am from the depths of my heart "** as you breathe into the heart.
> **"Embodies the Presence of Love,"** as you breathe out to the world.

Repeat several times, then say:

> **"I am the heart"** as you breathe in to the heart.
> **"Of Infinite Presence,"** as you breathe out to the world.

Practice formally alone, or as you go about your day, imbibing and spreading the energy of Love.

Letter "X." Traditionally, "X" always marks the spot! Physically, it distinguishes the navel point in the center of the body with the top arms (of the "X") indicating the physical arms/hands and the bottom representing the legs/feet. The navel-center marks the incoming of the life-force at conception and is the balancing point between earth energies from the feet and spiritual-interdimensional forces from the hands. "X" reminds us to ground our scattered mind and emotions through the feet, then the more mystical parts of us can manifest without stressing the physical body. The following breath assists the integration.

The "X" Breath. *There are two versions to his breath.* If necessary activate the hands and feet--rub your hands together and slap the bottoms of the feet, then lie on your back with your arms and legs spread-eagled...like an "X." First, to energize them, breathe in an out of your hands and feet in turn (tingling, means they're active!). Now simultaneously take the breath **in** through the hands and feet into the navel, hold the breath and "pulse" the energy at the navel, then breathe **out** through both hands and feet - as though flushing and clearing their channels. Your power center around the navel could become hot and energized, but If you get to the sensation of energy powerfully "streaming" through your limbs STOP - you've done enough!

In the second version you unobstusively become a cosmic "vacuum cleaner" to break-up dissention and other scattered energies in public places or gatherings. For this, you can be sitting, standing or walking; your hands and arms, legs and feet become antennae--again focusing in to the navel, but this time you discharge through the connecting rod of the spine....after breathing **in** to the navel, you simultaneously (with the **out** breath), ground half the energy into the earth through the tail-bone - and shoot the other half up the spine and out the crown Chakra. You've now become an "X" with a line drawn down the middle!! Experiment. See how the energy flows through you each time you do this in public, there's no

---

[8] Read "Opening the Heart Meditations" in Chapter 16.

guarantee you'll have the same experience twice, but you'll always be aware of moving and changing energy through your body-vehicle.

Letter "Y." Transformed, they have no desire (or need) to have power over others. To them, people no longer appear as "pawns" in games of gain or one-upmanship--but individuals, worthy of understanding and respect. **"Y's** now live like tigers with their claws sheathed. The sudden lashing power (intrinsic to their being), remains under gentle restraint and easy control for they have learned that they are **not** their emotions--it's easier and more comfortable to detatch from their anger/annoyance and "watch" it instead. They know how to motivate high performance in others--by their own inspiring example.

Letter "Z:" *the Collective Unconscious in the form of Fate.* Charles Jung (pioneer psychologist) said, "An individual is fated, to the degree that he or she is unconscious." A more modern therapist and revolutionary thinker Charles Ponce said, "Fate comes to you, you are without individual freedom, as long as you remain in the pool of the collective Unconscious." Therefore, you only *appear* helpless in the hands of inexorable outside forces! Unconsciousness, whether individual or collective, means minds lost in duality. **"Z"** represents the end of our present evolutionary and spiritual journey--and the beginning of a new one! The letter could be a symbolic "figure" of man on his knees, humbled by his uniqueness and awake at last within the Universal (Light) Consciousness.

PREPARING TO MEDITATE ON THE SACRED LETTERS

Mantras. In Sanskrit, the word mantra means "prayer" or "words of power." Mantras commonly find their place in the spiritual practices of Buddhists and Hindus and invoke traditional archetypal forces, or activate energy centers (Chakras) within the human body. The closest to mantras in our culture are the phrases from sacred texts (recited in ceremony or uttered as prayers), or the affirmations we might repeat to change old thought patterns. While the latter usually deal with mental, emotional and physical needs, mantras address the superconscious powers of higher Spirit and the Sacred Presence of All that Is. Later in this Chapter, you'll find meditative affirmations *and* mantras for each letter of the alphabet; their practice will bring you into a direct experience of your own Infinite Presence. You can use the accompanying large-print versions of the letters as visual meditations while sounding them or while reciting their affirmations and mantras. Although I employ the term "Infinite Presence" in the affirmations, if you prefer, you can substitute "the Christ within," or you might want to combine the two: "All the power that I am, flows from the Christ within - the Infinite Presence." *Simply know--whether Christian or otherwise--that in your essence-nature, you* ***are*** *this Presence - the mantra's function is to remind you of this, because in your conditioned state of duality--you appear to be separated!*

The Preparation.

Still yourself by relaxing and saying mentally several times:

"Soft eyes....inner-smile."

A melting feeling will flow from your eyes. Then softly follow the "inner-smile" as it floats like a feather down through your internal organs. Now take a series of gentle and loving breaths into your body. Feel the inner softness deepen as you experience a great loving tenderness towards yourself. Gradually, as you continue to breathe, the blissful energy of higher Spirit descends from the upper Chakras; this energy is love and the power of Infinite Life. Breathing ***without*** *awareness of Spirit only feeds the combustion-body, breathing* ***with*** *awareness activates the Chi and Light bodies. The subsequent flow of Chi (Ki) combined with higher Spirit energizes the cells and you feel it as heat, tingling and bliss. Take the breath down through the heart, then breathe it out* ***into*** *the Power Center at the solar plexus; from this point the energy will spread throughout the body.*

Do several of these breaths before beginning "The Practice" (next), in which the breath pattern changes direction and links you to your point of origin--the center of the galaxy (where the stillpoint in you corresponds to the point of no-time within it).

The Practice.

The eyes, the camera-lenses for outer sight, additionally serve as lenses for supernormal vision (called the inner-seeing), which like the breath, also strongly activates the blisses. In fact, all visible phenomena when acknowledged as "Divine Form," immediately feeds and calls forth the bliss energy (see Appendix 4). Try looking at one of the large letters of the alphabet, then close your eyes and recreate the image momentarily on your inner mind-screen--it will instantly result in the mild bliss. *I repeat: When you use the eyes like "shutter-lenses" and practice the shutter-action repeatedly, the bliss follows every time you close your eyes and re-see the image in your head. Open eyes--look! Close eyes--look within! Open--look--close--look within!!* You can do this with anything at all...the profile of a face, an ear, the side of a building, your big toe, a leaf, a flower, your pet--or someone sitting opposite you on the bus! When each is noted within the mind *as divine form,* bliss arises shuddering and rushing through you in mini-ecstasies! As soon as the ecstasy lessens, you do another "open--look--close--look" to keep the bliss flowing. Why raise the blisses?? Other than the fact that it's pleasantly sexual, bliss is good for you, it triggers the out-of-body Chakra energy (Prana or Chi) to nourish the cells and nervous system and when used with intention, becomes healing and rejuvenating. For instance**--healers try this:** next time you do a hands-on healing treatment, keep your hands perfectly still (on the other person's body); then observe any part of their physical form while you practice the 'shutter-eye' technique...you don't have to keep looking in the same place--shift your vision, but keep opening and closing the eyes and combine it with seeing inwardly what you've just been looking at outwardly; then, when you feel the bliss rippling through, direct it with your hands *into* the other person--you will both be amazed!

Another purpose of this Chapter: for you to discover how the inner bliss responds to the Sacred Symbols when you see *them* as divine form ("The Body"). Begin by meditating on your letter of choice, then use the galactic breath pattern[9] along *with* sound to quicken the energy. The sounds you use can be single or multiple intonations of the specific letter, or a mental mantra/affirmation *about* the letter. Experiment! Try sound and sight together: look steadily at the letter and either speak or sing it, then make your sounds together with the 'shutter-eye' effect. Other things to try: sound the letter by itself without trying to see it in your mind; or only use the seeing ('shutter-eye') of the letter--with no sound at all. Also experiment with making sounds 'mentally'- the bliss gets stronger!

At first, use the letters from your own name. Start with the vowels then proceed to the first and middle letters (which could happen to be vowels anyway!). If people call you by a nick-name, look up the meanings of the vowels in that name, then do the same for your *real* one. Accept your strengths *and* weaknesses! During the course of a day, try and alter your habitual reactions with a radical change of thought and behavior. Your sounding practice, affirmations--and **your thoughts and actions** must all go hand-in-hand for a balancing result.

For example: if your name is **Alex** - your personality drive comes from the **"A"** (which of course, is a vowel). Everyone's lessons vary with social conditioning plus what they came to learn this lifetime and indeed, another **"A"** person's lessons will vary for those same reasons, but you *both* will share some tendencies. If you're one of the powerful **"A's,"** your 'radical change' would mean stopping yourself every time you started being overbearing or controlling. The weaker **Alex'es**, would need to beef **up** their personal power, by standing ground instead of retreating when other people get officious and situations seem overwhelming. **"E"** is the second vowel in **Alex**, so don't neglect to look up what it means. The consonants (**"L"** and **"X"**--*look them up also*) act as experience-vehicles for the **"A"** and **"E"** and also shape the nature of their final expansion into the Sacred. For instance: with **"A"** and **"E"** sharing the **"L"** energy, you might "awaken" within a group situation, and subsequent enlightened public work (**"L"**) would find you communicating (**"E"**), and focusing your many interests (**"X"**) through the power of Spirit rather than your old ego and intellect.

The above gives you some idea of how to work with your own names.

---

9 See the Galactic Breath in Chapter 4, "Releasing The Voice."

The Sacred Symbol Alphabet.

Some final words about using the alphabet (on the turquoise pages) for personal name meditation.

1) Which ever letter you have chosen to work with, be sure you have read all the relevant information about it given in Chapters 6, 7, 8, and 9.

2) Look through the following pages and find your selected letter.

3) Seat yourself comfortably and prop the letter up in front of you.

Note: you'll notice the letters are printed on both sides of the page, so place a blank sheet of paper over the letter you are NOT contemplating - so it won't distract you.

4) Repeat the affirmation and/or Mantra mentally while you gaze at the letter of your choice.

5) Now close your eyes and "see" the image in your mind's eye. *Repeat several times.* If you cannot reproduce the letter in your mind, "draw" around the image on the page with your eyes...then close your eyes again and try and "see" it. *Repeat several times.* Finally, visualize a blackboard in your head and draw the image upon it.

6) Mentally repeat the affirmations/Mantra while observing the letter within you.

You may decide to continue with the above meditation, or you may choose to introduce sound.

1) Begin by speaking the letter in all of the 'voices' you can imagine. See what feelings and memories arise.

2) Change the speaking voice to sounding then sing the letter in many different ways.

3) Incorporate the sounding with the inner and outer 'seeing' of the letter.

4) Finish by combining the sounding of the letter with the Galactic Breath (from Chapter 4).

Remember:

Be aware
Of the awareness.
That which is lost
Is not lost.

It is already here.
It cannot be seen
Or understood,

Unless it is
Directly experienced
Through the body
As The Body.

Rinchenna K'hardo.

And deep within our various expanded states remains the 'still-point' of will..choosing to think or not to think--deciding into which mind mode to enter, or simply flowing in effortless emptiness...our Core-Essence of awareness playing in the field of the mind.

SUMMARY of SACRED AFFIRMATIONS and MANTRA

A.... (Voice of Spirit)...*"Oh..the power that you really are - if you would only believe it!"*
Affirmation: "All the power that I am - flows from the Infinite Presence."

MANTRA: **"Infinite Spirit, I am - I shine in the Body of Light."**

B.... (Voice of Spirit)...*"Feelings, feelings - listen to your feelings, they will take you home."*
Affirmation: "All that I sense and feel - reflects the Infinite Presence."

MANTRA: **"I am the Sacred Sound and Form - and all that is - is all I am."**

C.... (Voice of Spirit)...*"Such curiosity - and you really know everything!"*
Affirmation: "My passionate search to know - reveals the Infinite Presence."

MANTRA: **"I am the bright awareness - empty of thought, encompassing all."**

D.... (Voice of Spirit)...*"I am your authority and strength - trust me."*
Affirmation: "My authority rests in the Infinite Presence."

MANTRA: **"I am Warrior-Strength. I know that I know beyond knowing."**

E.... (Voice of Spirit)...*"Hush, hush!...listen deeply."*
Affirmation: "All that I freely express, flows from the Infinite Mind."
"I know the thoughts of others - I speak the Inner Word."

MANTRA: **"Thought and speech recede - the Infinite Mind arises."**
"I am the bright awareness - empty of thought, encompassing all."

F.... (Voice of Spirit).... *"Oh - how great I am - as you!"*
Affirmation: "My feelings of pride and accomplishment,
Dissolve into Infinite Presence."

MANTRA: **"I am the glory that is - and ever was."**

G.... (Voice of Spirit).... *"Tread lightly little one - tread lightly."*
Affirmation: "My passion for work becomes - the Infinite Presence of Play."

MANTRA: **"I am effortless work and magical play.**

H.... (Voice of Spirit).... *"Let's re-create the world of man."*

Affirmation: "My dreams of fortune and success - I offer to the Source of All.
"I see my work and discipline - as part of an amazing Plan."

MANTRA: "I am Vision without limit."

I...(Voice of Spirit) *"I dance within you, paint, sing, compose all manner of marvelous things -* ***let me!****"*

Affirmation: "My inspiration flows - from the Infinite Presence."

MANTRA: "I am Infinite creating, inspiring - showing, revealing."

J.... (The voice of Spirit)...*"Come fly with me to lands unknown - the inner realms of other worlds."*

Affirmation: "I align my will with the Infinite Presence - and the mystical inner journey."

MANTRA: "I point the way to realms within - the outer world I fill with joy."

K.... (Voice of Spirit) ...*"Be my passion-power of Life."*

Affirmation: "I light my flame from the Source of All."
"My body thrills in bliss - my soul in ecstasy."

MANTRA: "I am Eternal passion's Fire."

L.... (Voice of Spirit)... *"Let me be a light to others - a beacon on the hill."*

Affirmation: "I love to be with people, the Spirit shines in every face."
"Everyone I see - reflects the Sacred Presence"

MANTRA: "I am the Source in everyone - and everyone is me."

M.... (Voice of Spirit)...*"We are all one family."*

Affirmation: "I have found my home - in the Infinite Presence."
"I nurture myself - I nourish the world."

MANTRA: - "I abide within the Universal Family."

N.... (Voice of Spirit)...*"Don't pull things apart - bring them together."*

Affirmation: "All that I know and see - flows from Infinite Presence."
"I flow with the outer changes - within I am balanced and clear."
"My flame of service lights the way to inner planes of ecstasy.

MANTRA: "The knower and the known dissolve - the light remains, I am the Light."

O.... (Voice of Spirit)...*"Rest your aching heart in me."*

Affirmation: "All the emotions that come to me - I send them back as Love."
"All that delights my heart shows me the Sacred Presence."

MANTRA: "Dispassionate and empty - I am Infinite Compassion."

P.... (Voice of Spirit)....*"The Dove of Peace abides within you."*

Affirmation: "One with all things - I rest in the Presence."
"The still-point of Peace forms the core of my soul."

MANTRA: "All is the Sacred Space - and I am the Center, serene.

Q.... (Voice of Spirit)...*"Soul of yearning, striving, searching - do you search for me?"*

Affirmation: "My passionate quest for adventure - delights in the Infinite Presence.
"I have found thee in my heart - I have found thee everywhere."

MANTRA: "I am the object of the quest - the answer is myself."

R.... (voice of Spirit) *"I fill your thoughts with a thousand ideas - listen!"*

Affirmation: "All my thoughts and ideas unfold from the Infinite Presence."
"My inner mind opens to Infinite Wisdom - my outer mind listens."

**MANTRA: "Wise beyond words - I am the bright awareness
Empty of thought, encompassing all."**

S.... (Voice of Spirit)...*"Money, success, your place in the world - you might be disappointed!"*

Affirmation: "All that I accomplish comes through the Power of Spirit."
"I seize the day - as abundant opportunity."
"Success is empty of ego - it is merely something to do."

MANTRA: "I am the Essence of Abundance - fully in the world, yet not of it!

T.... (Voice of Spirit)...*"I call you in so many ways - why do you doubt my voice, my touch?"*

Affirmation: "All of my inner knowings flow from the Infinite Presence."
"All of my mystical senses expand to the realms beyond."

MANTRA: "I am the door within the doors - expanding all perception.

U.... (Voice of Spirit)...*"There is a balance - receiving and giving - becoming all of yourself!"*
Affirmation: "My need to expand and grow - I draw from the Infinite Presence.

MANTRA: **"Beyond the ordinary plane, of envy, hate and senseless gain,
Self, without self, expanded in form - empty of mind and open to wonder."**

V.... (Voice of Spirit)...*"Like some lost light, the hidden vision rises - brilliant and transforming!"*
Affirmation: "Bring forth the new creation - race and creed shall not divide us."
" Man shall join again in Spirit - we are really One."

MANTRA: "I fan the spark to flame - in every eye I see the One."

W.... (Voice of Spirit)...*"You are surrounded by such Love - how could you doubt it?"*
Affirmation: "All my need to impress - dissolves in the Infinite Presence."
"All of my friendly warmth - reflects the Source of All."
"All that I am from the depths of my heart,
"Embodies the Infinite Presence."
MANTRA: **"I am the heart of Infinite Presence."
"I am the way of the Heart."**

X....(Voice of Spirit)..*"How many times have I begged you to STOP, LISTEN and WAIT?"*
Affirmation: "Remind me to be still - and rest my mind in thee."
"I bring my every thought, to the Infinite Presence of peace."

MANTRA: **"Focused and Clear - I am the bright awareness
Empty of thought, encompassing all."**

Y.... (Voice of Spirit) "*Years have passed - where have you been? - it's time for us to work again.*
Affirmation: "I open my heart to the power within - the guiding Spirit of my soul."

MANTRA: "I am the charismatic Presence - self-contained and ever free."

Z.... (Voice of Spirit) *"All is made new - and I in you - have been within you all this time!"*
Affirmation: "Teach me to flow with every moving moment."
"And constantly know - there is a Master Plan!"

MANTRA: "Every breath I breathe - creates a new beginning."